*KYON is proud to support this important book
to assist veterinary professionals in their practice.*

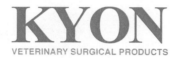

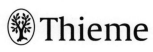

Diagnosing Canine Lameness

Daniel Koch, Martin S. Fischer

Contributor
Britta Dobenecker

Illustrations by Jonas Lauströer and Amir Andikfar
Translated by Corinna Klupiec

450 figures

Georg Thieme Verlag
Stuttgart • New York

Bibliographical data of the German National Library (Deutsche Nationalbibliothek)
The German National Library (Deutsche Nationalbibliothek) lists this publication in the German National Bibliography; detailed bibliographic information can be found on the Internet at http://dnb.d-nb.de.
Translated from the German 2nd edition "Lahmheitsuntersuchung beim Hund", 2019.

Your opinion is important to us! Please write to us at:
www.thieme.de/service/feedback.html

© 2020. Thieme. All rights reserved. Georg Thieme Verlag KG
Rüdigerstr. 14
70469 Stuttgart
Germany
www.thieme.de

Printed in Germany

Cover design: Thieme Group
Illustrators: Jonas Lauströer (www.jonas-laustroeer.de), Amir Andikfar (www.andikfar.de); Matthias Haab, Zürich, Schweiz; Karin Baum, Paphos, Zypern
Cover pictures: Gaby Ernst, Saland, Schweiz; Jonas Lauströer; Amir Andikfar
Videos: Videos in the chapters 3–6 originate from Tele D, Diessenhofen; videos in chapter 7 originate from Nicole Hollenstein, Tierfotografie
Copyediting: Stefanie Gronau, Haimhausen; (copyediting of the German edition: Katharina Schmalz, Wenzenbach bei Regensburg)
Translator: Corinna Klupiec, BVSc PhD Grad Cert Ed Stud (Higher Ed), Sydney, Australia
Typeset by L42 AG, Berlin, using Arbortext Advanced Print Publisher
Printing: Aumüller Druck GmbH & Co. KG, Regensburg

DOI 10.1055/b-007-170978

ISBN 978-3-13-243283-3   1 2 3 4 5 6

Also available as eBook:
eISBN (PDF) 978-3-13-243299-4

Foreword

The successful workup of an orthopedic disorder is predicated on a targeted, methodical lameness examination. In conjunction with general and neurological examinations, the orthopedic examination marks the beginning of a process that leads to a diagnosis, or to the development of an expanded diagnostic plan.

Different schools of thought and philosophies naturally give rise to varying strategies. In this book, we seek to teach a systematic approach.

Every lame dog is examined using the same process: history-taking, gait analysis, examination of the dog in the standing position, examination of the dog in recumbency. In each case, all of the limbs are assessed. Diagnostic imaging only comes into play at the end of the orthopedic examination. At first glance, this may seem anachronistic, since x-ray and ultrasound machines are readily available in virtually all veterinary practices, and computed tomography and magnetic resonance tomography have become affordable. Why not simply go ahead and scan a lame dog and see what this reveals?

In addition to the increased burden of exposure to radiation and anaesthesia, several factors highlight the paradox of failing to start with the best tool of all, namely the human brain, with its diverse range of sensors including the eyes, ears and fingers. The brain is faster than any machine, can use logic to arrange information appropriately on an intellectual meta-level, can use experience to distinguish the significant from the non-significant, can evaluate the relevance of aspects of the history and signalment with respect to the existing clinical presentation and, not least, can keep the client informed of diagnostic developments.

Thus, we are also providing instruction in an "art" – the art of the orthopedic examination. This art may not be new, but it deserves renewed attention, because our „sensors" are only as good as the knowledge that informs them.

This first English edition incorporates the latest findings from innovative locomotion research conducted at the Friedrich Schiller University Jena. In part 1 of the book, these insights provide a deepened functional understanding of the anatomy and physiology of the musculoskeletal system. In light of the close relationship between orthopedic and neurological disorders – in terms of anatomy as well as differential diagnosis - the first English edition provides a guide to both the orthopedic and neurological examinations, accompanied as required by relevant anatomy. While not presuming to serve as a therapeutic text, part 3 summarizes the most important orthopedic and neurological disorders.

Yet this book is not "only" a book; it is also a film. The accompanying URLs and QR codes enable the reader to use their tablet, mobile telephone or computer to view the entire examination process in video format.

Our book is intended for students of veterinary medicine, general practitioners, physiotherapists, osteopaths, chiropractors and other therapists with an interest in orthopedics, and also for inquisitive laypeople. It aims to create order in the sequence of diagnostic steps, to facilitate the use of observation and underlying anatomical and physiological fundamentals to establish an accurate clinical diagnosis, and to provide an overview of treatment.

Our thanks go in the first instance to Thieme Publishers Stuttgart, particularly to Dr Maren Warhonowicz and Ms Carolin Frotscher, for their capable and inspirational project leadership and realization of the textual, graphic and video content, and to Dr Martin Schäfer, previous Editorial Director of the Veterinary Medicine Program for commissioning this new book and for giving us his trust and support. Corinna Klupiec did an excellent job in translating our book. Her expertise even helped to improve the original German version. Most of the excellent graphics were painstakingly created by Jonas Lauströer and Amir Andikfar, to whom we owe a great debt of thanks. Without their richly informative images, the book would be worth only half as much. We also extend our gratitude to Matthias Haab for producing several of the graphics in part three. Particular thanks are due to Dr Roland Börner, whose initiative as a networker set this project in motion. We also offer sincere thanks to the sponsors, particularly to Heel (Biologische Heilmittel Heel GmBH).

The origins of the text by Daniel Koch go back to lectures by Professor Pierre Montavon at the University of Zurich. Dr Koch is thus especially grateful to his former teacher and intellectual father, who unfortunately passed away in September 2018. Martin S. Fischer thanks the Verband für das Deutsche Hundewesen (VDH), the Gesellschaft für kynologische Forschung (GKF) and Heel (Biologische Heilmittel Heel GmbH) for the many years of outstanding collaboration that have been the foundation of so many locomotion studies.

Then there are the numerous helpers who have consistently provided support, advice and editorial input. These include: photo- and film-star dog Leika and her owner Katharina Gasser, photo- and film-star dog Joyce and her owner Nicole Hollenstein, our proofreaders Dr Stefan Grundmann, Prof. Frank Steffen, Adjunct Professor Dr Manuela Schmidt, Dr Emanuel Andrada, Dr Barbara Happe and particularly Dr Christian Rode, whose many critically analytical comments helped to refine part one of the book. In addition, we thank the camera crew and editors at TeleD and Nicole Hollenstein Animal Photographer, the video actors, Indulab for supplying the examination table, colleagues who provided us with images and, finally, our families and wives, for granting us the freedom we needed while writing this book.

January 2019
Daniel Koch and Martin S. Fischer

Contents

Part 1

Basic principles

Part 2

Diagnostic Procedure

Part 3
Therapeutic Guidelines for Common Disorders

Part 4
Appendix

Addresses

Dr. med. vet. ECVS Daniel **Koch**
Kleintierchirurgie AG Überweisungspraxis
Ziegeleistr. 5
8253 Diessenhofen
Switzerland

Prof. Dr. rer. nat. Dr. h.c. Martin S. **Fischer**
Friedrich-Schiller-Universität Jena
Institut für Zoologie und Evolutionsforschung mit Phyletischem
Museum, Ernst-Haeckel-Haus und Biologiedidaktik
Erbertstr. 1
07743 Jena
Germany

Dr. med. vet., Dipl. ECVCN Britta **Dobenecker**
Fachtierärztin für Tierernährung und Diätetik,
Zusatzbezeichnung Ernährungsberatung (Kleintiere)
Ludwig-Maximilians-Universität München
Veterinärwissenschaftliches Department
Lehrstuhl für Tierernährung und Diätetik
Schönleutnerstr. 8
85764 Oberschleißheim
Germany

Amir **Andikfar**
www.andikfar.de

Jonas **Lauströer**
www.jonas-laustroeer.de

Authors Introduction

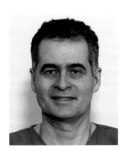

Dr. med. vet. **Daniel Koch** studied veterinary medicine at the Universities of Fribourg and Zurich. After successfully completing his final examinations in 1990, he furthered his education by completing a small animal internship at Utrecht University before working for two years in his family's general veterinary practice. In 1995, he undertook a residency at the Clinic for Small Animal Surgery, attaining his specialist qualification as a member of the European College of Veterinary Surgeons in 1999. He subsequently served in this clinic as associate professor, senior clinician and head of department. Since 2004, he has worked in a private small animal referral surgical practice in Diessenhofen (Switzerland), focusing on the fields of canine and feline orthopedics, upper airway disease and dentistry.

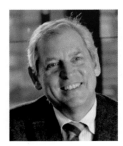

Prof. Dr. rer. nat. Dr. h. c. **Martin S. Fischer** studied biology and paleontology in Tübingen and Paris. After obtaining his doctorate in Tübingen, he worked at the at the University Hospital Frankfurt am Main, teaching human anatomy. He subsequently became a research assistant at the Zoologisches Institut in Tübingen. Upon completing his post-doctoral studies in Tübingen, he was appointed in 1993 as Professor of Special Systematic Zoology and Evolutionary Biology and director of the associated institute, as well as director of the Phyletisches Museum. He is a member of the scientific advisory board of the Verband für das Deutsche Hundewesen (VDH). His research focuses on the functional morphology and evolution of terrestrial vertebrates. In 2006, he commenced the Jena study of canine locomotion, subsequently authoring the book „Dogs in Motion", together with Dr Karin E. Lilje. In 2018, he was awarded the title of Honorary Doctor by the Faculty of Veterinary Sciences of the Justus Liebig University Giessen.

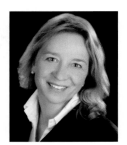

After completing her studies in veterinary nursing, Dr. med. vet. **Britta Dobenecker** studied veterinary medicine at the University of Veterinary Medicine Hanover. She completed her doctorate at the Institute for Physiological Chemistry Hanover and the Institute for Animal Nutrition and Dietetics at the Ludwig Maximilian University Munich (LMU). Since then, she has been working actively in teaching and research at LMU, currently serving in the roles of senior lecturer and acting director. Since 1994, she has provided advice on the nutrition of companion, farm and zoo animals. In 1997 she became a specialist in animal nutrition and dietetics. In 2000, she attained the additional qualification of nutritional consultant (small animals) and, in 2001, became a diplomate of the European College of Veterinary and Comparative Nutrition. Her key research areas include the effect nutrition on skeletal health (particularly in growing dogs), kidney health, energy analysis, chondroprotection and canine sports physiology.

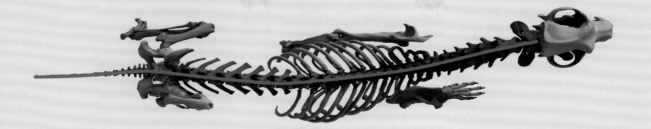

Source: Jonas Lauströer, Amir Andikfar

Part 1
Basic principles

1 Physiology and Anatomy of the Locomotor Apparatus of the Dog

Martin S. Fischer, Daniel Koch, Britta Dobenecker

1.1

Introduction

Martin S. Fischer, Daniel Koch

Wolves and other large canids are adapted in specific ways for sustained pursuit of large prey. Dogs possess a similar degree of endurance, as demonstrated by the daily experience of every dog owner when their dog returns home from a walk full of energy, regardless of the distance covered. Due to their exceptional endowment with fatigue-resistant muscle fibers and their use of energy-sparing mechanisms, wolves and, thus, also dogs usually use less than 10% or, in rare cases up to 20%, of their daily energy requirement for the purpose of locomotion.

In recent years, our understanding of canine locomotion has been fundamentally revised by sophisticated monitoring techniques and intensive investigation by research groups around the world. This has revealed that variation between individuals is greater than that between breeds. In other words, while ten great Danes each have an individual running gait, the average values for great Danes and Dachshunds are surprisingly similar.

A further key finding of recent studies is that, in all gaits, dogs systematically exploit gravity to recover energy from gravity-induced movements. Tendons and muscles undergo passive stretching, muscles frequently contract isometrically or perform negative work, and overall there is considerably less movement in the joints of the limbs than previously thought. With the exception of the hip joint, which contributes most to propulsion, the joints of the limbs always undergo the least possible deviation during cyclic locomotion. The task of the joints is to translate movement occurring at the highest possible pivot point in the limb. In the forelimb, this pivot point is always located in the upper third of the scapula. During walking and trotting, the most proximal pivot point in the hindlimb is in the hip joint; in the various types of gallop, it also incorporates an extensive portion of the lumbar spine. The compliance of the limb is adjusted according to the terrain.

In the dog, as in all terrestrial mammals, the developmental homology between the upper arm and thigh has been replaced by a functional analogy between the scapula and femur. In addition, it has recently been demonstrated using comprehensive three-dimensional kinematic measurements that movement of the limbs during locomotion is not limited to the parasagittal plane; in the stifle, for example, there is also a substantial amount of cyclic torsion.

This new perspective on the skeleton also necessitates a revised view of the muscles. Physicians studying anatomy have long regarded muscles in a purely topographical sense, learning their insertion, origin and innervation. In the veterinary field, the presumptive function of muscles was adopted from human medicine. The triceps brachii or gastrocnemius muscles were thus considered extensors, even though they only act as extensors in the dog when the animal stretches its legs while in dorsal or lateral recumbency. Through detailed electromyographic studies, investigation of the inverse dynamics of canine locomotion and analysis of the internal structure of muscle, a different picture of the function of the musculoskeletal apparatus has emerged. In the aforementioned example, the putative extensors have been shown to act against gravity-induced flexion while simultaneously storing elastic energy. A further example is the latissimus dorsi. The activity of this muscle ceases on touch down when the dog is moving on level ground, serving in this situation purely to brake the forelimb as it swings forward, and to change its direction of movement. Only when the dog is moving on an upward plane does the latissimus dorsi contribute to limb retraction during the stance phase.

An understanding of lameness and its diagnosis requires an appreciation of the effective functional relationships of the limbs, the extent of rotation and translation of the scapula during each step, the limited intervertebral movement in the lumbar vertebral column, the action of individual muscles during locomotion and the three-dimensional kinematics of the limbs.

1.2

Movement, Kinematics, Energetics and Biomechanics

Martin S. Fischer, Daniel Koch

The canine musculoskeletal system is responsible for locomotion and for several other movements that are important for quality of life (e.g. stretching, scratching and playing). Since all movements involve close interaction between active (muscles, nerves) and passive structures (bones, joints tendons and ligaments), it is important to consider these components in a collective sense in order to better understand dysfunction. Our knowledge of canine movement is largely limited to locomotion. Moreover, movements unrelated to locomotion are of relatively little significance in diagnosing lameness. Such movements, that are directed towards the dog's own body or towards other dogs, are referred to as non-locomotor movements ("idiomotion").

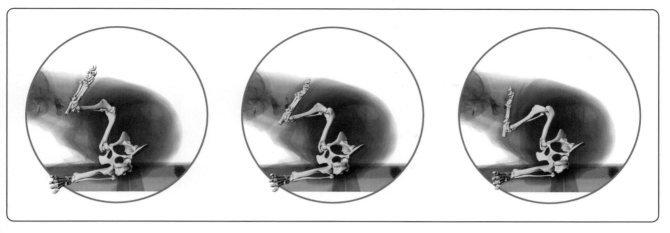

▶ **Fig. 1.1** Illustration of a dog scratching its ear, using three pictures from an animation based on high frequency biplanar fluoroscopy. Note the marked rotation of the right femur around its longitudinal axis. (source: Martin S. Fischer, Lisa Dargel, Institut für Zoologie und Evolutionsforschung, Friedrich-Schiller-Universität Jena)

In a study conducted at the Friedrich Schiller University Jena, researchers investigating the three-dimensional kinematics of grooming movements made the surprising observation that, during ear scratching, the femur rotates up to 50% on its longitudinal axis (▶ **Fig. 1.1**). During locomotion, only a narrow segment of the head of the femur is weight-bearing, irrespective of gait. Thus, from a functional perspective, the spherical shape of the femoral head is perhaps based more upon its contribution to idiomotor movements. In all canine gaits, the femur typically rotates about two axes (forward-backward movement in the sagittal plane and abduction-adduction in the frontal plane during change in direction), with the hip acting as a universal joint. However, idiomotor movements also require rotation around the longitudinal axis, whereby the hip acts as a ball and socket joint. This may be a significant consideration in the early detection of joint disease, as restrictions of joint movement may be evident during grooming before they affect locomotion. Also at Jena, recent 3-D kinematic studies of canine locomotion have demonstrated a feature particular to French Bulldogs. In this breed, considerable longitudinal rotation of the outwardly deviated leg is also observed during locomotion, with up to 40° rotation during a step in the trot. Further studies have shown that grooming necessitates a high degree of mobility of the shoulder joint; here again, the range of movement exceeds that occurring during locomotion.

1.2.1 Canine Locomotion

In the largest scientific study of canine locomotion to date, sagittal motion parameters exhibited a high degree of consistency across the 32 examined breeds [25]. The central objective of this study, conducted at Friedrich-Schiller University Jena, was to examine similarities and differences in the locomotion of different breeds of dog. Gait analysis in the sagittal plane was performed on ten dogs per breed during walking, trotting and galloping. Locomotion was recorded using three different techni-

ques: high frequency videography, marker-based motion analysis (Qualisys®) and high frequency biplanar fluoroscopy. Care was taken during breed selection to represent a diverse range of sizes and body shapes. In the subsequent "Heel study of joint dynamics", three-dimensional movements (thus, also including ab- and adduction and long-axis rotation) were examined in dozens of dogs and combined with ground reaction force measurements. This approach permits calculation of "inverse dynamics" in dogs ([2],[24]).

Although most dogs today are on an excessive plane of nutrition, their use of metabolic energy is economical. This reflects their descent from wolves, which exhibit particular endurance in running over large distances. The same energy-sparing mechanisms also operate in dogs. The common assumption that locomotion is at all times achieved through strenuous muscle activity has thus been proven wrong.

1.2.2 Energetics of Cyclic Locomotion

In all gaits, the intrinsic joints of the limbs - other than the hip - exhibit surprisingly little movement (▶ **Fig. 1.2**, ▶ **Fig. 1.4**). In fact, during walking, the joints remain so rigid that the functional limb length hardly changes (▶ **Fig. 1.3**). Functional limb length is defined as the distance between the proximal pivot point of the limb and the point of touch down. The proximal pivot point thus rises and falls during walking; the limbs act as essentially rigid pendulums that exert a lever action on the components of the body in chronological sequence.

The existence of such a pendulum mechanism has been demonstrated during walking in bipeds. In this process, kinetic energy is converted into potential energy, and vice versa. An egg rolling end-over-end serves as a useful analogy. When the egg rolls onto one point, its forward motion slows and its potential energy increases; as it rolls on, the potential energy decreases and the egg rolls more quickly. In the walking biped, this cyclic transformation ensures that part of the energy of motion is

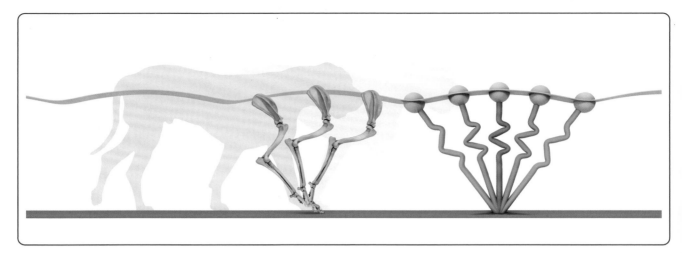

▶ **Fig. 1.2** The spring-mass model describes the course of the body's center of gravity. During walking, the limbs act as rigid struts; the center of mass rises until the middle of the stance phase then falls back to its starting position. (source: Martin S. Fischer, Jonas Lauströer, Amir Andikfar)

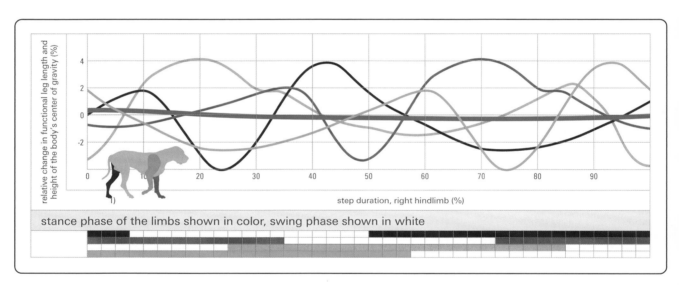

▶ **Fig. 1.3** Changes in functional leg length and resulting oscillation of the body's center of gravity. The center of gravity (green line) only follows the vertical deviations of the limbs to a limited extent because vertical displacement is equalized across all limbs. (source: Martin S. Fischer, Jonas Lauströer, Amir Andikfar)

conserved and does not need to be constantly generated and exhausted. Dogs potentially also benefit from this mechanism, when one considers the individual limbs and the body parts to which they are attached (▶ **Fig. 1.3**). However, in contrast to bipeds, dogs and other quadrupeds can simultaneously restrict the movement of their center of mass (body's center of gravity) almost to a horizontal line (▶ **Fig. 1.3**, thick green line), a phenomenon also seen in cars. For dogs, this makes walking very comfortable and results in a stable field of vision. The center of mass (body's center of gravity) is the point through which the resultant of gravitational forces experienced by the parts of the body acts. If the body were suspended by this point, it would be in equilibrium. In the standing position, the center of mass

of the dog is located caudal to the sternum, at the level of the ninth intercostal space.

When the limbs swing in unison, thus with the same step length and step frequency (as seen in the trot), vertical movement of the body's center of gravity can be used specifically for storing elastic energy. Maneuvers such as acceleration, braking and changes in direction and jumping require additional muscle work.

In the dog, the limbs only remain rigid during slow walking. Bending of the limbs begins to occur at fast walking speeds. Breed-related variation is evident in this regard, and differences have been observed between the front- and hindlimbs. During walking in certain breeds (Bedlington Terrier, Bearded Collie), the front limbs are rigid while the hindlimbs are flexible.

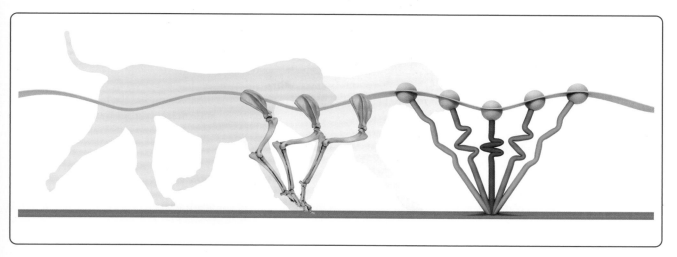

▶ **Fig. 1.4** The spring-mass model describes the course of the body's center of gravity. During trotting, the limbs are compliant; the center of mass falls until the middle of the stance phase and then rises again, primarily through recovery of elastic energy. (source: Martin S. Fischer, Jonas Lauströer, Amir Andikfar)

In the trot and pace, the „running" gaits, the body's center of gravity behaves differently. From the beginning to the middle of the stance phase, the center of gravity drops and slows down. In the second half of the stance phase, it rises and accelerates. Sparing of energy via the rigid pendulum mechanism is no longer possible, as potential and kinetic energy simultaneously rise and fall. The center of gravity follows a wave-like course. The limbs are flexible, bending and subsequently straightening during each gait cycle. Thus, in these gaits, the limbs act as springs. The spring-mass model developed by Blickhan (1989; [5]) provides a surprisingly simple explanation of the movement of the center of gravity of bipeds under the influence of gravity, and the corresponding forces exerted by the legs on the ground.

Here, a new energy-sparing principle comes into effect. In a manner resembling a rubber ball, tendons, ligaments and intrinsic muscle elasticity are used during the stance phase to recover energy. At the same time as potential and kinetic energy are decreasing in the first half of the stance phase, the leg undergoes flexion and elastic energy stores are replenished (i.e. through stretching); in the second half of the stance phase, the leg is extended and the temporarily stored elastic energy is transformed back into kinetic and potential energy (▶ Fig. 1.4). In this process, an important and frequently underestimated role may be played by titin, the molecular spring of the sarcomere [58]. As vertical ground reaction forces are higher in the forelimbs (60%), these remain more rigid than the hindlimbs, which exhibit greater flexion (▶ Fig. 1.4).

In the gallop, the two previously mentioned energy-sparing mechanisms act in combination; potential energy is converted into kinetic energy through the relative rigidity of the forelimbs, resulting in a ca. 15–30% "saving" in energy output, and recovery of elastic energy is even more efficient [30].

When a body performs, or is subjected to, work, its energy changes. In the trot and gallop, the work performed and energy recovered is highly unevenly distributed across the individual joints in a gait-specific fashion. As a fundamental principle, negative work is performed at the distal joints during bending of the limb in the stance phase, as the direction of force is opposite to the direction of movement. In the gallop, 81% of the total negative work occurring in the forelimb takes place at the carpal joints; in the hindlimb, up to 98% occurs at the tarsus. However, it is precisely these two joints that, through bending, are able to recover considerable elastic energy in strong tendons such as the common calcaneal tendon, thus helping to reduce the high cost of concentric muscle work. In contrast, the heavy, proximal extensors of the hip joint only perform positive work. In this case it is not possible to reclaim energy. Accordingly, these predominantly fleshy muscles have long fascicles and only short tendons; see Functional Myology (p.55). In the elbow joint, the proportion of positive work that can be recovered from elastic energy is up to 96% in the trot, and less than 60% in the gallop; in the shoulder, the equivalent figures are 38% for the trot and 49% for the gallop. Major gait-related differences are evident in the stifle joint, in which the potential recovery is 60% for the trot and less than 5% for the gallop (all values taken from [30]).

Canine locomotor mechanisms are heavily geared towards minimizing energy consumption. Modelling analyses have shown that, in a 9 kg dog, the trot is the most energetically efficient gait up to a speed of approximately 13 km/h; at higher speeds, it is the gallop [48]. Maneuvers such as acceleration, braking and also changes in direction and jumping require additional muscle work.

Energy used for locomotion constitutes only a small portion of total daily energy consumption. A walk on a lead accounts for just 5% of daily energy consumption; even with extended exercise, this figure rarely reaches 20%. Around 70% of daily energy consumption is used primarily for the production of heat.

As heat loss is dependent upon the ratio of volume to surface area, which becomes more favorable as body size increases, it follows that energy consumption in kilocalories per kilogram body weight decreases with increasing body size. The energy requirement of small dogs is 3–4 times that of large dogs and from 30 kg body weight onwards the energy requirement remains almost constant [45]. Castration reduces the energy requirement by 12–15%; advancing age results in a further reduction of similar magnitude. Obese dogs have the additional problem that fat acts as an insulator, thus restricting heat loss and further reducing the energy requirement. Weight loss in dogs is difficult to achieve, since a reduction in food intake of 50% produces a decrease in body weight of just 1% per week. As a general rule, half rations for 4 months result in only a 15% reduction in body weight!

1.2.3   Dynamic Stability

In humans and quadrupedal mammals, perturbation of a motion sequence is followed by a return to cyclic locomotion, i.e. locomotion is dynamically stable [6], [23]. Rather than requiring elaborate steering and significant input from the brain, regular cyclic locomotion is probably based upon intelligent mechanics. Such a system can negotiate disturbances, like unevenness in the terrain, and can guarantee dynamically stable movement without the need for additional energy. In this context, dynamic stability refers to a model in which a stable recurring cycle is produced purely by feedback mechanisms within the "mechanics of the limb". The bipedal spring-mass model for walking and running shows that, depending on speed, stable

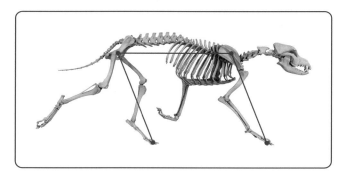

▶ **Fig. 1.5** Touch down angle of the fore- and hindlimbs. The touch down angle is the angle between the supporting surface and a line drawn from the proximal pivot point to the point of touch down. The pivot points of the front- and hindlimbs are usually at the same height. (source: Martin S. Fischer, Jonas Lauströer, Amir Andikfar)

movement can be explained using just two parameters: angle of attack of the limbs and limb stiffness [28]. The angle of attack is the angle between the supporting surface and a line drawn from the center of gravity of the body to the point of touch down. Although a model has not been developed for the dynamics of the dog, the observation that the touch down angle is consistently between 68° und 70° in all breeds examined to date suggests that dogs make use of similar mechanisms (▶ **Fig. 1.5**).

1.2.4   Generating Propulsion

During locomotion, a dog transfers forces to the ground in order to support the body and propel it forward. Force transfer is distributed almost evenly over the paw, with minimal variation in the center of pressure between the front and hind paw, and between the inside and the outside of the paw [8]. The forces exerted by the dog are transformed into ground forces, referred to as ground reaction forces. Over the last 40 years, numerous researchers have used force plates to measure ground reaction forces for various gaits in over 20 dog breeds and in many mixed breed dogs. Ground reaction forces occur in all three directions in space. The vertical force holds the body above the ground. Horizontal forces acting in the direction of motion result in braking or acceleration of locomotion. Forces acting perpendicular to the latter horizontal forces bring about sideways movements.

Ground reaction forces are dependent on the following general factors (▶ **Fig. 1.6**):
- the distribution of body mass over the front- and hindlimbs: depends on the actual distribution of body mass (e.g. large or small head) and the distance between the point of touch down and the center of mass;
- speed and, thus, the duration of the stance phase: on average, the vertical force produced must always be equivalent to the weight force; the shorter the stance phase compared to the suspension phase, the higher the vertical force;
- the stiffness or compliance of a limb.

All four of the dog's limbs participate in propulsion. During steady, cyclic locomotion (horizontally oriented forces), the contribution of the forelimbs to propulsion is minimal. As their touch down point is located in front of the center of mass for most of the stance phase, the front limbs can only pull the body. Since the front feet are not anchored to the ground by the claws, pulling by the forelimbs depends upon the friction of the footpads. It is not until the end of the stance phase that the

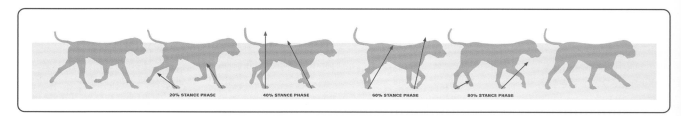

▶ **Fig. 1.6** Direction and relative size of force, represented by ground reaction force vectors. (source: Martin S. Fischer, Jonas Lauströer, Amir Andikfar)

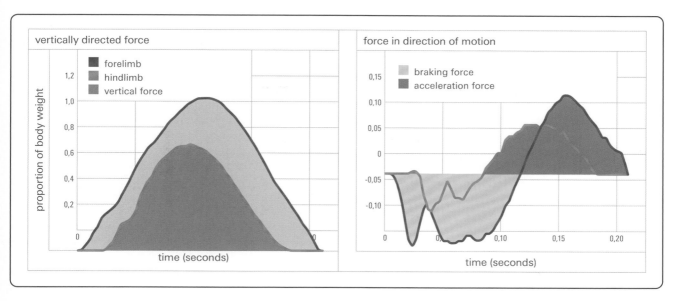

► **Fig. 1.7** The vertical ground reaction force is around 50% higher in the forelimb than in the hindlimb. The maximum horizontal force is reached after the mid-point of the stance phase in the forelimb, but considerably earlier in the hindlimb. Braking is stronger and more protracted in the forelimb than in the hindlimb, which is already generating propulsion after the first third of the stance phase. (source: Martin S. Fischer, Jonas Lauströer, Amir Andikfar)

forelimbs generate forward-acting forces and thereby advance the body.

Indeed, during walking and trotting, braking forces often dominate in the forelimbs, with propulsion coming primarily from the hindlimbs, particularly from the hip joint. In spontaneous movements, such as rapid acceleration and the like, the contribution of the forelimbs to propulsion increases. Changes in direction are initiated exclusively by the front legs.

Surprisingly, in contrast to humans, dogs do not loose speed when sprinting around a bend. For the paw to maintain an immovable point of contact, the body must turn around the fixed paw and the antebrachium must be able to rotate passively in both an external and - to a point beyond its normal alignment – internal direction.

Maximum vertical forces are 50% higher in the forelimbs than in the hindlimbs (► **Fig. 1.7**). This can be simply explained by the mass of the head and neck, which causes the center of mass to lie more cranially. During standing and walking, 30% of the dog's weight is carried by each forelimb and 20% by each hindlimb. Accordingly, the front paws are also larger than the hind paws. The force in the front limb increases during trotting, becoming greater than just the weight of the body; in the gallop it rises to more than double the body weight. In small breeds of dog, the maximum ground reaction force based on body weight is higher than in larger breeds. As body weight increases, there is a relative decrease in maximum ground reaction force. Vertical forces measured upon landing after jumping over a typical agility course obstacle have been shown to exceed body weight by a factor of 2.5. Similar values have been observed during sprints in Greyhounds with very short ground contact times (duty factor 20%); see Gait parameters (p. 23).

1.2.5 Pivot points of the Limbs

The simplest way for the limbs to swing in unison, and to move forward with the same stride length and stride frequency, is for the pivot points of the fore- and hindlimbs to be aligned at the same height above the ground. In the walk, trot and pace, these pivot points are located in the hip (hindlimb) and in the upper third of the scapula (forelimb). Execution of limb movement at an elevated pivot point produces the greatest possible stride length with the least possible displacement.

The pivot point of the scapula is not a true joint. The scapula and the trunk are connected by a system of muscles in what is referred to as a force-driven joint. Since the forelimb is suspended only by muscles, it moves around a so-called instantaneous center of rotation, rather than around a fixed point. In kinematics, an instantaneous center of rotation is defined as a point where the motion of a body is represented as a superimposition of translation and rotation. Extensive translation of the scapula along the thorax is observed at the end of the stance phase. The instantaneous center of rotation can be localized with a high degree of accuracy to the upper third of the scapular spine.

In contrast to the femur, which is the main generator of propulsion, the scapula serves to secure an elevated pivot point through which the trunk is "pushed" over the forelimbs. Thus, the specific role of the forelimbs is to carry the body at the appropriate height, via pre-defined bending and corresponding displacement of the body's center of gravity. A further important function is the absorption by the shoulder girdle muscles of the load produced upon landing after a jump. Although the power required to generate kinetic energy is the same for take-off and landing, landing occurs more quickly than take-off. Thus, the forces are correspondingly higher in the forelimbs.

1.2.6   Main Components of Movement

Only through the evolution of mammals has the scapula become a functional component of the forelimb. Whereas the shoulder girdle previously served as a skeletal attachment between the arm and the torso, it has been "liberated" from this task, particularly in mammals that lack a clavicle, such as the dog. During the course of evolution, the scapula has become aligned with the upper and lower arm, giving rise to a new functional analogy in which the scapula is equivalent to femur. The proximal bones of both limbs now operate concordantly. The scapula rotates through 30–40° (► Fig. 1.8) and the femur through 40–50°. In the gallop, sagittal flexion and extension of the back contribute to the work performed by the hindlimbs; together these serve as an integrated propulsive unit.

In the dog, the scapula lies alongside the trunk, to which it is attached by the extrinsic muscles of the shoulder (► Fig. 1.9). Only the thoracic part of the serratus ventralis (► Fig. 1.41) acts exclusively to suspend the trunk; the other muscles (cervical part of the serratus ventralis, pectorals, rhomboid) are responsible for pro- and retraction of the forelimbs and stabilization of the pivot point of the scapula. Except at the gallop, both portions of the rhomboid are continuously active. The cervical part of the serratus ventralis is active from the middle of the swing phase to the middle of the stance phase. Conversely, the superficial pectoral is active from the middle of the stance phase to the middle of the swing phase. In all gaits, the deep pectoral is only active in the second half of the swing phase. The cervical part of the trapezius has three phases of activity: in the first half of the stance phase, at the end of the stance phase and at the beginning of the swing phase. The thoracic part exhibits greatest activity in the first third of the swing phase. The primary action of the trapezius is to stabilize the pivot point of the scapula. At times, the activity of the muscles is low, suggesting that only small torques are generated at the pivot point of the scapula in a relatively sagittal plane of motion.

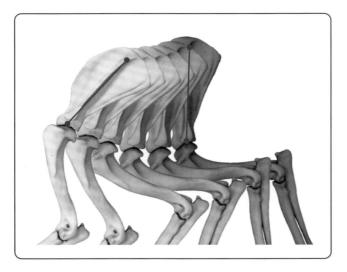

► **Fig. 1.8** In the stance phase, the scapula rotates (usually through 35–40°) around an instantaneous center of rotation located in the upper third of the bone. At lift off, the scapula is oriented vertically. At larger step lengths, the end position of the scapula may be 10° past the perpendicular. (source: Martin S. Fischer, Jonas Lauströer, Amir Andikfar)

1.2.7   Limb Kinematics

Movement during the stance phase involves uniform retraction of the three-segment limb at an almost constant angular velocity. In this process, the first and third segments, comprising the scapula and forearm, and thigh and hindfoot, remain parallel to one another (► Fig. 1.10). This locomotor principle is referred to as matched motion . In technical terms, the mechanism is described as a constraint linkage, in which the biarticular muscles (long head of the triceps brachii and the gastrocnemius muscles) form the actuating variable (► Fig. 1.11). As in a pantograph, a once frequently used drawing device, displacement of the first segment of the limb (scapula, femur) is transferred in amplified form to the third segment (antebrachium, hindfoot). The degree of amplification is determined by the length and angulation of the second segment. In all breeds, the two second segments (upper arm, lower leg) are of almost equal length, thus the angulation of the middle segments is also the same. The ratio of the length of the first segment to that of the third segment determines the force required to move the other respective segment. Thus, the same mechanical principle applies in the forelimb and the hindlimb. Appreciation of the parallel orientation of the first and third segments is particularly helpful in identifying the position of the scapula and femur beneath the skin and musculature; the orientation of the antebrachium during touch down and lift off provides a good approximation of the position of the scapula. This also applies when the dog is in a standing position (► Fig. 1.12).

The main action during the stance phase is rotation of the fore- and hindlimbs, with the first and third elements in parallel alignment, from the touch down position (50 to 60°) to a vertical lift off position. Although the scapula and femur undergo retraction until the end of the stance phase, a protraction torque is present at both bones for approximately half of the stance phase in the front limb, and 85% of the stance phase in the hindlimb (► Fig. 1.39, ► Fig. 1.40) [2]. This means that, as the limb in retraction undergoes braking, protraction of its proximal elements by the corresponding muscles has already commenced. Protraction of the hindlimbs is initiated by flexion of the hip joint and dorsiflexion of the foot. Retraction of the tibia continues into the swing phase. Plantar flexion does not occur in the hindlimb. At lift off, the scapula rotates cranially and the elbow joint flexes. In contrast to the hind foot, the front foot undergoes palmar flexion. The carpal joint is of particular significance at lift off. During the stance phase, a substantial torque is generated in the direction of palmar flexion, during which energy is absorbed and the flexor tendons are "loaded". Immediately after lift off, the carpus is catapulted towards the flexor aspect and is abducted, propelling the limb forward. During the swing phase, the effective length of the fore- and hindlimbs is reduced in a gait-dependent manner, whereas the duration of the swing phase is independent of gait and is remarkably constant.

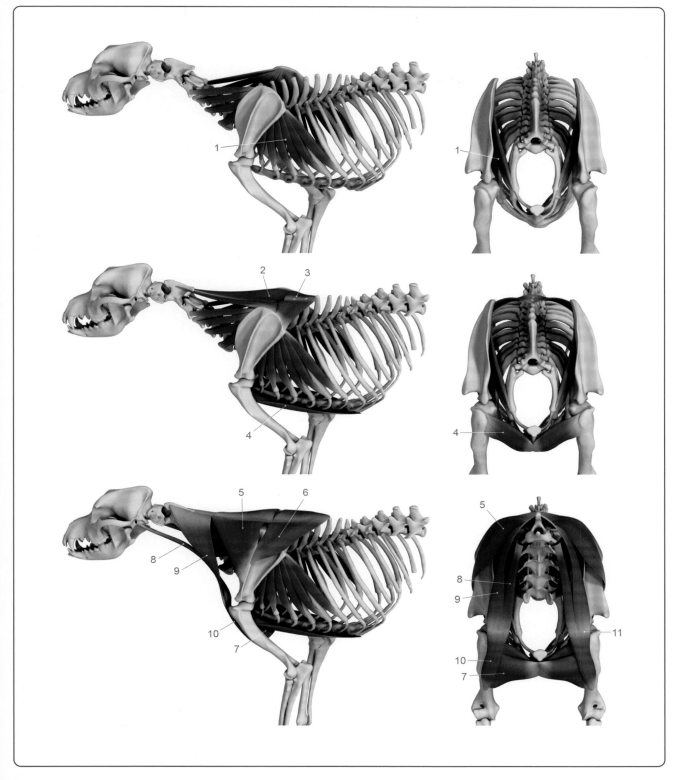

▶ **Fig. 1.9** Extrinsic muscles of the shoulder. 1 m. serratus ventralis, 2 m. rhomboideus cervicis, 3 m. rhomboideus thoracis, 4 m. pectoralis profundus, 5 m. trapezius pars cervicalis, 6 m. trapezius pars thoracica, 7 m. pectoralis superficialis, 8 m. brachiocephalicus pars cleidomastoidea, 9 m. brachiocephalicus pars cleidocervicalis, 10 m. brachiocephalicus pars cleidobrachialis, 11 tendinous intersection. (source: Martin S. Fischer, Jonas Lauströer, Amir Andikfar)

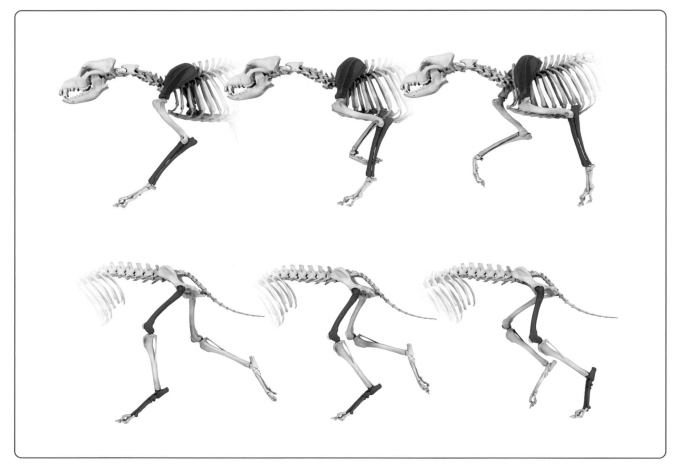

► **Fig. 1.10** The first and third segments move in matched motion because of the constraint linkage formed by the middle segments. (source: Martin S. Fischer, Jonas Lauströer, Amir Andikfar)

In addition to pro- and retraction, there is abduction, adduction and rotation on the longitudinal axis, particularly in the proximal long bones. These movements exhibit a high degree of breed-related variability (► **Fig. 1.13**) [24].

The following rules apply to touch down in the forelimb:
1. Touch down usually occurs directly beneath the ear.
2. The point of touch down lies on a line extending through the pivot point of the scapula and the glenoid cavity.
3. The humerus is always angled caudally; the shoulder is never extended so far that the humerus is oriented vertically.
4. The carpus extends from the antebrachium at almost 180°.

The following applies to lift off in the forelimb:
1. The angle of lift off is the same in the walk and the trot.
2. The scapula and the antebrachium are aligned vertically at lift off; rotation beyond this alignment results in lifting of the limb.
3. The brachium is oriented almost horizontally.

The following applies to touch down in the hindlimb:
1. The femur is already in retraction at touch down, the tibia is almost vertical, the foot is oriented parallel to the femur.

The following applies to lift off in the hindlimb:
1. The angle of lift off is the same in the walk and the trot.
2. The femur and the hind foot are vertically aligned at lift off; rotation beyond this alignment results in lifting of the limb.
3. The alignment of the tibia is almost horizontal.

By examining the difference between maximum angular movement (difference between the maximum and minimum joint angle in the stance phase) and effective angular movement (difference in the angle of the joint between touch down and lift off), it is possible to determine whether the movement of a joint is optimized for stride length or height adjustment. The smaller the difference, the greater the contribution of the joint to stride length. Effective angular movement of the hip joint and the dorsal edge of the scapula is greater than 90%. In contrast, the effective angular movement of the shoulder and elbow joints, and stifle and tarsal joint, is surprisingly small (5 to 20°). The primary function of the latter joints is height adjustment during the stance phase (e.g. during movement over uneven terrain; akin to having two shock absorbers in each limb), and flexion and extension during the swing phase, where the total amplitude is much greater.

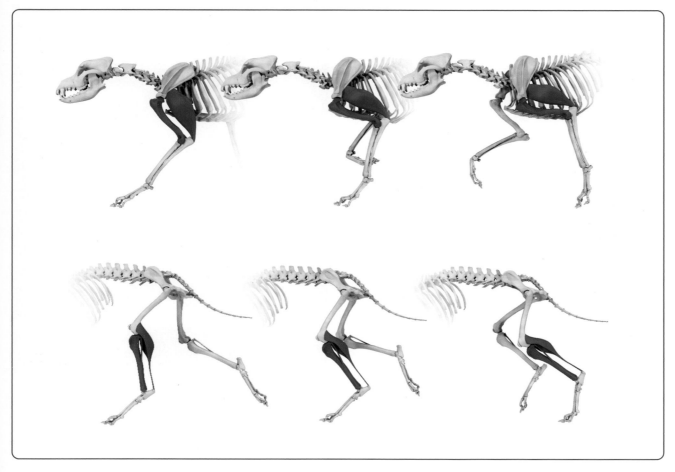

▶ **Fig. 1.11** The biarticular muscles (m. triceps brachii caput longum, mm. gastrocnemii) and the „middle" bones (humerus, tibia, fibula) constitute the actuating variable in the constraint linkage system. (source: Martin S. Fischer, Jonas Lauströer, Amir Andikfar)

In the swing phase, the limb moves at low velocity at the beginning and end of the phase, and at high velocity in the midsection. Thus, in contrast to the stance phase, angular velocity is not constant. Irrespective of gait, the average duration of the swing phase is 0.25–0.3 sec. The limb moves fastest in the middle third of the swing phase when, sharply angled, it swings forward like a short pendulum. Protraction begins with forward rotation of the scapula and thigh, which are already moving forward while the brachium and crus are still in retraction. Maximum extension of the limbs is reached in the last quarter of the swing phase, i.e. not at touch down.

In most of the joints of the limbs, the muscles act against the gravitational force and are thus referred to as „anti-gravity muscles" (▶ Fig. 1.41, ▶ Fig. 1.42). Contraction in biarticular anti-gravity muscles (long head of triceps brachii, gastrocnemius muscles) is largely isometric. The force of a muscle depends on both the degree of its activation and its length; optimum muscle length is 90 to 110% of its resting length. The long head of the triceps brachii and the gastrocnemius muscles are active in the first two thirds of the stance phase, not while the elbow and tarsal joints are undergoing extension. While these muscles contribute to axial limb strength in the stance phase (thus would be designated in the classic sense as leg extensors),

their contribution to limb extension in the swing phase is passive at best.

Control of flexion and extension permits dogs to react quickly and "intelligently" to depressions and elevations in the ground, especially on uneven terrain. The compliance of the joints, and thereby of the limbs, is a prerequisite for smooth locomotion in the field. A further division of labor is observed within each limb: the more distal their location in the limb, the more the muscles serve to store elastic energy and, in a functional sense, to make adjustments in height. In accordance with this biomechanical observation, Pitbull Terriers, which are bred for stability, have more muscle mass in the antebrachium and crus than Greyhounds, which are specialized for running [53]. Greyhounds also have a greater capacity for storing elastic energy, particularly in the common calcaneal tendon.

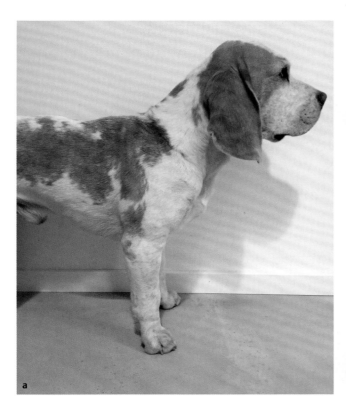 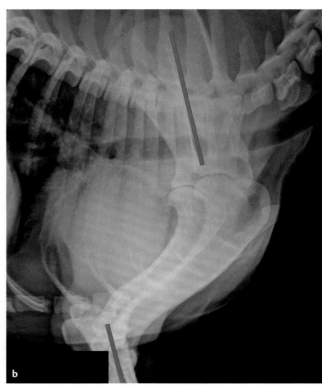

▶ **Fig. 1.12** When the dog is in a standing position, alignment of the scapula and the antebrachium is almost parallel.

a When the dog is in a standing position, the almost completely straight alignment of the antebrachium is obvious externally. (source: Dr. Alexandra Keller, Frankfurt am Main)

b In a radiograph of the same dog, the parallel alignment of the scapula and antebrachium is clearly evident. (source: Dr. Alexandra Keller, Frankfurt am Main)

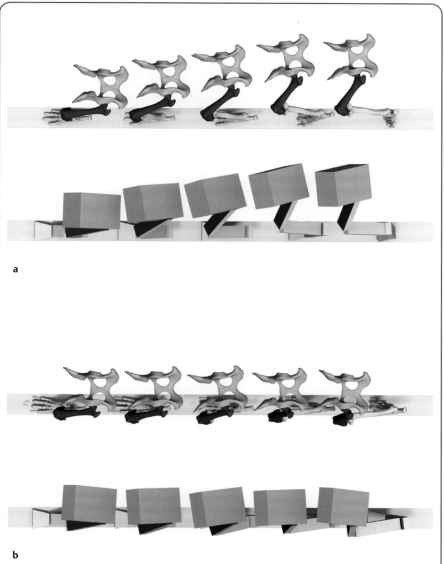

▶ **Fig. 1.13** Abduction and rotation of the femur in the French Bulldog and the Whippet.
a In the French Bulldog, abduction and rotation of the femur leads to pronounced medial displacement and twisting of the pelvis. (source: Martin S. Fischer, Jonas Lauströer, Amir Andikfar)
b In the Whippet, the largely parasagittal movement of the limbs results in only limited movement of the pelvis. (source: Martin S. Fischer, Jonas Lauströer, Amir Andikfar)

1.2.8 Movement of the Trunk

All gaits involve movement of the back. Movements between the individual vertebrae, particularly between the lumbar vertebrae in the gallop, give rise to large-scale excursions manifesting as flexion and extension of the back and, therewith, forward and backward movement of the pelvis.

Movement of the back is less obvious during walking and trotting than during galloping. This is largely because, in the walk and trot, the main purpose of the back muscles is to prevent movement. Back movements can be summarized according to two principles. In the trot, the middle of the body moves side to side and up and down, while the ends of the trunk, near the limbs, remain stationary (▶ Fig. 1.15).

During walking, on the other hand, a traveling wave, resembling the movement of a snake, passes over the back from front to rear (▶ Fig. 1.14). Movement of the back in the gallop can also be described as a traveling wave, based on the sequential flexion or extension of the intervertebral joints from front to rear.

1.2.9 Gait Parameters

Speed is a function of stride length and stride duration. The number of strides per second determines the stride frequency. Thus, dogs can increase their speed by lengthening their stride, increasing their stride frequency or by a combination of these factors. In all breeds examined to date, an increase in speed is achieved through alteration of both stride length and stride frequency.

Increased stride frequency at higher speeds is achieved exclusively by shortening the duration of the stance phase. The duration of the swing phase is completely independent of speed and gait, except in the Bernese Mountain Dog, in which minor variations are observed. Swinging limbs are similar in principle

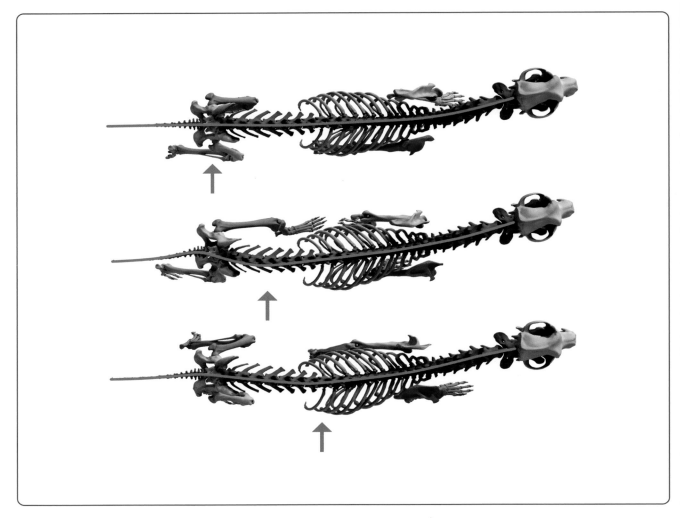

▶ **Fig. 1.14** In the walk, the back moves in a traveling wave. (source: Martin S. Fischer, Jonas Lauströer, Amir Andikfar)

to a pendulum. The duration of the swing phase thus depends on relative limb length and the distribution of mass over the limb, which is similar within and between breeds. In all breeds except the Tibetan Terrier, changes in stride length are brought about by altering the distance covered during the swing phase.

The term „duty factor" refers to the percentage of total stride duration that is taken up by the stance phase. A duty factor of 50% means that the stance phase and swing phase are of equal duration; a value of greater than 50% indicates that the stance phase is longer than the swing phase. Running gaits (trot, pace) have a duty factor of < 50%. Generally, for a particular gait, the duty factor is the same for the fore- and hindlimb.

1.2.10   Gaits and Footfall Patterns

The term gait is used to describe a regularly recurring sequence of limb movements. Dogs exhibit individual variation in the speed of locomotion within each gait; thus, one dog is already trotting while another of the same breed is still walking. Transitioning from one gait to another differs from changing gears in a car, in that dogs can move directly from a standing position into a high-speed gait. The transition between gaits is usually completed within two steps.

The walk (▶ Fig. 1.16), pace and trot are referred to collectively as symmetrical gaits, as the limbs on one side of the body move with the same temporal rhythm, and in the same way, as those on the contralateral side, just in a staggered fashion. Within these symmetrical gaits, the gait type is determined by the temporal offset between the fore- and hindlimb on one side of the body. In the pace, the fore- and hindlimbs on one side touch down at the same time (▶ Fig. 1.17). Touch down is offset by about a quarter of a gait cycle in the walk and half a gait cycle in the trot (▶ Fig. 1.18). The symmetrical gaits represent a continuum that includes both pace-like walking (also referred to as fast walking) and trot-like walking. It has recently been shown in horses that just a single gene (DMRT3) is responsible for the ability to pace [1]. Specialized nerve cells formed in the presence of the DMRT3 gene connect the left and right sides of the locomotor apparatus and, in mice, are responsible for coordination. Interestingly, during swimming, dogs exhibit a gait that is not used in terrestrial locomotion. This fast, diagonal single footfall or dog paddle, is a four-beat gait in which each foot

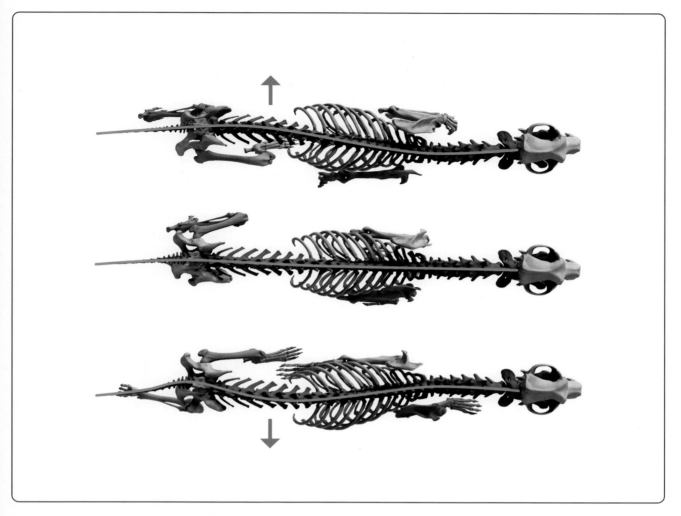

▶ **Fig. 1.15** In the trot, the movements of the back resemble a standing wave. (source: Martin S. Fischer, Jonas Lauströer, Amir Andikfar)

strikes the "surface" individually [21]. This gravity-free form of locomotion is further distinguished by greater angular movement in all joints.

'Gallop' is an overarching term for the various types of this gait. The gallop is described as an asymmetric gait, as the fore- and hindlimbs do not touch down consecutively on the same side of the body. Instead, the limb pairs (either both forelimbs or both hindlimbs) touch down one after another. As these touch downs are not simultaneous, a distinction is made between the limb that touches down first (trailing) and the one that touches down second (leading). The trailing limb always takes considerably more body weight than the leading limb, particularly upon touch down immediately after the suspension phase. This form of interworking of the hind- and forelimbs enables the back to participate in lengthening the stride. When both forelimbs are on the ground and the hindlimbs are in the air, the lumbar vertebral column is arched, causing the hindlimbs to be brought further forward; upon contact with the ground, the lumbar spine extends.

Dogs exhibit the slow gallop, also termed the canter, and both types of fast gallop, the diagonal and rotary gallop. In the

canter, there are alternating phases of unipedal and tripedal support; a suspension phase is short or absent (▶ **Fig. 1.19**). In the diagonal (▶ **Fig. 1.20**) and rotary gallop, there is at least one period of suspension, often followed by a second at higher speeds. When two suspension phases are present, the gait is referred to as a double-suspension gallop. In the diagonal and rotary gallops, the suspension phase is followed by unipedal, bipedal and sometimes even tripedal support phases. In the rotary gallop, the limbs strike the ground in a clockwise or anticlockwise sequence (▶ **Fig. 1.21**). Grounding of the second hindlimb is followed by landing the ipsilateral forelimb. In the diagonal gallop, grounding of the second hindlimb is followed by landing of the diagonally opposite forelimb.

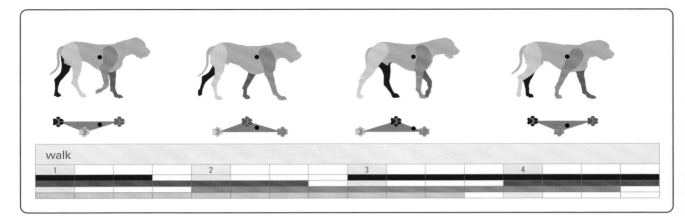

▶ **Fig. 1.16** In the walk, there are alternating phases of bipedal and tripedal support. This has the advantage of keeping the body's center of gravity in the region where the body is supported by the grounded limbs. (source: Martin S. Fischer, Jonas Lauströer, Amir Andikfar)

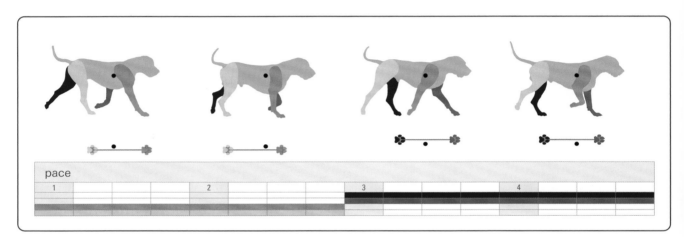

▶ **Fig. 1.17** In the pace, the body is supported by the ipsilateral fore- and hindlimbs. The body's center of gravity is not located on this axis of support, thus the trunk "sways". (source: Martin S. Fischer, Jonas Lauströer, Amir Andikfar)

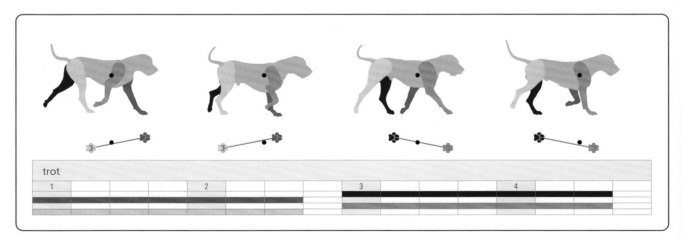

▶ **Fig. 1.18** In the trot, the body is supported by diagonally opposite limb pairs. The stance phase alternates between the right forelimb and left hindlimb and the opposite respective limbs, sometimes with a period of suspension between the changeover. Ideally, the body's center of gravity during the trot remains on the axis of support between the grounded limbs. (source: Martin S. Fischer, Jonas Lauströer, Amir Andikfar)

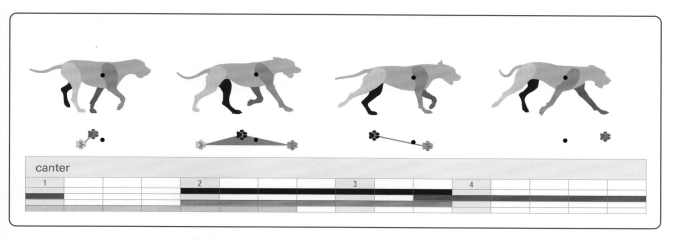

► **Fig. 1.19** The canter is the slowest form of gallop. There is no suspension phase. A unipedal support phase alternates with a tripedal support phase. The support base for the body's center of gravity may lie on a line, within a triangle or, during the unipedal support phase, on a single point. (source: Martin S. Fischer, Jonas Lauströer, Amir Andikfar)

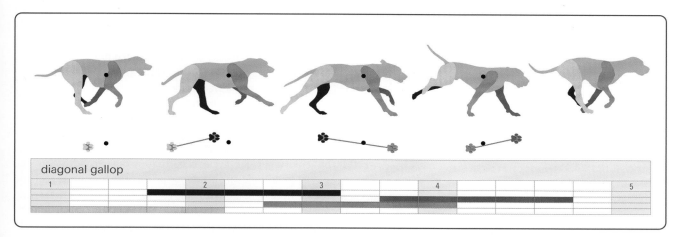

► **Fig. 1.20** In the diagonal gallop, grounding of the second hindlimb is followed by landing of the diagonally opposite limb. The fore- and hindlimbs that land first are located on the same side of the body. (source: Martin S. Fischer, Jonas Lauströer, Amir Andikfar)

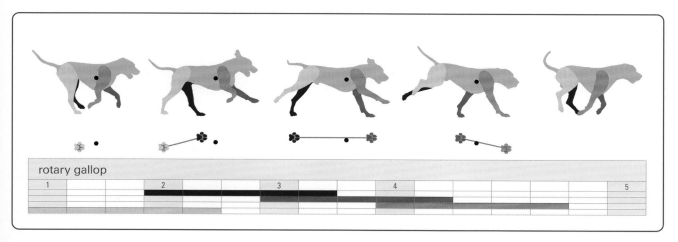

► **Fig. 1.21** In the rotary gallop, the limbs strike the ground in a clockwise or anticlockwise sequence. Grounding of the second hindlimb is followed by landing of the ipsilateral forelimb. (source: Martin S. Fischer, Jonas Lauströer, Amir Andikfar)

1.2.11 Muscle Activity in the Walk and Trot

The descriptions of muscle activity in this chapter are based on electromyographic studies of various functional muscle groups. Electromyography measures changes in electrical activity of muscle; muscle activity at the measurement site is recorded in the form of an electromyogram (EMG). In early electromyography techniques, the electrical signal was transmitted from individual needle electrodes inserted into the muscle at different depths. More recent studies using surface electrodes have shown that a muscle is rarely activated as a whole. In some cases, waves of activation are observed in individual muscles, exemplified by the sequential activation of different regions of the triceps brachii during cyclic locomotion. Alternatively, the EMG may reveal only very small regions of activation when, in the course of cyclic locomotion, small regions of muscle rich in type I fibers are active, while regions dominated by type II fibers are inactive; see Muscle Fiber Types (p. 37).

Of particular note are the following muscles or muscle groups, for which actions deduced from topographical anatomy are partly incorrect. The latissimus dorsi does not draw the forelimb backwards during the stance phase. Instead, it is only active during the second half of the swing phase. Its task is to brake the swinging limb and to retract it until the point of touch down. At touch down, its activity ceases. This applies to motion on a level surface.

Only few muscles are active during the entire stance phase (supraspinatus, acromial part of the deltoid, flexor digitorum profundus); these muscles work against gravity. The infraspinatus, triceps brachii, extensor carpi ulnaris and flexor carpi ulnaris are active from touch down until the middle of the stance phase and similarly act to counter gravity-induced flexion. In the second half of the stance phase, the teres major, deltoid (scapular part) and flexor carpi radialis act to support retraction of the forelimbs. The biceps brachii is active in the last third of the stance phase and initially counteracts passive extension of the elbow, to which this joint is subject as soon as the point of support has passed the elbow joint. During the swing phase, it acts to lift and protract the forelimb. This action is also initiated by the brachiocephalicus, brachialis and flexors of the carpal joint. During trotting and galloping, the activity of the flexors, particularly the brachialis and biceps brachii, is greater than during walking, as the limbs are lifted higher from a usually lower starting position against the trunk. The activity of the muscles that counteract gravity-induced flexion after landing is also greater in the trot and the gallop.

Three muscle groups are responsible for pro- and retraction of the hindlimbs. Hindlimb retraction and thus propulsion of the body is brought about largely by the croup muscles (cranial part of the biceps femoris, gluteals, semimembranosus and adductor magnus). The activity of these muscles begins at the end of the swing phase and usually lasts until midstance. During running on an incline, the activity of the retractors can increase severalfold (at just a 10% incline the increase is already 20-fold). The caudal part of the biceps femoris, semitendinosus and gracilis are active from towards the end of the stance phase until early in the swing phase and are thus responsible for lifting the hindlimbs. In situations where additional force is needed for propulsion, such as running uphill or pulling on a lead, these muscles are activated early and serve as retractors. The hindlimbs are swung forward primarily by the action of the iliopsoas, tensor fasciae latae and sartorius, and also the rectus femoris, which exhibits biphasic activity in the symmetrical gaits.

The stifle join (p. 67)t, in which there is little effective angular movement during the stance phase, is stabilized against gravity-induced flexion by the vastii. For the tarsal joint, this task is performed by the gastrocnemii which, like the aforementioned muscles, are active at the end of the swing phase and the beginning of the stance phase. Their contraction is essentially isometric and serves to counteract gravity-induced load rather than to extend the limb. Subsequent flexion of the tarsal joint at lift off is produced by the action of the tibialis cranialis and extensor digitorum longus.

As in other mammals, the back muscles of the dog consist of three longitudinal systems: the transversospinalis, longissimus and iliocostalis systems. The muscle segments of the longissimus and iliocostalis span several vertebrae, while the transversospinalis system consists of long and short segments. Adjacent vertebrae are connected primarily by deep muscles lying close to the bone (e.g. the rotatores). For a long time, the action of the back muscles during locomotion remained unclear. To date, EMG recordings have been made for just three of the canine back muscles: multifidus lumborum, longissimus thoracis et lumborum and iliocostalis thoracis et lumborum.

In the walk and trot, these three muscles exhibit two phases of activity per gait cycle, occurring in the second half of the stance phase and in the swing phase. Thus, activation of the same muscles has two different effects. During the swing phase, muscle contraction results - as expected - in lateral flexion of the trunk. This does not occur in the stance phase, in which the muscles serve to stabilize the trunk. In this way, the back muscles establish a static base for the work performed by the limb muscles that originate from the trunk, and compensate for the torques that pass into the trunk. In the walk and gallop, the cranial portions are activated earlier than those located caudally, resulting in sequential activation along the back. In contrast, all portions are activated concurrently in the trot.

In the gallop, recorded muscle activity can be readily reconciled with observed movement of the vertebral column. On both sides of the body, the muscles exhibit a concurrent phase of activity per gait cycle. This commences in the suspension phase, shortly before touch down of the first hindlimb, and results in extension of the back during the course of the stance phase. The activity of the back muscles and extension of the back ceases when the trailing hindlimb (first to strike the ground) lifts off.

1.3

Bones, Joints and Muscles

Martin S. Fischer, Daniel Koch

1.3.1 Bones

Bone is a form of connective tissue. The cells are embedded in an extracellular matrix, the composition of which determines the mechanical properties of the bone. In all vertebrates, the matrix contains collagen fibers that are mineralized through deposition of hydroxyapatite. Bone is a living, dynamic tissue that undergoes constant remodelling. Old bone is resorbed and new ossification takes place. In humans, 5–10% of bone is replaced in this way per year. Bone responds to changing mechanical demands, accumulating at appropriate locations under load and breaking down relatively quickly when mechanical stress is absent. With increasing age, bone density decreases due to reduced perfusion, and associated reduction in calcium supply, and altered hormonal influences. The extent of the reduction in bone density varies in different bones. Life-long loading is essential for stimulation of the processes involved in bone formation and resorption. Frequency of loading is more important than the magnitude of the load. Remodelling is dependent on dynamic and non-static load. In addition to its supportive function, bone is the largest repository of calcium and phosphate in the body. It also stores fat, produces hormones (osteocalcin), and stores growth factors (e.g. IGF) and cytokines, among many other substances. In the process of mammalian evolution, storage of phosphate is considered to have become a basic function of bone.

Bone is resorbed by multinuclear, amoeboid giant cells referred to as osteoclasts. Osteoclasts initially lyse bone within resorption lacunae (Howship's lacunae), via active proton transport (H^+ion secretion) in an acid environment, and then break down the organic matrix with the aid of proteolytic enzymes. Osteoblasts are usually found directly underneath the periosteum. These cells produce mostly type I collagen and contribute to mineralization. Osteoblasts that have „walled themselves in" become osteocytes. These cells are interconnected by long cytoplasmic processes (osteocyte-bone lining cell system) that are able to detect local changes in loading. This triggers the release of messenger substances, including the important signalling molecule nitrogen monoxide (NO).

Structurally, bone consists of substantia corticalis (or substantia compacta; compact bone) and substantia spongiosa (spongy bone). Compact bone constitutes over three quarters of bone tissue. Spongy bone is distributed irregularly in bones, with bone trabeculae oriented along lines of tension and compressive stress. In the adult mammal, compact bone occurs as lamellar bone, which resembles plywood in its lightweight construction while also incorporating space for capillaries. The fewest possible materials are used to create the greatest possible strength; bone is able to withstand tensile and compressive loads of 10 kg and 15 kg/mm² respectively. Woven bone (containing irregular collagen fibers) grows faster but has considerably less strength; in adult dogs it occurs only in the early

stages of fracture healing. Woven bone is always replaced by lamellar bone.

The periosteum is a layer of fibrous connective tissue that surrounds the compact bone and from which circumferential growth of bone takes place. It contains blood vessels, nerve fibers, osteoblasts and osteoclasts, and plays an important role in fracture healing.

Bone is composed of inorganic material (> 50%), organic material (about 25%) and water. The inorganic components consist of calcium phosphate as hydroxyapatite (up to > 90%), calcium carbonate, magnesium phosphate and calcium fluoride. The proportion of hydroxyapatite determines the hardness of the bone. Crystalline hydroxyapatite develops from amorphous calcium phosphate. In a preliminary stage of development, 1 nm sized domains acting as precursors for calcium phosphate are suspended in the matrix without undergoing mineralization. In the presence of an appropriate surface, these begin to aggregate, initially forming amorphous structures and eventually crystallizing into mineralized calcium phosphate. More than 90% of the organic ground substance of bone consists of collagen fibers (type I collagen). The remainder is composed of proteoglycans and glycoproteins that serve to bind water.

Bone is also a hormone-producing organ. Mice lacking osteocalcin become overweight and develop diabetes, reflecting a hormonal communication between adipose tissue and bone. In addition, osteocalcin increases the production and effect of insulin within the body. Moreover, osteocalcin enhances reproductive capacity in male mice, particularly by influencing the survival of male gametes – an unexpected relationship between bone and fertility [51].

The spaces between the trabeculae of spongy bone contain red or yellow bone marrow. In long bones such as the femur and tibia, the medullary cavity of adult animals is filled with yellow, fat-rich marrow that lacks the capacity to produce blood cells. In flat and short bones, such as the scapula or carpal bones, the interior is completely filled with spongy bone, in which the spaces between the trabeculae are packed with red bone marrow. Bone tissue is well vascularized. The arterial blood supply arises from the medullary cavity, whereas venous blood drains from outside to inside. Within compact bone, the arteries pass through osteons that are about 10 cm long, but only around 200 µm wide.

As body size increases or decreases, surface area and volume change by a power of 2 and 3 respectively. This means that volume changes exponentially compared with surface area. Since the strength of bone is a surface area-based property, growth would be limited unless there was a disproportionate increase in surface area and diameter (allometry). Nevertheless, large dogs have relatively narrow bones.

The feedback systems for load-dependent adjustments of bone morphology are not limited to local mechanisms. As is the case with evolutionary adaptations, selective breeding practices impact on all elements of the locomotor apparatus, even when the intention is to influence only one component. Consequently, two developmental directions (functional trade offs) are observed with respect to canine body structure, one optimized for strength and other for speed [11], [33]. Surprisingly, pelvis shape (narrow or broad) is correlated with limb

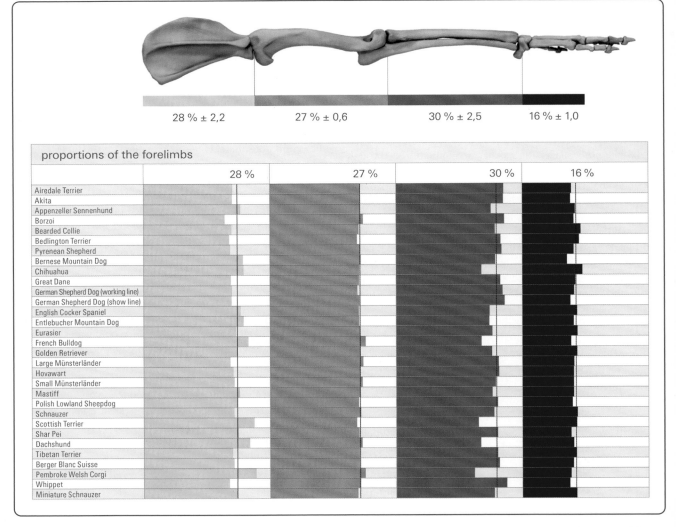

28 % ± 2,2   **27 % ± 0,6**   **30 % ± 2,5**   **16 % ± 1,0**

proportions of the forelimbs	28 %	27 %	30 %	16 %
Airedale Terrier				
Akita				
Appenzeller Sennenhund				
Borzoi				
Bearded Collie				
Bedlington Terrier				
Pyrenean Shepherd				
Bernese Mountain Dog				
Chihuahua				
Great Dane				
German Shepherd Dog (working line)				
German Shepherd Dog (show line)				
English Cocker Spaniel				
Entlebucher Mountain Dog				
Eurasier				
French Bulldog				
Golden Retriever				
Large Münsterländer				
Hovawart				
Small Münsterländer				
Mastiff				
Polish Lowland Sheepdog				
Schnauzer				
Scottish Terrier				
Shar Pei				
Dachshund				
Tibetan Terrier				
Berger Blanc Suisse				
Pembroke Welsh Corgi				
Whippet				
Miniature Schnauzer				

▶ **Fig. 1.22** Proportions of the forelimb. In all species examined to date, the proportional length of the humerus is almost identical. Shortening of the antebrachium in chondrodystrophic breeds is counterbalanced by an increase in the relative length of the scapula. (source: Martin S. Fischer, Jonas Lauströer, Amir Andikfar)

bone shape (elliptical or round) and the shape of the skull (long or broad). Try as one might, it is not possible to breed a Greyhound that has the powerful head of a Pitbull. The same correlation has been demonstrated in silver foxes, suggesting the existence of a fundamental underlying control mechanism, at least in canids. The differentiation between strength- and speed-oriented body types is accompanied by an observable change in the shape of the thorax and the associated positioning of the limbs. Alterations also occur in the distribution of body weight over the fore- and hindlimbs, the relationship between wither height and body length, and the legginess index.

Whether a dog is large or small, the length of the long bones is related isometrically to body mass, though in smaller dogs (femur length less than 12.5) the metacarpals are comparatively long, and the metatarsals relatively short. Comparison of the anatomical length of the fore- and hindlimbs reveals that the forelimbs are slightly longer in all dogs. The same anatomical length relationships are observed in both lines of German Shepherd Dogs, which also have the relatively longest forelimbs.

Mathematical simulations have shown that the proportions (▶ Fig. 1.22, ▶ Fig. 1.23) of the three-segment leg have a substantial influence on the mechanical function of the limb in terms of its dynamic stability [66]. In leg models, the greater the dynamic stability (p. 16) of the leg, the faster it returns to a stable trajectory following perturbation of the motion sequence. This is an important component of intelligent mechanics. The length of the middle leg segment (humerus, tibia) is particularly important; this should not be less than 40% of total leg length. The more unequal the length of the first and third segments, the greater the potential range of stiffness of the joints, which in turn promotes dynamic stability While optimal leg proportions are not always observed in nature, the hindlimbs have been found to follow this mechanical principle more closely, with a relative tibia length of 37% ± 1.3%. The hindfoot is always shorter than the femur. In the forelimb, dissimilarity of the length of the first and third segments is increased by lengthening of the metacarpal bones and the straightness of their connection with the antebrachium. The humerus exhibits the least variation in relative length (27% ±

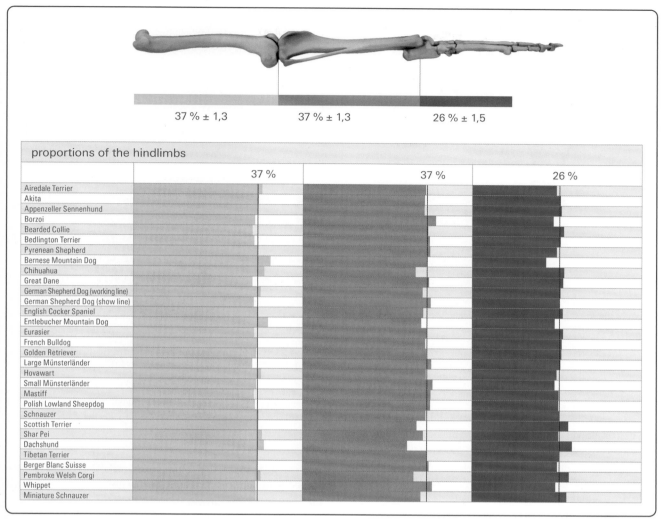

proportions of the hindlimbs	37 %	37 %	26 %
Airedale Terrier			
Akita			
Appenzeller Sennenhund			
Borzoi			
Bearded Collie			
Bedlington Terrier			
Pyrenean Shepherd			
Bernese Mountain Dog			
Chihuahua			
Great Dane			
German Shepherd Dog (working line)			
German Shepherd Dog (show line)			
English Cocker Spaniel			
Entlebucher Mountain Dog			
Eurasier			
French Bulldog			
Golden Retriever			
Large Münsterländer			
Hovawart			
Small Münsterländer			
Mastiff			
Polish Lowland Sheepdog			
Schnauzer			
Scottish Terrier			
Shar Pei			
Dachshund			
Tibetan Terrier			
Berger Blanc Suisse			
Pembroke Welsh Corgi			
Whippet			
Miniature Schnauzer			

37 % ± 1,3   37 % ± 1,3   26 % ± 1,5

▶ **Fig. 1.23** Proportions of the hindlimb. In general, the thigh and crus are equal in length. (source: Martin S. Fischer, Jonas Lauströer, Amir Andikfar)

0.6%). Investigations in Beagles have shown that these leg segment length ratios are present in the early stages of ontogenesis.

1.3.2 Joints

A joint is a moveable connection between two or more skeletal components. True joints, or diarthroses (▶ Fig. 1.24, ▶ Fig. 1.25) are those incorporating a joint space between two articular surfaces lined with cartilage. Synarthroses occur where bones are connected by osseous fusion, as in the sacrum (synostoses), by cartilage, as in the sternum (synchondroses) or by connective tissue as seen in the sacroiliac joint (syndesmoses). Whereas forces acting on true joints are transmitted as pressure and tension, synarthroses are subjected to shear, i.e. they experience shear stress [38]. Furthermore, the rotational axis of diarthroses is relatively fixed, while in synarthroses it moves in accordance with the forces acting on the joint.

True joints are hermetically enclosed by a joint capsule composed of connective tissue (capsula articularis). The outer layer (stratum fibrosum) varies both within and between joints. The thin, inner layer (stratum synoviale) of the capsule produces and reabsorbs the synovial fluid . Blood vessels pass between the layers; free nerve endings and mechanoreceptors are also found in this location. Depending on the joint, the volume of synovial fluid is less than 1 milliliter to just a few milliliters. This highly viscous fluid acts to lubricate the joint, nourish the articular cartilage and prevent direct contact between the two cartilaginous surfaces under normal load bearing conditions. Synovial fluid is an ultrafiltrate of blood plasma with a high concentration of hyaluronic acid as well as proteoglycans (such as aggrecan or lubricin). Lubricin has an extremely low coefficient of friction, allowing the joint surfaces to glide easily over one another for long periods. Synovial fluid has a small population of cells, including macrophages (63%), lymphocytes (25%), neutrophils (7%) and synovial cells (4%), that contribute to repair and immune defense. Synovial fluid also serves to remove the end products of metabolic processes occurring in the articular cartilage and the menisci.

The articular surfaces of diarthroses are lined with cartilage, a viscoelastic material composed of cartilage cells (chondrocytes) and a specialized extracellular matrix. Cartilage matrix is produced by chondrocytes in a process that progresses very

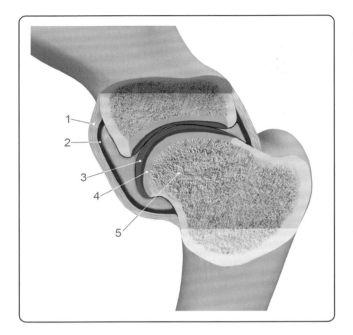

▶ **Fig. 1.24** Section of a true, synovial joint. Joint capsule with 1 stratum fibrosum und 2 stratum synoviale, 3 articular cartilage, 4 subchondral bone, 5 spongy bone. (source: Martin S. Fischer, Jonas Lauströer, Amir Andikfar)

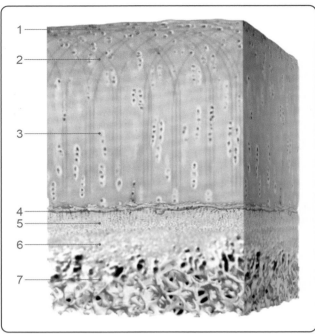

▶ **Fig. 1.25** Components of a true joint. Based on the shape of the chondrocytes, the orientation of collagen fibers and the composition of the ground substance, articular cartilage is divided into four zones: the tangential (1), intermediate- (2) and radial (3) zones and, below the tide mark (4), the calcified zone (5). Located deep to the cartilage is subchondral bone (6) and spongy bone (7). (source: Martin S. Fischer, Jonas Lauströer, Amir Andikfar)

slowly. Through secretion of cytokines, chondrocytes also break the matrix down. Chondrocytes only constitute around 5% of the total cartilage volume; 70–80% of the intercellular volume consists of water and just 20–30% comprises solid components, primarily collagen (10–30% of the wet weight) as well as proteoglycans (5–10%) and minerals.

Collagen gives cartilage tensile strength. Constituting over 90% of the collagen in the articular cartilage, type II collagen is the most important type of collagen found in this tissue. Its fibers extend throughout the articular cartilage as a three-dimensional network. In the superficial tangential zone, the collagen fibers are arranged tangentially, providing maximum strength and, thereby, uniform distribution of load. Within the transitional or intermediate zone, the fibers are arranged in crisscrossing arcades. In the radial zone, which makes up around 40–60% of the thickness of the articular cartilage, the radially arranged collagen fibers are thickest and the water content is lowest. Sometimes a deeper layer can be distinguished, in which 2–6 chondrocytes are arranged radially in small columns. The radial collagen fibers extend through the tide mark and a cell-poor layer of calcified cartilage (calcified zone) into the subchondral bone.

Proteoglycans are responsible for the compressive resilience of articular cartilage. Aggrecan molecules account for 90% of the proteoglycan content. These molecules interact with hyaluronic acid to produce large proteoglycan aggregates in a highly ordered spatial arrangement. The aggregates are able to bind large quantities of water. As the proteoglycan aggregates and interstitial fluid are not compressible, deformation of the articular cartilage is based on changes in volume and egress of water into the joint space (▶ Fig. 1.26). Thus, as load increases the cartilage becomes firmer. As a side effect of water moving

into the joint space, the volume of synovial fluid between the loaded joint surfaces increases, further reducing direct contact between them.

During growth, articular cartilage is directly supplied by blood vessels extending from the bone. With continuing development of the layers beneath the tide mark (▶ Fig. 1.25), this source of nutrition is significantly curtailed and the cartilage becomes a bradytrophic tissue, devoid of blood vessels, nerves and lymph vessels. Due to its unique metabolic situation, it must derive its nutrition from the synovial fluid by diffusion and convection, i.e. through the carriage of dissolved substances by a moving fluid (synovial fluid). Deformation of the cartilage under load subjects not only the cartilage matrix but also the chondrocytes to alternating forces of suction and pressure. Under load, fluid is pressed from the extracellular matrix into the joint cavity; when the load is removed, the cartilage absorbs synovial fluid containing nutrients and oxygen. Thus, a constantly changing load is required for continuous nourishment of the cartilage. Even the synthetic capacity of the chondrocytes, which is fueled by anaerobic glycolysis, adapts to the prevailing mechanical conditions, whereby the demand for biosynthesis increases under dynamic load and decreases when the load is static. Without periodic loading, individual regions of cartilage become undernourished and the cartilage transforms into so-called fibrocartilage, with different biochemical and mechanical properties, or undergoes calcification. The fibrocartilage occurring in discs and menisci contains 70% Type I collagen fibers in parallel arrangement and is more pliant. Car-

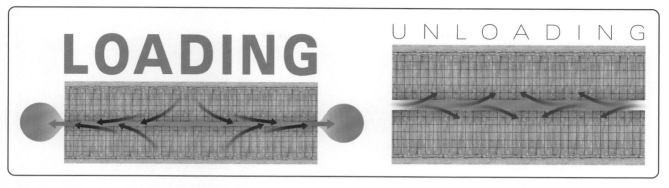

▶ **Fig. 1.26** Schematic representation of cartilage deformation during application and release of a load. When a load is applied, small amounts of fluid pass from the cartilage into the joint space. When the load is removed, the cartilage absorbs fluid like a sponge. (source: Martin S. Fischer, Jonas Lauströer, Amir Andikfar)

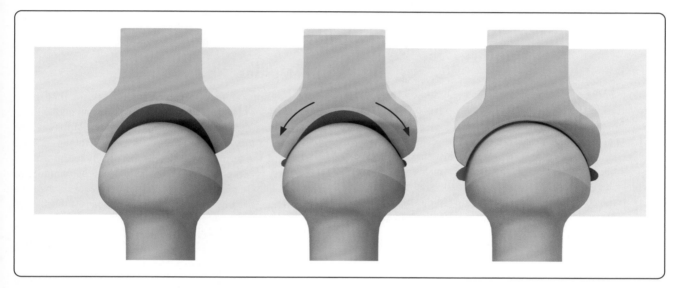

▶ **Fig. 1.27** Behaviour of an incongruent joint under load. With increasing load, the synovial fluid is displaced to the periphery of the joint. Load is greater there than at the center and the peripheral cartilage is correspondingly thicker. Tensile loading (arrows) occurs in the bone beneath the layer of articular cartilage (subchondral bone). (source: Martin S. Fischer, Jonas Lauströer, Amir Andikfar)

tilage that has been destroyed cannot regenerate! Lesions are merely covered with inferior scar tissue. It follows, therefore, that dynamic and varied load is essential for the health of articular cartilage and, thereby, the joint. In view of the limited effective movement of the joints of the limbs during locomotion (p. 62) (in the elbow joint, for example, the difference between the angle of touch down and the angle of lift off is often less than 10°), it is important to emphasize the role of the varied movements that dogs can only perform during off-leash activity in preserving the health of articular cartilage.

Cartilage is 10 times more deformable than spongy bone, which in turn is 10 times more deformable than cortical bone. However, since it is thin, cartilage makes only a limited contribution to shock absorption. The subchondral bone layer, measuring a few millimetres in thickness, and the underlying spongy bone work together with the muscles to serve as the primary shock absorber. The subchondral bone is thicker and more extensively mineralized at locations subjected to substantial load. In the shoulder joint of the dog, it is 6 times thicker on the concave side of the joint than in the head of the humerus. As early

as 1963, Pauwels had already identified subchondral bone density as a material representation of stress, i.e. as a record of lifetime load [54].

Anatomy has always adopted terms from mechanical engineering. Accordingly, the elbow joint is described as a hinge joint and the shoulder and hip joints as ball and socket joints. Joint function is nonetheless much more complex, and the image of joints as closely interlocking hinges or ball joints requires further differentiation. Today, based on the work of Felix Eckstein (now at Paracelsus Private Medical University, Salzburg) and Johann Maierl and his research group at the Ludwig-Maximilians-University Munich, all joints, including those of the limbs of dogs, are predominantly regarded as physiologically incongruent [17], [43]. In a congruent joint, small forces cause the corresponding articulating surfaces to come largely or completely into contact. In physiologically incongruent joints that are not under load, a tight fit between the articular surfaces is lacking, and there is only limited contact. (▶ Fig. 1.27). As load increases, the areas of contact between the joint surfaces enlarge and pressure is distributed over a larger surface. Conse-

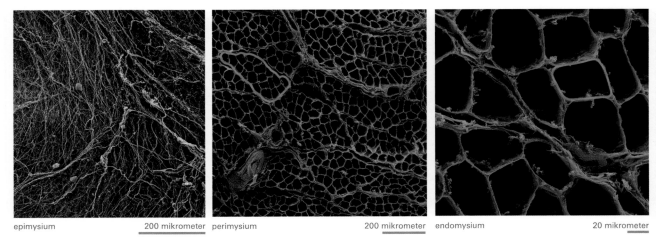

epimysium   200 mikrometer   perimysium   200 mikrometer   endomysium   20 mikrometer

▶ **Fig. 1.28** The connective tissue sheaths surrounding the muscle are subdivided into the epimysium, perimysium and endomysium. (source: Nadja Schilling, Institut für Zoologie und Evolutionsforschung, Friedrich-Schiller-Universität Jena)

quently, the load per unit of surface area decreases or remains the same as the degree of force increases. Based on the radius of curvature of the concave surfaces, two types of incongruity are recognized. Convex incongruity occurs when the concave side has a greater radius than the convex articular surface (e.g. shoulder joint), leading to a bell-shaped distribution of pressure over the concave side. In the case of concave incongruity (e.g. hip joint), the concave side has a smaller radius of curvature than the convex side, initially resulting in bicentric peripheral pressure distribution and, under greater load, in uniform distribution of pressure across the entire joint surface.

Physiological incongruity should not be confused with the term used in veterinary medicine to describe the pathological formation of a step within the elbow joint. Physiological incongruity optimizes the distribution of stress by evenly distributing pressure in the joint, while the concave portion of the joint surface is subject to tensile stress. Particularly the peripheral regions are incorporated into pressure distribution when the joint is loaded. Under larger loads, the concave joint surface is stretched and the convex counterpart is pushed in deeper. The pressure-transmitting surfaces are enlarged, avoiding localized pressure peaks that would form in a congruent ball joint with centrally distributed pressure. This elastic surface enlargement is made possible by the properties of the cartilage.

Cartilage thickness is an indicator of lifelong load. It varies both between and within joints. The cartilage of physiologically incongruent joints is generally thicker than that of congruent joints, as focal forces occurring in incongruent joints are distributed over a larger surface, especially to the peripheral regions. Accordingly, the subchondral bone layer is also thicker at the periphery than at the center of the joint. An understanding of these relationships has led to thorough investigation of the thickness of cartilage and the subchondral bone layer in dogs, enabling conclusions to be drawn about long-term joint stress. These findings are referenced in the descriptions of individual joints (p.62). An interesting example is the greater thickness of the cartilage near the medial coronoid process, compared with the lateral side.

1.3.3 Muscles

In the dog, muscle mass accounts for 50–60% of total body weight. Muscles play a significant role in almost all bodily functions including digestion, gland emptying and maintenance of body temperature. As this book deals only with the skeletal musculature, the term 'muscle' refers specifically to this muscle type. Muscle is composed of two tissue types: dense connective tissue and muscle fibers. Muscle fibers generate force; the connective tissue, with its high tensile strength, is responsible for force transmission.

Irregular dense connective tissue covers the entire muscle (epimysium), each muscle fascicle (perimysium) and individual muscle fibers (endomysium; ▶ Fig. 1.28). Regular dense connective tissue (aponeuroses and tendons) attaches the muscle to the bone. The term „fascia", a vaguely defined form of connective tissue, is currently attracting strong media interest. At present, the term fascia incorporates aponeuroses (with their well-known capacity for transient storage of mechanical energy), tissues found in the subcutis, and tissues that „connect" muscles and contain sensory receptors (for which a role in force transmission during locomotion has not been demonstrated). The tubular sarcolemma forms the cell membrane of the muscle cell.

Entheses (attachment zones) are areas where tendons, and also ligaments and joint capsules, integrate with, and transmit tensile forces to, the bone. Entheses occur in fibrous and fibrocartilaginous forms. In the former, the connective tissue attaches indirectly via the periosteum, which is joined to the bone by Sharpey's fibers or by connective tissue fibers that pass directly into the bone. Fibrous entheses are found at diaphyses and metaphyses. Fibrocartilaginous entheses occur at the epiphyses and apophyses of long bones (▶ Abb. 1.29). In this form of enthesis, the connective tissue transitions into initially unmineralized and then mineralized fibrocartilage, whereby the various elastic moduli (Young's moduli) of tendons and bone are evened out.

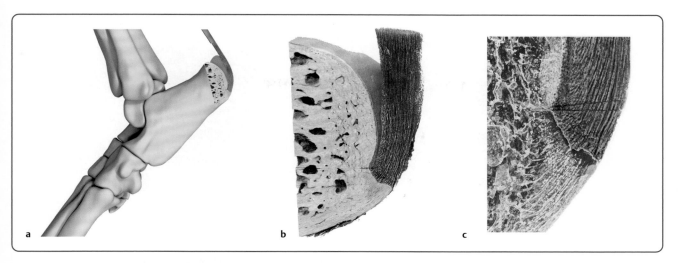

► **Fig. 1.29** Fibrocartilaginous entheses are areas of transition between tendon fibers and bone, via uncalcified fibrocartilage (dark blue) and calcified fibrocartilage (light blue). **a** The common calcaneal tendon inserts at the distal portion of the calcaneal tuberosity. The tendon fibers enter the bone at right angles to the direction of tension. **b** and **c** Semi-schematic illustrations based on micro-CT imaging of the calcaneal tuberosity of a rat. (source: Martin S. Fischer, Julian Sartori, Institut für Zoologie und Evolutionsforschung, Friedrich-Schiller-Universität Jena)

During muscle contraction, chemical energy is converted into mechanical energy. A muscle always generates force in the same direction. When it shortens, it performs positive work (e.g. when the foot lifts off from the ground). When a muscle lengthens, it performs negative work (e.g. when a leg takes on load while running). Since the muscle can only pull in one direction, muscles are arranged around joints as agonist-antagonist pairs. The processes involved in force generation occur at the molecular level. The following quote gives at least some indication of the molecular processes that transpire during a simple movement: *It takes about 2 trillion myosin molecules to provide the force to hold up a baseball. Our biceps have a million times this many, so only a fraction of the myosin molecules need to be exerting themselves at any given time.* (© RCSB Protein Data Bank).

The arrangement of similar structural elements in series and in parallel allows the degree of muscle shortening and the force of contraction to be scaled. The sarcomere, comprising two half-sarcomeres, is the smallest functional unit of a muscle (► Fig. 1.30). Muscle shortening, and the associated visible thickening of the muscle, result from the action of many serially connected sarcomeres. A 1 cm long muscle fiber (ca. 5000 sarcomeres) can shorten a muscle by 5 millimeters. A leg muscle contains 300 muscle fibers per mm², which extrapolates to around 50000–90000 fibers in the whole muscle. Since the muscle moment arm is shorter than the resistive moment arm, muscles must be very strong. The quadriceps femoris muscle of humans, for example, can generate a force of 7000 N (equivalent to supporting up to 700 kg against gravity).

When muscle contracts, actin and myosin filaments slide over one another. Force is generated in the process by myosin heads, which temporarily connect the filaments and undergo reconfiguration, resulting in very small movements (5 nm). When an active muscle is subjected to stretching, it can generate greater force than when it is shortened. In addition to this classic force generation mechanism, current muscle research

suggests that an important role is played by titin. Spanning half a sarcomere, thus approximately 1 µm in length, titin is the largest protein in the mammalian body. Titin was originally identified as a structural protein that plays an important role in cell assembly and ensures that muscle returns to its resting state after stretching. Recent research has demonstrated that it contributes to the elastic properties of active muscle. In muscle that is actively stretched, titin adheres to actin filaments (e.g. [58]) and generates force during the stretch-shortening cycle by acting as a spring. When muscle contracts to short lengths, titin may perform a preparatory function in the recently proposed model for the intermeshing of myosin filaments by centering these filaments [59] (► Fig. 1.30). Limb stiffness observed during locomotion is thus not only attributable to the elastic properties of tendons and the associated activation of muscle fibers, but also to elastic characteristics of the muscle.

The structural components of muscle are listed in ► Table 1.1.

This book focuses on the topography and function of muscles. As a rule, muscles are characterized by their origin and insertion, and by their innervation (Nomina Anatomica Veterinaria). Every muscle has a Latin name which, when present in humans, also applies in human nomenclature, from which the name was originally derived. Even when the muscle looks different in dogs, has a different origin or insertion, or is otherwise modified, it bears the same name as in human anatomy, i.e. it is „homologized“ with the human muscle. In humans, the biceps brachii has two heads, as indicated by its Latin name, whereas the equivalent muscle in the dog has only one. In the dog, the triceps brachii has 4 heads, rather than 3. The anatomical names can thus be misleading.

The action of a muscle in a particular movement is not easy to determine. The origin and insertion provide an initial indication; from these it can be established which joint the muscle can flex or extend. However, as there is a degree of redundancy (this applies, for example, to 40 of the leg muscles), the action of a muscle during locomotion becomes clearer when it is

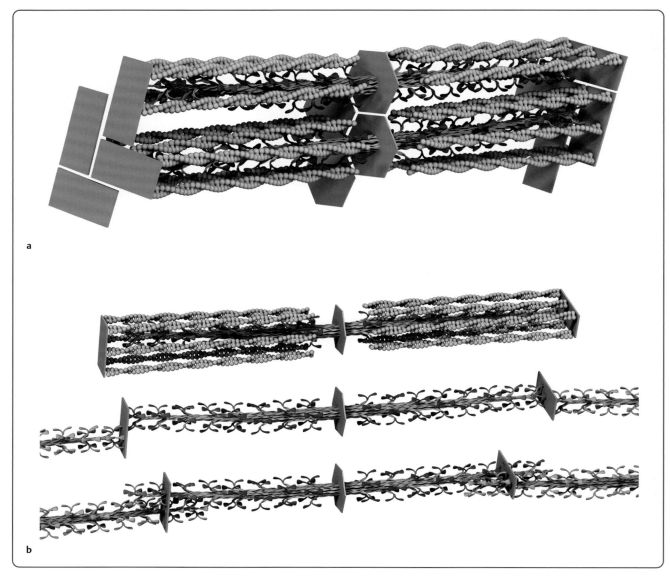

► **Fig. 1.30** Muscle contraction.
a Portion of a sarcomere with actin (pink) and myosin (grey) filaments. (source: Martin S. Fischer, Christian Rode, Jonas Lauströer, Amir Andikfar)
b When the muscle is activated, myosin heads (red) undergo cycles of binding to, and pulling on, actin filaments, causing the filament lattices to slide past each other like two brushes. At the Z disc (left and right) the actin filaments are attached tetragonally. In the middle, they are arranged hexagonally. During contraction, the myosin filaments probably slide through the Z disc for a short distance ([59]). (source: Martin S. Fischer, Christian Rode, Jonas Lauströer, Amir Andikfar)

► **Tab. 1.1** Structural components of muscle.

Component	Diameter
actin filaments	8 nm
myosin filaments	15 nm
myofibrils	1–3 μm
muscle fibers	10–100 μm
muscle fiber bundle = fascicle	0.5–5 mm

known when that muscle is active. The situation becomes more complex with biarticular muscles. Through interactions with other muscles or ligaments, a biarticular muscle may cause the extension of a joint that it actually flexes (Lombard's paradox).

The action of a muscle can also be modified by alteration of the lever arm ratio in different limb configurations. In a further example, hip extension in the frog can result in extension of the whole leg due to biarticular interconnection of adjacent joints. Moreover, skeletal muscles may perform other functions, such as stabilization of the vertebral column, depending on how they are arranged and embedded within the musculoskeletal system. A current topic of interest in this regard is the influence of lateral forces on muscle forces acting along the line of pull between the origin and insertion (e.g. [70]).

Ultimately it is the orientation of the muscle fascicles that determines the force transmission vector. A muscle fascicle incorporates 20 to 50 muscle fibers that are oriented parallel to one another, thus predefining the direction in which force is developed. In contrast, individual muscle fascicles within a muscle may be oriented in different directions. They are only rarely aligned in parallel or in the direction of pull of the muscle. This is necessary, since a muscle seldom has a single point of origin or insertion, thus forces must be transmitted to tendons or bones in various directions. In many muscles, the fascicles are oriented at an angle to the longitudinal axis. Since it resembles an avian feather, this arrangement is described as pennate. In reality, the arrangement of fascicles in pennate muscles is considerably more complex. Moreover, when the muscle contracts, the fascicles both shorten and change their angle of orientation, making it even more difficult to identify the primary direction of force transmission.

Muscle Fiber Types

Muscle fibers represent the cellular level of muscle. The muscle fibers found in vertebrates are classically defined as „tonic" fibers (do not exhibit twitching) and „phasic" fibers (exhibit twitching). As the skeletal muscle of dogs, like that of all mammals, is composed entirely of the latter type, only these twitch-type fibers are described in the following text. Twitch-type muscle fibers contain thousands of nuclei. Interestingly, the diameter of muscle fibers is independent of body size, being influenced instead by various factors such as oxygen and nutrient transport pathways or the ratio of fiber volume to fiber surface area. The cross-sectional area of a muscle fiber depends on fiber type, the position of the fiber in the muscle and the particular muscle. Individual training status also determines cross-sectional fiber size. Training increases the sectional area, while the number of fibers remains unchanged. Training and nutrition are the factors that have the greatest influence on muscle fiber size. Development of new muscle fibers from stem cells only occurs during regeneration after injury.

Classification of twitch-type fibers is based on metabolism, the presence of different types of myoglobin proteins and the contractile properties of the fiber (► Fig. 1.31). Type I fibers are characterized by sustained, slow contraction and oxidative metabolism. Type II fibers contract fast and are more prone to fatigue; their metabolism may be purely glycolytic or oxidative-glycolytic. The type of innervation also varies between these muscle fiber types. The branches of nerves supplying type I fibers penetrate the muscle from one side, course parallel to the muscle fibers and, at regular intervals, send perpendicular side branches to the muscle fiber. In the case of type II fibers, the nerve arborises on both sides, perpendicular to the direction of the muscle fibers.

Force generation is dependent upon the cross-section of the muscle fiber, not on its contractile properties. Type II fibers frequently have a greater cross-sectional surface area than type I fibers ($2–3\,\mu m^2$ vs $1–2\,\mu m^2$). Thus, in absolute terms, type II fibers often generate more force than type I fibers.

A distinguishing feature of dogs is the absence of purely glycolytic type IIb fibers [73]. In place of type IIb fibers, dogs have an additional mixed fiber type designated as type IIa/X or, in abbreviated form, type IIX. The presence of type IIX fibers instead of purely glycolytic type IIb fibers is a key factor in dogs' capacity for endurance. In contrast to almost all other mam-

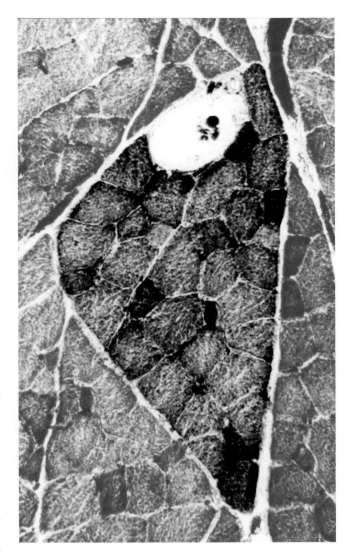

► **Fig. 1.31** Representation of muscle fiber types using an enzyme reaction. The colored area corresponds to a muscle fascicle surrounded by perimysium.

mals, dogs can recruit all of their muscle fibers for endurance work. In addition, an abundance of capillaries provides muscle fibers with a rich supply of blood. The absence of type IIb fibers virtually eliminates the risk of muscle hyperacidity. In dogs, the muscles continue to use oxidative metabolism even during very prolonged locomotion and do not fatigue under normal external conditions, except during extreme sprints.

The distribution of different muscle fiber types varies greatly from one muscle to another. Except for Greyhounds, which have a higher proportion of fast-twitch type II fibers, individual and breed-related variation in muscle fiber distribution is very limited. Generally, the proportion of type I fibers is higher in the muscles of the forelimb than in those of the hindlimb. Yet there are no two muscles in which fiber distribution is the same. In a study examining the distribution of type I and II fibers in all muscles of the fore- and hindlimbs in 3 mixed breed dogs, Armstrong et al. found that the proportion of type I fibers in individual muscles ranged from 14 to 100% [3]. Fibers were also distributed unevenly within a given muscle. In almost all of the muscles examined, the population of type I fibers increased from the outside to the inside. Considerably more type I fibers were found near the bone than in the more superficial portions of the muscle. Compared with fibers situated close to the bone, the outer fibers have a longer lever arm; thus, the quickly contracting type II fibers are located externally.

Force Generation

As well as being determined by the number of active muscle fibers (Hennemann's size principle) and the frequency of stimulation, the isometric force generated by a muscle depends on the zone of overlap between the muscle filaments. In non-isometric contraction, force is modulated by the relative speed of the filaments and also by titin. The number of hemi-sarcomeres arranged in series has no influence on force. Every filament has the same number of myosin heads, so the force of a muscle is proportional to the number of its filaments. The higher the number of filaments, the greater is the generation of force. The physiological cross-section of a muscle, which is calculated from the cross-section of individual muscle fibers, gives a very good approximation of the number of sarcomeres connected in parallel. Muscles with long fibers can contract quickly due to the large number of serially arranged hemi-sarcomeres; muscles with short fibers are particularly strong. For a given muscle length, the pennation angle increases with decreasing fiber length. The pennation angle reduces the speed of contraction and the amount of force that can be generated. This is taken into account in the architectural index, the modified quotient of muscle fiber length and total muscle length. In the Greyhound, the index is 0.07–0.14 for the powerful calf muscles (medial and lateral gastrocnemius) and 0.7–0.88 for the fast semitendinosus and semimembranosus muscles (in which the fibers are up to 10 times longer) [84], [85]. The forelimbs are also connected to the trunk by fast muscles with long fibers (rhomboid and latissimus dorsi, index 0.97). The digital flexors (flexor digitorum muscles: 0.06), with their extremely short fibers (0.8 cm fiber length at 13.8 cm muscle length) are the relatively strong muscles [68].

Some muscles are adapted to suit their primary action. For example, for muscles involved in lengthening-shortening cycles, it is important to be able to generate large forces, i.e. a large physiological cross-sectional area is required. This allows muscle activity to be adjusted so that the work takes place primarily in the tendons. Muscles that mainly perform negative work, i.e. that contract eccentrically, are more likely to have a smaller physiological cross-sectional area. At an equivalent cross-sectional area, muscles that perform positive work tend to have longer fibers.

The power of a muscle is proportional to its volume. Muscle volume is calculated by dividing muscle mass by muscle density. In practice, maximum muscle power is based on muscle mass, as muscle density is very close to 1. The biceps femoris is by far the most powerful muscle in the hindlimb (mass approximately 500 g, maximum isometric force 940 N, maximum power 50 W [84], [85]). Whereas the flexor digitorum superficialis generates more force than the biceps femoris (1260 N vs 940 N), its power output is smaller (6 W vs 50 W) [84], [85].

The strongest and most powerful muscle in the forelimbs is the long head of the triceps brachii muscle. Its values for force and power (1475 N and 58 W) exceed those of the biceps femoris muscle. Comparison of muscle mass also reveals the large differences between individual muscle groups at the level of different joints.

Transmission of muscle power depends not only on the characteristics of different muscles, but also on the relationships of the moment arm. The muscular moment arm is the perpendicular distance between the line of action of the muscle and the pivot point (e.g. joint center of rotation). The moment arm changes during movement and modulates the torque generated by the muscle (muscular force × length of moment arm). At the same time, the resistive moment arm modulates the required torque in the joint. At 30% of the way through the stance phase, the gastrocnemius muscles must generate almost twice as much force as at 70%, purely because of changes in moment arm ratio (force × length of moment arm [distance to the joint], ▶ Fig. 1.39). Here, it is evident that the resistive and muscular moment arms change in phase, reducing the impact of moment arm variation during locomotion.

Muscle Spindles

Muscle is also an important sensory organ. Muscle spindles provide information about the length of muscle fibers and their speed of contraction; this can be used in reflex reactions for regulating the activity of the muscle itself, or that of other muscles.

Muscle spindles are modified muscle fibers with thin muscle fibers in their interior. The length of the muscle spindle is determined by the contractile state of the internal fibers. The spindle has a maximum length of 3 mm and is surrounded by a connective tissue sheath, through which it is tightly connected to surrounding muscle fibers. The number of muscle spindles varies from muscle to muscle. The highest density of muscle spindles, around 1 spindle per mm^2, is found in the short muscles of the paw (interflexorii, lumbricals). The biceps brachii contains 1 spindle per 7 mm^2, whereas the density in the long head of the triceps brachii is only 1 spindle per 50 mm^2.

In addition to the spindles present in muscle, there are specialized nerve plexuses in the tendons. Referred to as Golgi tendon organs, these plexuses send signals about tension in the tendon, and thus muscular force, to the spinal cord. Golgi tendon organs are enclosed in connective tissue capsules measuring around 1 mm in length and 0.1 mm in diameter.

The intrinsic sensory system of muscle is an important feedback mechanism for rapid correction and fine tuning of systems such as rhythm generators in the spinal cord. Instantaneous acquisition of information about the underlying surface via changes in muscle length (e.g. stretching of muscle when a dog steps in a hole) facilitates coordination and correction of limb movement at spinal cord level. The long head of the triceps brachii, in particular, is at the center of a regulatory loop in the forelimbs. Mapping of its Ia afferent fibers through measurement of the excitatory postsynaptic motor neuron potentials has shown that the triceps brachii sends signals proximally and distally, indicating that this muscle performs a controlling function in the forelimb [10].

Muscle in Metabolism

In recent years, an additional function of muscle has become increasingly apparent, namely its role in metabolism and in physical and mental well-being. The benefits of exercise that we perceive in our own bodies surely, and perhaps particularly, also apply to dogs. To date, almost 400 different hormone-like messenger molecules have been identified in muscle („myokines"), shedding ever more light on the biomechanical basis for the contented state of a dog (and its owner) at the end of a long walk.

Muscles only utilize blood glucose when they are active. While they are consuming energy, muscles are receptive to the hormone insulin, which is needed for the uptake of glucose by muscle fibers. When activity is lacking, glucose is converted into fat. Thus, there is a direct association between activity and diabetes. Overweight dogs frequently have one main problem – inactivity. This leads to muscle wastage, in itself a natural consequence of aging, and accumulation of fat. The relationship between breakdown of fat in subcutaneous connective tissue and the activity of the underlying muscles has now been demonstrated biochemically. Locally active messenger molecules, hormone-like proteins known as interleukins, are released during muscular activity. Interleukin 6 has been shown to regulate fat metabolism and also to have an anti-inflammatory function. Moreover, an intrinsic muscle protein (MIP) participates in regulation of calcium levels in the body. Through this mechanism, muscle influences changes in bone density associated with aging and activity.

1.4
Role of Nutrition

Britta Dobenecker

1.4.1 Overview

Provision of a balanced, adequate supply of nutrients is the basis for a healthy musculoskeletal system. As well as causing specific diet-related disorders, nutritional deficiencies can exacerbate the severity and clinical manifestations of musculoskeletal diseases of non-nutritional origin. A prime example is the chronic oversupply of energy, resulting in overweight. **At every stage of** life, excess weight places a burden on the musculoskeletal system and can turn even minor changes into processes that are painful for the dog.

The growth phase is a particularly sensitive period for the health of the canine skeleton. During this phase, various factors can play a role in the occurrence of skeletal malformation and developmental orthopedic diseases (DOD). The term DOD embodies a complex of diseases including osteochondroses, joint dysplasia, osteodystrophy and bone deformities. One reason for the development of such disorders is a high capacity for growth, particularly in large breeds (expected adult

weight ≥ 25 kg). The greater vulnerability of rapidly growing animals to development of musculoskeletal disorders is also recognised in other species.

Pet owners, and also veterinarians, frequently ask why the diet of a dog should be balanced so precisely, when this is not something they do for themselves or for their children. The answer becomes clear when one considers that growth occurs over 15–17 years in humans, compared with around one year in dogs. In other words, in growing dogs, a much higher proportion of the daily nutrient intake is needed for tissue accretion than for maintenance. In the case of a dog and a human with an identical actual body weight during growth and an identical expected adult weight of 70 kg, the daily calcium requirement is 7 times higher in the dog than in the child. Recent findings indicate that humans also have more efficient processes for counteracting dietary shortfalls in calcium, whereby absorption of calcium from the food is increased through higher digestibility and utilization. An increase in active Vitamin D levels is one way to achieve this. It has recently been demonstrated that these adaptive mechanisms are virtually non-existent in the dog [42]. In contrast to humans, the proportional uptake of dietary calcium remains constant in the dog, irrespective of the calcium content of the food. Thus, dogs are unable to protect themselves against excessive calcium absorption when there is a dietary oversupply. Conversely, lack of calcium in the diet can manifest very rapidly as inadequate skeletal mineralization. Thus, an inappropriate supply of nutrients, particularly calcium and phosphorus, is the other major problem area in terms of nutritionally induced DODs, alongside overly rapid growth due to excessive energy intake.

Since most of the dog's body mass develops in the first year of life, and its phylogenetic origins as a predator have not compelled it to cope with a low-calcium diet, inappropriate intake of a key nutrient for just a few weeks is likely to be far more damaging in this species than in humans, in which growth occurs over two decades and nutrient utilization can be adapted more efficiently to the supply. **Consequently, periods of inadequate nutrition have a disproportionately greater impact on puppies and young dogs than on children and youths.** Just a few weeks of deficient intake of calcium and phosphorus, the most important minerals for bone formation, can result in significant derangements such as angular limb deformities, joint incongruity and abnormal ossification at growth plates, with associated pain and lameness. The extent of these changes is influenced by the degree of nutrient deficiency, breed, rate of weight gain and management factors such as type and intensity of exercise and activity. Whereas pronounced, clinically relevant changes may develop within 4 weeks in one dog, other young dogs may exhibit only mild, indistinct lameness, even after 2–3 months of inappropriate nutrition. Dietary errors are more commonly observed in growing dogs with DODs, compared with those in which skeletal development is normal.

Determination of an optimal nutrient supply requires information about the nutrient content of the food and ration components, respectively, as well as valid data regarding the requirements of the animal. The latter is complex, particularly during the growth phase, as the nutrient requirements depend on body weight relative to age and on the expected adult body weight. Thus, while the recommended intake of calcium, for example, is influenced by the expected adult weight and thereby indirectly by breed, the amount changes during the period of development. **Consequently, there is no fixed value for all puppies and young dogs, and no simple formula that is suitable in all cases for calculation of an animal's calcium requirement.** The minerals that are intended to meet the daily requirements must be present in the food in sufficiently available form. This is influenced by the chemical form of the mineral [16], and the concentration of other elements (e.g. utilization of phosphorus is reduced by high calcium concentrations in chyme; [42]). The digestibility of the whole food is also important. High fibre content, found for example in rations high in vegetables, various „light" formulations and also in poor quality ration components, is associated with increased fecal excretion of calcium and phosphorus, reducing the utilization of these minerals by the body [35]. Even the amount of acidifying and alkalizing components in the food (the so-called cation-anion balance) affects the utilization of dietary minerals. Foods with alkalizing properties increase intestinal calcium losses [36]. In addition to the animal's requirements, and its ability to absorb nutrients from the food, the concentration of the various nutrients in the food clearly plays an important role. Whether a particular product or type of food is high or low in certain nutrients is another area in which misjudgments are often made. Foods considered to be calcium-rich in the context of human nutrition may, for dogs and particularly puppies, be regarded as containing moderate or even low levels of calcium, rendering it inadequate for meeting the animal's needs. In the preparation of home-made diets, especially for growing dogs with high mineral requirements, green vegetables and milk products are unsuitable sources of calcium. Only bones or suitably formulated mineral feeds can deliver appropriate quantities (in the gram range), though the use of bones (p. 43) also has disadvantages that are described below. The use of milk and milk products as a calcium source results in varying degrees of deficiency that can very quickly lead to abnormal skeletal development in animals prone to DODs. Even in adults, ongoing calcium deficiency can cause serious problems, though the time taken for clinical signs to develop ranges from months to 2–3 years, depending on the level of deficiency.

Yet not only a lack of calcium can lead to negative outcomes. More frequently, damage results from an **excess of calcium**, caused for example by supplementation of adequate and balanced complete foods or by excessive bone content in BARF products (BARF = bone and raw food). Undesirable consequences of oversupply are particularly likely to result in abnormalities during the growth phase. In contrast, adult dogs are relatively tolerant. Potential adverse effects of excess calcium also include substantially reduced availability of other minerals including phosphorus and zinc, which can lead to a secondary deficiency of these nutrients.

Preventing nutritionally induced skeletal abnormalities, and avoiding burdening of the skeletal system through poor nutrition, is of paramount importance. Accordingly, every owner should be informed in a timely manner about optimal nutrition for their dog and about the importance of feeding a ration that is balanced and consistent with the animal's needs. This applies particularly to periods of specific nutritional demand, such as the growth phase, pregnancy and lactation. If abnormalities have already been diagnosed, immediate transition to a suitable diet is essential, even though a complete recovery is not always possible. In the management of nutritionally based disorders, and also orthopedic abnormalities of non-nutritional origin, an optimal diet provides the necessary foundation for successful medical or surgical therapy. Prompt correction of inappropriate nutrient supply in puppies and young dogs may even lead to remission of early-stage DODs.

> **⧉ Practical Application**
> - The growth phase is a particularly sensitive period for healthy skeletal development in the dog. During this phase, various factors play a role in the occurrence of skeletal malformation and developmental orthopedic diseases (DOD). One reason for the development of such diseases is a high capacity for growth, particularly in large breeds (expected adult weight ≥ 25 kg).
> - In young dogs, inappropriate intake of a key nutrient for around 8 weeks is likely to be far more damaging than in humans, in which growth occurs over two decades and nutrient utilization can be adapted more efficiently to the supply.
> - There is no fixed value for all puppies and young dogs, and no simple formula for calculation of an animal's calcium requirement. The amount of calcium required at a given point in time depends on actual body weight and the expected adult weight of the dog.

1.4.2 Growth

Healthy growth with optimal musculoskeletal development is the basis for long term health of the locomotor system. During growth, it is important not only to avoid clinically apparent abnormalities, but also to prevent damage to bone and cartilage that could subsequently lead to abnormalities and lameness that reduce the animal's quality of life. Of particular significance in this regard is the supply of energy, calcium, phosphorus, Vitamins A and D and the trace elements zinc and copper.

Energy

Daily energy intake affects the growth rate of puppies and young dogs. Particularly in dogs with a high capacity for growth, an oversupply of energy results in a steep growth curve, rather than obesity. In young dogs, especially in large breeds, metabolic processes use surplus energy for accelerated growth, not for storage of energy as fat. This leads to a situation that is often regarded as paradoxical: the animal may be thin to very thin, yet weigh too much for its age. Thus, the body condition scoring system (BCS) is clearly not useful for assessing nutritional status in growing dogs. The appropriate method in this case is to compare the animal's body weight with the recommended growth curve (▶ Fig. 1.32). An oversupply of calories can of course be determined by the presence of excess body fat, but the converse does not apply, i.e. the energy intake of a dog that appears very thin cannot be assessed by visual inspection

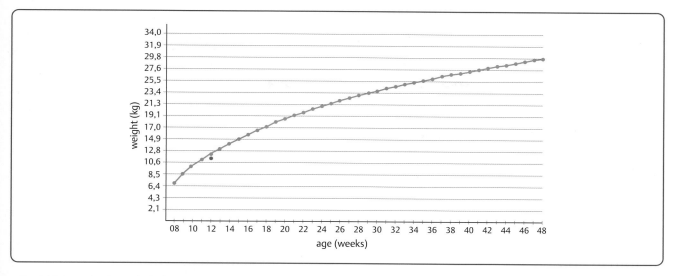

▶ **Fig. 1.32** Example of an individual growth curve. A suitable program, in this case Diet Check Munich©, is used to calculate the recommended growth curve based on the parameters „actual weight", „date of birth" (age) and „expected adult weight" (estimated based on the ideal weight of the parent of the same sex, breed standards etc.). The dog should be weighed weekly by the owner (if/as appropriate, by calculating the difference between the owner themselves and the owner carrying the dog) and the weight marked on the printed graph. The aim is for the weight to be on or just under the line. If the weight does deviate from the target, weight loss or intensive „feeding up" are not recommended. If the puppy or young dog is too heavy, its weight should be maintained for a certain period, or limited to a small increase, so that it gradually approaches the curve. If the dog is markedly underweight, the aim should be to achieve a rate of gain that is parallel to the curve – in this case, it will take longer to reach the adult weight, but the risk of abnormal skeletal development is reduced. With young dogs of indeterminate breed, for which it is difficult to estimate an adult weight, the recommended approach is to make careful estimates and to adjust these as required during the growth phase. In the context of skeletal development, it is always safer to underestimate, than to overestimate, the adult weight!

or palpation! The best approach is to weigh the dog regularly (preferably weekly) and to plot the weight on a graph (▶ Fig. 1.32). This method requires estimation of the expected ideal adult weight of the dog, for which the best guide is the actual ideal weight of the parents. For the parents, the BCS is suitable for assessing nutritional status. If the BCS is over 4 to 5, an estimate of ideal weight should be used. It is preferable to underestimate the adult weight of the young dog to some degree, rather than to overestimate. Using a graph of the recommended growth curve, actual weight can be compared with the recommended weight. This allows any necessary adjustments to be made promptly, noting that a degree of underachievement of the recommended weight is tolerable, while (marked) excesses should be avoided. It has been shown under large-scale experimental conditions that dogs are significantly more likely to be overweight or to develop musculoskeletal abnormalities if they have experienced a period of excessive weight gain during the growth phase (crossed > 2 centiles) [27].

The normal values given in most reference materials for energy requirements during the growth phase are relatively high. These are often based on data from trials involving dogs housed in groups. More recent studies have identified considerably lower average daily caloric requirements during the growth phase in the dog. These new, lower values are derived from studies involving privately owned dogs, and dogs kept under experimental conditions in which growth rates were managed according to the recommendations described above [16], [37]. Thus, strict adherence to the feeding recommendations given on complete foods is not necessarily recommended. These feeding instructions can serve as an initial indication, but it is im-

portant to then be guided by the weight gain of the individual animal: if a young dog is growing too quickly, the daily calorie intake should be reduced sufficiently to avoid exceeding the recommended weight (▶ Table 1.2). Feeding of treats, rewards, snacks and chews should be cut back first, before reducing intake of a balanced complete food. Regular weight monitoring is useful for checking the success of energy restriction – if the animal's weight remains above the target, further limitations must be imposed. The average daily energy requirement of growing dogs can be estimated by the following equation [37]:

$$\text{ME intake (MJ)} = \left(1.063 - 0.565 \times \frac{\text{actual BW}}{\text{expected mature BW}}\right) \times \text{actual BW}^{0.75}$$

Deformities and developmental abnormalities are caused not only by excess body weight during the period of incomplete bone mineralization, but also by a combination of overweight with well-developed musculature and elevated levels of hormones (growth hormone, thyroid hormone) and specific chemical messengers. By influencing the level of hormone secretion (including GH, IGF-I, insulin, T3/T4), energy intake affects bone and cartilage metabolism, leading to increased cartilage proliferation and a higher rate of bone remodeling. Thus, ad libitum feeding, provision of excessively energy dense food/rations, additional feeding of rewards and treats etc. (all of which result in a calorie overload for most individually homed puppies and young dogs) can pose a considerable risk to healthy skeletal development. The possibility that alterations of joint formation also occur at this early stage, leading to arthritis/arthrosis that

▶ **Tab. 1.2** Recommended body weight in kg [45].

Month (middle of)	Adult body weight 5 kg	Adult body weight 10 kg	Adult body weight 20 kg	Adult body weight 35 kg	Adult body weight 60 kg
1	0.5	0.7	1.1	1.5	2.1
2	1.2	1.9	3.1	4.7	6.6
3	1.9	3.3	5.9	9.6	13.2
4	2.6	4.8	8.9	14.5	20.4
5	3.5	6.5	12.2	19.8	30.0
6	4.0	7.5	14.0	22.8	36.0
12	5.0	9.5	19.0	30.8	48.0

causes lameness and other problems later in life, cannot be excluded.

In the converse situation, young dogs weighing substantially less than their target weight, according to the recommended growth curve, should not under any circumstances be „fed up", i.e. their weight should not be increased quickly to be near the optimum value. Although the dog is underweight, an overly intense period of growth can lead to the problems described above. Thus, the growth curve of an underweight puppy or young dog should only be brought into alignment with recommended values very gradually. **It is important to note that the body size of the adult dog is genetically determined. Only profound feeding errors (e.g. substantial protein deficiency) can, to a limited extent, influence body size.** The effect of the growth curve being below the recommended values is that the dog will reach its adult weight slightly later, as opposed to its adult size being smaller. In terms of healthy skeletal development, restricting growth according to recommended values is certainly preferable to acceleration of growth by feeding of high energy rations.

Since daily energy requirements are modulated by a number of factors, only average values based on the actual and expected body weight of the adult animal can be established. The required calorie intake is influenced particularly by activity level and housing conditions. Thus, a relatively placid, long-haired dog in a single dog household has a below-average requirement for energy/food intake. In contrast, group-housed, young, active, short-haired dogs have a greater than average demand for energy and must therefore consume more of the same food for growth to occur normally. Thus, the same food can result in a different nutrient supply in two different types of young dog due to differences in their energy requirement. To avoid dietary deficiencies or overweight in a young dog with below-average energy requirements, the food/ration must have a relatively high nutrient/energy ratio. Conversely, a food with a relatively low nutrient concentration is required for a very active, growing Great Dane in a multi-dog household during the winter months. **Thus, there can be no single food that is ideally suited to the energy and nutrient requirements of all puppies and young dogs.**

In addition, the level of energy intake during the growth phase, and the proportion of adipose tissue accretion during this period, can influence the energy requirement and thereby, indirectly, the nutritional status of the adult animal. Dogs with excessive fat accretion during growth have a lifelong tendency to be overweight. Thus, monitoring of growth by regular weighing and checking against recommendations is also important for dogs in which excess energy tends to be used for fat depostion, rather than accelerated growth. Throughout its lifetime, a dog that has grown up lean has a lower risk of developing certain diseases.

It is important to include rewards, treats, snacks and chews etc. when calculating daily energy intake. The nutritional composition of such products rarely corresponds to a dog's requirements, particularly when it is growing. If they remain part of the diet, either the total calorie intake increases or the amount of normal food is reduced accordingly. The latter results in a concurrent reduction of the intake of important nutrients; the ration is no longer balanced and does not meet requirements. Malnutrition due to nutrient dilution occurs more quickly in dogs with a below average energy requirement.

Practical Application

During the growth phase, excess energy intake tends to result in a steeper growth curve, rather than deposition of fat, particularly in animals with a high capacity for growth. To assess the energy supply, the expected ideal adult weight of the dog should be estimated, so that the actual weight can be compared with the optimal growth curve. Expected ideal adult weight is based on the actual ideal weight of the parents. A degree of underestimation is preferable to overestimation.
The normal values given in most reference materials for energy requirements during the growth phase are relatively high. Based on more recent data, showing that energy requirements during the growth phase are lower, these recommendations will presumably be adjusted downwards in years to come.

Protein

As stated previously, the increase in body weight, or the rate of weight gain, of a puppy or young dog depends on its daily energy intake. If the daily food (and thus energy) supply for an individual dog is adjusted so that weight gain follows the recommended rate, the proportion of protein in the diet is irrelevant in this regard. This assumes, of course, that the protein requirements of the animal are met, as a severe deficiency of protein/ amino acids can lead to growth retardation, a higher percentage of fat in gained tissue and developmental disorders. It is often stated that excess protein has a detrimental impact on skeletal development, but this has no factual basis. The origin of this persistent claim dates back to experiments conducted in the 1980's [31] that laid the foundations for our current understanding. In these studies, a group of growing Great Danes was fed an adequate amount, while animals in another group received larger quantities of the same food. At the time, it was hypothesized that the extensive abnormalities of skeletal development observed in the group fed higher amounts was caused by an excess of all nutrients – energy, protein, minerals and vitamins. In all likelihood, however, these malformations resulted from rapid growth due to high energy and nutrient intake. This interpretation is supported by the work of Nap et al. [49], [50]. In standardized trials, these authors found that the level of protein intake had no impact on skeletal development in growing dogs. Since the investigations of nearly 40 years ago, numerous experiments and case studies have established that the main nutritional causes of abnormal skeletal development are surplus energy and a deficienct or excessive supply of calcium and phosphorus.

> ⚡ **Practical Application**
> It is often stated that excess protein has a detrimental impact on skeletal development, but this has no factual basis.

Calcium

One of the primary roles of the mineral calcium is formation and maintenance of the osseous skeleton. Based on the functional and regulatory relationship between calcium and the element phosphorus, **calcium and phosphorus intake must always be considered together**. As well as meeting absolute requirements, intake of these minerals must ensure that the Ca/P ratio lies within the recommended range of 1/1 to 2/1. Ideally, the extremes of this spectrum are avoided, the optimal range comprising 1.3/1 to 1.8/1. Deviation from the ideal ratio can result in abnormal average rates of mineral utilization. For example, a calcium surplus leading to a very high Ca/P ratio of > 2/1 can decrease the digestibility of phosphorus, resulting in secondary phosphorus deficiency.

The amount of a particular nutrient required by the body each day, i.e. the quantity that the body must be able to access, is referred to as the net requirement. Since a portion of the consumed quantity of nutrient is lost in the feces, rather than being absorbed by the body, recommendations are made for gross daily intake (gross requirement), taking into account average digestibility. For a nutrient with an average digestibility of 50 %, an animal requiring 100 mg of this nutrient per day should be given 200 mg in its daily ration. Nutrient requirement standards generally give recommendations on the gross amount of a nutrient in the feed; depending on the nutrient, the net requirement is lower, to a greater or lesser extent, than the recommended intake. A certain safety margin is usually also included. Losses based on digestibility and availability are also considered. Poorly digestible foods (e.g. poor protein quality, vegetarian/vegan foods or other foods very high in fibre) are associated with low calcium utilization [35]. Overall, the regular calcium supply should be kept close to the actual requirement, particularly in growing dogs, even when a (purportedly) highly available source of calcium is used. If the limited capacity of dogs for regulation of calcium availability (described above) also applies to growing dogs, as is likely to be the case, then it is not possible to rely on the significant increases in calcium utilization seen in humans and other animals, facilitated by factors such as Vitamin D and PTH. The minimum requirement should therefore be provided on a daily basis as part of the food ration, factoring in also the availability of other minerals. On this basis, it is necessary both to meet demand and to ensure that the nutrient content of the diet is balanced, in order to maintain average levels of availability.

A deficient calcium supply leads to suboptimal ossification of the growing skeleton and possibly even increased bone breakdown. At a certain level, calcium deficiency gives rise to secondary nutritional hyperparathyroidism, resulting in generalized fibrous osteodystrophy. Possible consequences range from angular deformities, bone malformations and altered bone structure through to spontaneous fractures.

Conversely, **excess calcium** can lead to secondary phosphorus deficiency if high levels of calcium are supplied in isolation, e.g. through supplementation with calcium carbonate in the form of powder or egg shells. Phosphorus deficiency can cause profound derangements of skeletal development; refer to section on Phosphorus (p. 44). Utilization of minerals such as zinc and copper is also poorer in the presence of excess calcium, potentially also impairing skeletal development. In animals susceptible to DODs, surplus calcium can also restrict longitudinal growth of the long bones of the limbs, presumably due to premature closure of the growth plates. Furthermore, a causative role of excess calcium has been proposed in the development of wobbler syndrome.

Consequences of altered cartilage metabolism and ossification caused by inappropriate calcium supply (deficiency or excess), including angular deformities (radius curvus, carpus valgus), hypertrophic osteodystrophy and ostechondrosis dissecans, often result in very painful changes in the juvenile skeleton that manifest as shifting lameness and reluctance or inability to move. The latter in turn impacts detrimentally on the developing skeleton, since tensile and compression forces provide important stimuli for appropriate bone remodeling and formation. Even in adults, immobility is known to cause skeletal bone resorption.

It should be noted here that **a highly irregular supply** of calcium, e.g. through feeding of bones only once per week, **is not recommended**. Rather than providing the equivalent of the daily requirement (weekly feeding divided by 7 days), this equates to 6 days of deficiency and one day of massive excess. Healthy, appropriate development and mineralization of the skeleton is unlikely to occur under these conditions. Bone feeding is also inadvisable for other reasons, including hygiene and the risk of injury and constipation. Furthermore, the dose delivered this way is very inexact, as the calcium and phosphorus content of bone varies with species and age (e.g. calf vs ox) and also with location in the body. Moreover, when bone fragments are broken off and swallowed, a much greater proportion of the minerals is excreted in the feces, than would be the case if the bone was fed in ground form.

> **▣ Practical Application**
> An **insufficient calcium supply** leads to suboptimal ossification of the growing skeleton and may even cause increased bone breakdown.
> **Excess calcium** leads to secondary deficiencies of other minerals such as phosphorus, zinc and copper, which has detrimental impacts on the development of the musculoskeletal system; in animals predisposed to DODs it may restrict longitudinal growth of the long bones of the limbs, presumably due to premature growth plate closure. A causative role of excess calcium in development of wobbler syndrome has also been proposed. Consequences of cartilage metabolism and ossification due to inappropriate calcium levels (deficiency or excess), including angular deformities (radius curvus, carpus valgus), hypertrophic osteodystrophy, ostechondrosis dissecans, often result in very painful changes in the juvenile skeleton that manifest as shifting lameness and reluctance or inability to move.

Phosphorus

A deficient supply of phosphorus can result from an absolute deficiency in the food, or from suboptimal utilization, e.g. due to an excessively high Ca/P-ratio of > 2/1. This is especially likely to occur with home-made foods lacking added minerals or supplemented exclusively with calcium (e.g. CaCO3). Generally, just a few weeks of phosphate deficiency can lead to reduced appetite, diminished overall health with decreased activity/longer rest periods, exercise intolerance, a dull coat and scaly skin. Ongoing deficiency may lead to abnormalities of the locomotor system including hyperextension of the carpal and tarsal joints and angular limb deformities. This can result in abnormal joint mobility and bowing of the forelimbs; very rapid progression of such changes can be an indicator of phosphorus deficiency. When caused by phosphorus deficiency, as opposed to other nutritional aberrations, angular limb deformities can manifest clinically and worsen within just a few hours. This is because they result from abnormalities of the muscles and supporting structures, rather than from bone deformation – at least at this early stage. Initially, changes resulting from phosphorus deficiency are neither painful nor detectable as osseous abnormalities (i.e. bone malformation) on x-ray [34]. This is presumably because the stability and strength of the muscles and connective tissue supporting structures are affected to begin with, rather than bone development. At this stage, the changes can be reversed by correcting the phosphorus content and Ca/P ratio of the food; even though the limb deformities appear dramatic, this situation is less critical for puppies and young dogs than the consequences of inappropriate calcium intake. Some sources refer in this context to „carpal laxity syndrome", which can be greatly improved by adjusting the nutritional content of the food [14]. The diet should certainly be assessed in these cases, and promptly corrected if necessary, since continued selective deficiency of phosphorus is likely to cause abnormal ossification, as seen with calcium excess/deficiency. The prospects

for achieving a full recovery by optimizing the diet are much poorer under these circumstances.

> **▣ Practical Application**
> Ongoing phosphorus deficiency may lead to abnormalities of the locomotor system including hyperextension of the carpal and tarsal joints. When caused by phosphorus deficiency, as opposed to other nutritional aberrations, angular limb deformities can manifest clinically and worsen within just a few hours. This is because they result from abnormalities of the muscles and supporting structures, rather than from bone deformation. These clinical signs can be reversed by prompt correction of the diet.

Further Important Nutrients

Malnutrition involving other nutrients is less frequently identified as a cause of DODs. It is not clear whether this is because deficiencies or excesses are less common in general feeding practice, or whether their effects are less dramatic. Nevertheless, the same principle applies: an effort should be made to optimize the supply of all nutrients because, in particular, Vitamins A and D and the trace elements copper, zinc, manganese and iodine are essential components of the diet, alongside energy, calcium and phosphorus. Deficiencies of these other nutrients can lead to suboptimal development and can exacerbate existing problems. Of greatest practical relevance are deficiencies of fat-soluble vitamins and copper.

Vitamin D plays a central role in bone metabolism and, in conjunction with calcitonin, PTH and other messenger substances, has a substantial influence on calcium and phosphorus metabolism. A deficiency of active Vitamin D_3 during growth leads to rickets with thickened growth plates, thin bone cortices and corresponding consequences for skeletal development (especially hypertrophic osteodystrophy, mainly affecting the carpal joints, and angular limb deformities). In dogs, as in cats, cutaneous synthesis of Vitamin D from precursors in the presence of UV radiation occurs only to a limited extent. Thus, Vitamin D must be consumed in the diet. Natural sources include animal tissues (especially fat, liver, blood, certain fish), but also Vitamin D_2 of plant origin. Vitamin D_3 is hydroxylated in the liver and kidney to produce the active form ($1,25(OH)_2D_3$). If a commercial diet constitutes at least part of an animal's diet, or if liver or vitamin and mineral supplements are added to home-made rations, development of DODs due to Vitamin D_3 deficiency is unlikely. Substantial overdosing with Vitamin D, e.g. by adding Vitamin D supplements to a complete food, can cause severe abnormalities of endochondral ossification that lead to angular deformities.

Vitamin A is also an important factor in bone metabolism, as its influence on osteoclasts plays a crucial role in bone remodeling. Both a deficiency and surplus of Vitamin A should be avoided, particularly during the growth phase, though the impacts of abnormal intake are less critical than for Vitamin D. In a relatively recent study involving growing Beagles, even levels of Vitamin A distinctly exceeding requirements had no measurable effects, including on concentrations of markers of bone turnover [46]. Far greater excesses of Vitamin A can result in reduced food intake, retarded growth, joint pain, premature growth plate closure and general derangements of bone metabolism. Thus, the dietary content of Vitamin A should not exceed 100000 IU per 4184 kJ (1000 kcal) metabolizable energy. Noteworthy in this context is the teratogenic effect of Vitamin A: in bitches, it is particularly important to prevent excess Vitamin A intake during early gestation. The Vitamin A content of natural food sources such as liver and cod liver oil depends on the diet of the source or prey animal and can be highly variable. If these are included in the diet, it is particularly important to avoid regular and excessive supply. Since liver is a delicacy for most dogs, the amount of liver in home-made rations, and also in commercial foods, can be quite high in some cases. The level of active Vitamin A is reduced to some extent by heating, sterilization and storage. Hypovitaminosis A should also be avoided, as this affects bone metabolism (abnormal remodeling due to reduced rate of bone resorption) and has other consequences such as impaired immune defense, reduced appetite, weight loss and ataxia.

Copper is required for the development of strong connective tissue, particularly during the growth phase. Substantial undersupply of copper due to absolute dietary deficiency or decreased utilization (e.g. due to excess calcium or zinc) can lead to hyperextension of the carpal and tarsal joints and osteoporotic bone lesions, as well as malformation of limb bones and even fractures. Cases of DODs caused exclusively by copper deficiency are relatively rare, though the use of certain foods, such as milk products, vegetables and grain, as the principal dietary component can result in a significantly deficienct supply.

Iodine is required by the thyroid gland for synthesis of the hormones T3 and T4, which are essential for healthy skeletal development. The manifold consequences of iodine deficiency include abnormal development of bone and cartilage, which may manifest clinically as reduced growth.

Concluding Remarks

It is recommended that all aspects of the diet be assessed and optimized, with emphasis on provision of an adequate and balanced supply of energy, calcium, phosphorus, copper, iodine, Vitamins A and D and other essential nutrients. This serves to prevent nutritionally induced DODs and allows optimal nutrition to be used, where possible, to mitigate risks posed by genetic predisposition, overtraining and trauma.

> **Practical Application**
> **Feeding Recommendations for Growing Dogs**
> - Key factor: energy intake!
>   - Compare actual weight with growth curve.
>   - Adjust energy intake (reduce calorie intake if weight is above the curve, and vice versa).
>   - As a general rule: too little energy is better than too much.
>   - Exercise caution with respect to extra calories from snacks, rewards etc.
> - Adjust nutrient/energy ratio (for below-average energy requirement, increase the nutrient concentration).
> - Ensure that the nutrient supply is adequate and balanced. In particular:
>   - Provide sufficient calcium and phosphorus to meet absolute requirements.
>   - Maintain calcium/phosphorus ration in the recommended range of 1/1 to 2/1 (optimally 1.3–1.8/1).

1.4.3 Maintenance Requirement (Adult Dog)

Once the growth phase is complete, and the dog has entered a state of maintenance metabolism, the implications of malnutrition for the skeletal system are considerably less critical. Although the demand for nutrients such as calcium and phosphorus remains high in the dog, compared to humans, deficiencies and excesses do not affect adults as quickly or severely as puppies and young dogs.

Nevertheless, there are several reasons for aiming, where possible, to provide a diet that closely approximates the animal's needs. Although it may not be possible to identify disparities between demand and supply in a timely and definitive manner, the health of the locomotor apparatus is still best served by a balanced diet that meets the nutritional requirements of the adult dog.

Energy Supply

Excess body weight and obesity have a profound impact on bone and joint health. The state of being overweight, per se, plus secretion of proinflammatory mediators and other metabolic influences can have detrimental effects or can cause existing changes to become clinically relevant. Increasing prevalence of overweight and obesity – currently 35 to 50% in dogs, depending on region – indicates that prevention and treatment are important from an orthopedic perspective.

In contrast to growing dogs, adult dogs routinely respond to a chronic excess of energy by laying down surplus fat. Deposition of fat to levels that affect the dog's health occurs gradually and is relatively inconspicuous during daily contact with the animal. At ≥ 10% above its normal or ideal weight, a dog is considered to be overweight. At 130% or more of its normal weight, the dog is classified as obese. It is important to note that a yo-yo effect, as seen in humans, is also recognised in dogs. If, after a successful weight reduction program, a previously overweight animal does not receive a lower-energy maintenance diet, and does not get more exercise, just a small oversupply of calories is enough to return the animal to its original overweight state.

This increased food efficiency can make successful dietary management increasingly difficult. Clearly, prevention of obesity is the best approach. In adults, as in young dogs, monitoring is facilitated by regular weighing. If the dog is weighed regularly, ideally on a weekly basis, and its weight recorded, necessary steps can be taken quickly, before significant changes occur.

As nutritional status is frequently misjudged by pet owners, assessment should be based on body condition scoring. This involves visual inspection and palpation of particular body regions to quantify the levels of fat tissue. Using such a system, e.g. a 9 point system in which 1 = cachectic, 4/5 = normal and 9 = morbidly obese, nutritional status can be assessed objectively, avoiding preconceptions and personal bias, and can be communicated more easily to the owner (▶ Table 1.3).

Overall, there is a causal link between the increasing frequency of overweight and physical activity. Changes in the living conditions and habits of people have brought about a decrease in activity in the everyday life of dogs. Pain and lameness further reduce activity, resulting in decreased energy expenditure and increased body weight, unless caloric intake is restricted. The demand for energy also declines with age, presumably due to decreasing physical activity. The very high palatability of most currently available complete foods is not particularly helpful in this regard. The energy requirement of the animal, and thus its daily food ration, is subject to variation and must be constantly adjusted. In addition, severe, painful diseases frequently lead to substantial loss of muscle mass. Recorded body weight may thus change relatively little, while the

▶ **Tab. 1.3** 9-point BCS system. This clinically tested system for assessment of body fat based on visual inspection and palpation allows conclusions to be drawn about nutritional status. It is important to distinguish between muscle and fat deposits; this makes it easier to distinguish between a „skinny fat" dog (under-muscled, high proportion of body fat, „normal" body weight) and a muscular, well-conditioned dog with normal amounts of body fat but above-average body weight. (source: Nestlé Purina, Body Condition System)

Scale	Description	
1 = cachectic	Ribs and tuber coxae clearly visible. No palpable subcutaneous fat, prominent abdominal tuck. Obvious reduction of muscle mass.	very thin
2 = very thin	Ribs and tuber coxae clearly visible. No palpable subcutaneous fat. Clear abdominal tuck.	
3 = thin	Tuber coxae and waist discernible on visual inspection. Small amount of fat detectable on flat palpation of the ribs.	thin
4 = under-weight	Fat detectable on flat palpation of the ribs, abdominal tuck evident. Waist clearly discernible. Minimal fat palpable over the abdomen.	
5 = normal	Animal is well proportioned, waist evident, ribs covered with thin layer of fat. Minimal fat deposits palpable over the abdomen.	**normal**

► **Tab. 1.3** continued

Scale	Description	
6 = overweight	Ribs difficult to palpate due to increased fat coverage. Waist no longer clearly evident. No clear abdominal tuck, underline passes almost horizontally towards the stifle.	overweight
7 = very over-weight	Ribs barely palpable under a layer of fat, waist poorly discernible, abdomen seems filled out, palpable fat deposits over the abdomen.	
8 = obese	Ribs covered in thick layer of fat. Waist absent, increasing fat deposits in the abdominal region forming a paunch. Additional fat deposits evident around the hips.	obese
9 = morbidly obese	Continued development of substantial fat deposits around the hips, pronounced pot belly with accumulation of fat (visible and palpable). Waist not visible. Ribs not palpable beneath layer of fat.	

The Body Condition Score system was developed at the Nestlé Purina Center and validated in the following publications:
- LaFlamme DP. Development and Validation of a Body Condition Score System for Cats. A Clinical Tool. Feline Practice 1997; 25: 3–17
- LaFlamme DP, Hume E, Harrison J. Evaluation of Zoometric Measures as an Assessment of Body Composition of Dogs and Cats. Compendium 2001; 23 [Suppl gA]:88

proportion of body fat markedly increases. For these patients, assessment of the muscle score should be included when assessing nutritional status.

Minerals

Discrepancies between nutrient intake and requirement are better tolerated in the fully-grown dog. Development of clinically significant changes is preceded by a substantial grace period. This is explained by the relatively low maintenance requirements of adults and the ability of the body to compensate to some extent for deficiencies of a certain magnitude or duration. Depending on the type of nutrient, suboptimal intake can be counteracted by increased utilization or exploitation of body reserves; if intake exceeds requirements, storage reservoirs can be filled, or excretion can be increased. The duration and efficiency of compensation depends on various factors. Yet even when dogs appear to be highly resilient, malnutrition can result in significant skeletal abnormalities. Thus, the diet of adult dogs should also account for their nutritional requirements, albeit not necessarily as strictly as that of puppies and young dogs.

Over several months, calcium deficiency in adults dogs (e.g. due to inadequate mineral content in home-made rations prepared from meat, grain and vegetables) can result in demineralization of the skeleton, even to the point at which spontane-

ous fractures occur. Adult dogs appear to tolerate surplus calcium much better than growing dogs. In contrast to skeletal abnormalities, frequently reported consequences of excess calcium in growing dogs include obstipation and urinary calculi. An excess of phosphorus and phosphate is more commonly described as having negative impacts on kidney health than on the skeletal system.

Reproduction in the Bitch

Reproduction in the bitch presents a special case. During pregnancy, the demand for calcium and phosphorus is greatly increased, due to the development of fetal skeletal tissue. The requirement for these minerals increases further during lactation, according to the size of the litter. Here again, there are obvious differences between humans and dogs; the dog is multiparous and produces considerably more milk relative to its body weight, precluding a simple comparison between the two species.

Since the calcium concentration in milk is constant, and only the milk yield declines over the course of lactation, nutritional deficits must be counterbalanced by the breakdown of maternal bone tissue. Although a certain degree of bone loss during the lactation period is considered normal, it is important to provide breeding bitches with an adequate supply of calcium and phosphorus to avoid excessive bone resorption. This applies particularly for bitches that have multiple litters. By the second half of gestation, the demand for calcium is already double the maintenance requirement. During lactation, bitches require 2–7 times the amount needed for maintenance, depending on the size of the litter.

Renal Insufficiency

The prevalence of chronic renal insufficiency is greater in older animals. Nutrition is important in this context for countering the development of osteorenal syndrome due to renal secondary hyperparathyroidism. As the capacity of the kidneys to excrete phosphate declines, phosphate retention increases. In response, secretion of PTH is increased to stabilize calcium and phosphorus homeostasis. Without effective intervention, the various consequences of these changes can include increased bone resorption, whereby complications can arise from calcification of soft tissues, particularly the kidneys. Thus, control of hyperphosphatemia is essential for slowing the progression of renal insufficiency. It is particularly important to correct excesses by adjusting dietary phosphate intake, culminating in reductions to below recommended levels, in order to control serum phosphorus concentrations. As calcium has an osteoprotective effect, the supply of calcium should not be reduced. This can lead to an increase in the calcium/phosphorus ratio in the food to beyond the normal range of 2/1. In this situation, the increased ratio is not only well tolerated, but is also beneficial through its depressive effect on phosphate utilization. Reduction of dietary phosphorus is achieved by decreasing mineral sources of phosphorus and increasing the calories derived from fat/fat-rich food components.

1.4.4   Diagnosis

It is often impossible to trace the cause of clinical abnormalities of skeletal development back to a particular event. Whether the clinical signs are of uni- or multifactorial origin can seldom be determined. Radiography can be used to identify clinically relevant aberrations (though this often occurs at a relatively late stage, particularly with widespread bone changes such as generalized fibrous osteodystrophy), while the etiology remains unclear. It is advisable though to identify specific causes, also to rule out the influence of genetics, husbandry and nutrition.

Ideally, it would be possible to use simple laboratory method such as a blood test to diagnose nutritionally induced DODs, or at least to identify nutritional inadequacies. However, this is very rarely the case. Blood concentrations of most nutrients are poorly correlated, if at all, with oral intake because they are closely regulated, can be supplemented by bodily reservoirs and exhibit diurnal or phasic variation, and because inadequate intake can be masked in other ways. Blood calcium is a case in point; concentrations are maintained in a very narrow range, as hypo- or hypercalcemia has significant consequences for the health of the animal. Parathyroid hormone, calcitonin and Vitamin D are the most important and well-recognised regulators of blood calcium. If insufficient calcium is consumed in the diet, the body attempts to minimise renal and fecal losses and calcium is liberated from the bone. Blood concentrations of Ca^{2+}

and total calcium may be within normal ranges while the skeleton is substantially demineralized. This can result in severe bone malformations or fractures, even though blood values remain within the reference range. Similar principles apply in the case of calcium excess. Normal blood values for calcium and phosphorus are by no means a guarantee that the supply of these minerals is adequate, though small deviations from the reference range may be observed periodically. The relatively high levels of blood phosphate in growing animals, compared with adults, may be slightly reduced if intake of phosphorus is substantially deficient. If at all, an increase or decrease in average blood calcium or phosphorus levels in a group of animals (e.g. in a research study) may be informative, though even here the observed values may be normal. For individual animals, measurement of blood values is an unsuitable diagnostic technique. Although relatively laborious, determination of blood PTH-concentrations may have diagnostic value for detecting secondary nutritional hyperparathyroidism induced by calcium deficiency. Yet even in this case, large fluctuations and circadian regulation may result in detection of low values. To avoid misinterpretation, it is necessary to perform multiple tests, which is often cost-prohibitive.

Ration calculation remains the **gold standard** for timely, accurate diagnosis. This is predicated on comprehensive and accurate appraisal of the feeding history and growth rate data. Daily nutrient intake is compared with individual requirements. As well as being the most reliable means of detecting nutritional inadequacies, this approach allows deviations from required daily values to be quantified, thus permitting targeted optimization of the food ration. The use of a rough estimate to correct suspected nutrient deficiencies, without nutritional analysis, is not recommended under any circumstances.

⚡ Practical Application

Ideally, it would be possible to use a simple laboratory method such as a blood test to diagnose nutritionally induced DODs, or at least to identify nutritional inadequacies. However, this is very rarely the case. Blood concentrations of most nutrients are poorly correlated with oral intake because they are closely regulated, can be supplemented by bodily reservoirs and exhibit diurnal or phasic variation, and because inadequate intake can be masked in other ways. Blood calcium is a case in point; concentrations are maintained in a very narrow range, as hypo- or hypercalcemia has significant consequences for the health of the animal.

Normal blood values for calcium and phosphorus are by no means a guarantee that the supply of these minerals is adequate, though small deviations from the reference range may be observed periodically.

Assessment of Feeding

An adequate and balanced supply of nutrients can be achieved using a variety of diets. Commercial complete foods can be just as effective as home-made rations created from cooked or raw ingredients. Conversely, nutritional inadequacies can arise with both of these approaches, either through the use of unsuitable ingredients and/or quantities, or through lack of, or inappropriate, supplementation with minerals and vitamins. In both cases, problems can also arise from nutrient dilution due to additional feeding of (calorie-rich) poorly balanced foodstuffs. Feeding of treats, rewards, snacks, table scraps and purpose-specific supplements (e.g. oil for improving coat condition, mineral preparations containing chondroprotective substances) leads to nutritional aberrations that can have detrimental effects on skeletal health. Similarly, problems can result from supplementation of balanced diets with selected, individual nutrient sources. This includes feeding of calcium carbonate for prevention of calcium deficiency, a common practice among puppy owners. In addition to calcium oversupply, and its aforementioned potential consequences, this can result in secondary deficiencies of important nutrients and trace elements such as phosphate, zinc and copper.

Thus, it is essential to undertake a thorough and detailed evaluation of the animal's existing diet. Is the animal strictly fed a complete food, or is this supplemented or combined with other food sources? Which mineral preparation is added to a home-made diet based on meat and grain, and in what quantity? Preparations used to supplement calcium and phosphorus must contain appropriate amounts of these minerals, i.e. 10–20% calcium and 5–10% phosphorus. Is the mineral supplement actually being consumed with the food? Mineral preparations are usually less palatable than the other components of the ration, and less desirable dietary constituents tend to be used in ever decreasing amounts. It has proven useful to have the owner write down the types and quantities of each food component that are used. Family members that were not present at the consultation can also contribute to this activity. Useful information about actual food intake can also be gleaned by ascertaining how long a bag of food lasts.

In some cases, particularly when many food components are used, and their nutrient content is not known, additional methods are required to assess the adequacy of the nutrient supply. In this case, ration calculation should be conducted. It is possible, though, to identify suspected cases of incorrect feeding in advance. Whether it is an un-supplemented home-made ration, a complete food supplemented with minerals or a complete food given to an animal with below-average energy requirements, the ration should be assessed and optimized with the aid of dietary analysis. This can be facilitated by the use of specialised software such as Diet Check Munich©. Referral to specialists, particularly veterinarians with additional nutritional qualifications, certified veterinary nutritionists or European Specialists in Veterinary and Comparative Nutrition (EBVS) of the European Colleges of Veterinary and Comparative Nutrition ECVCN, is also recommended, especially in challenging cases.

1.5 Functional Anatomy of the Locomotor Apparatus

Martin S. Fischer, Daniel Koch

1.5.1 Functional Osteology and Skeletal Development

Vertebral column

As in almost all mammals, the canine vertebral column is conventionally divided into cervical, thoracic, lumbar, sacral and coccygeal regions. There are 7 cervical vertebrae, 13 thoracic vertebrae, 7 lumbar vertebrae, 3 sacral vertebrae and a variable number of coccygeal vertebrae. In terms of function, this regional subdivision only reflects the organization of the axial skeleton to a limited extent. Functional anatomical analysis using biplanar fluoroscopy has confirmed earlier findings, based upon which the cervical vertebrae were divided into three sections: atlas–axis, C3–C5 and C6–C7. According to these observations, the vertebrae C3–C5 do not contribute to motion in the sagittal plane, which involves only the atlantooccipital, atlantoaxial and C6/C7 intervertebral joints. Lateral and axial rotation are limited to the atlas and C3–C5. The vertebrae C1 and C2, and also C6 und C7, have characteristic anatomical features that distinguish them from C3–C5.

In the lumbar vertebral column (▶ **Fig. 1.33**), the anatomy of the vertebrae changes gradually from caudal to cranial (e.g. the angle of inclination of the facet joints [syn. intervertebral joint, articular process joint or zygapophysis]). While the greatest joint movement occurs at S1/L7 and L7/L6, there is less movement in the walk and trot, compared to the gallop. The cranially progressive reduction in movement results primarily from the stabilizing effect of the epaxial musculature, which counteracts the forces transmitted from the limbs to the trunk during locomotion. Thus, intervertebral movement is also actively restricted in all gaits.

In-vivo measurements of movement during walking and trotting differ considerably from values recorded for sagittal motion using vertebral column specimens derived from German Shepherd Dogs [9]. Measurements obtained using anatomical specimens – 3° between L3 und L4 increasing in a caudal direction to 12° at L6/L7 and 32° (even > 40° in some specimens) in the lumbosacral joint (S1/L7) – have so far not been confirmed in live animal studies. A significant difference was also observed between males and females in the anatomical preparations, with movement in the lumbosacral joint found to be around 9° greater in females.

The degree of movement of the lumbar vertebral column, and the demonstrated increase in mobility towards its caudal end, are reflected in the structure of the intervertebral discs. Whereas the thickness of the discs increases by 58% from L4–L5 to L7–S1, the cross-sectional surface area only rises by 20%, resulting in an increase of 32% in the cross-sectional thickness to surface area ratio. This is an indicator of markedly increased mobility, because the greater the relative thickness of an intervertebral disc, the greater is the capacity for flexion and exten-

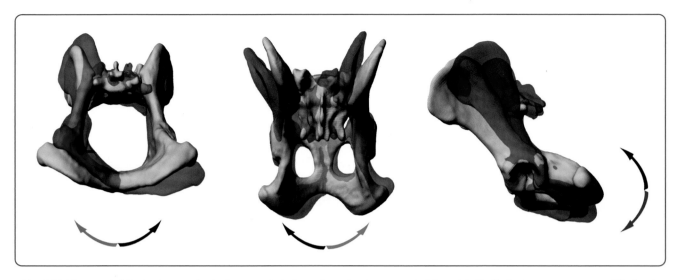

▶ **Fig. 1.33** Movement of the lumbar vertebral column results in three-dimensional movement of the pelvis. Red indicates movement around the longitudinal axis, green represents lateral movement and blue denotes movement in the sagittal plane (after [80]). (source: Martin S. Fischer, Katja Wachs, Jonas Lauströer, Amir Andikfar)

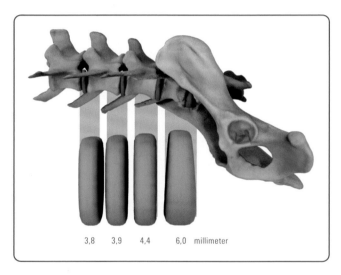

3,8   3,9   4,4   6,0 millimeter

▶ **Fig. 1.34** Increasing intervertebral disc thickness from lumbar vertebra 4 to the lumbosacral joint (after [4]). (source: Martin S. Fischer, Jonas Lauströer, Amir Andikfar)

sion (▶ **Fig. 1.34**). Whereas the intervertebral discs of the lumbar vertebral column are consistent in shape, the lumbosacral intervertebral disc is shaped like a club with is expanded section directed ventrally.

This is consistent with the observation that, during walking and trotting, there is compression of the intervertebral discs of the last presacral joints at the point of touch down and lift off, and in the middle of the stance and swing phases, of the hindlimbs. Using touch down of the right limb as an example, this is because the pelvis is maximally anteverted, yet the lumbosacral joint is in maximum flexion.

In the sacrum, the transverse processes and the rudimentary accessory processes of three vertebrae are completely fused, leaving only openings through which the spinal nerves exit. Osseous fusion generally occurs within the first 18 months of life. The connection between the sacrum and the pelvis, the sacroiliac joint, consists of two components: a true synovial joint and a taut ligament (syndesmosis). Movement of the sacroiliac joint is very limited. This joint serves mainly as a buffer and transmits forces from the limbs to the trunk. In a study of 145 adult and 45 juvenile dogs, ranging from Yorkshire Terriers to Rottweilers, Breit and Künzel found that a 7-fold increase in body weight is accompanied by just a 6-fold increase in the surface area of the sacroiliac joint [7]. Consequently, there is disproportionately higher tensile and compressive loading of the sacroiliac joint in large breeds, reaching 2.7 times the body weight of the animal. In noting that the shape of the joint also varies, the authors made the interesting observation that the joint is concave in certain breeds, specifically the Rottweiler, Bernese Mountain Dog and German Shepherd Dog. The angle of inclination and ossification of the sacrum are age- and breed-dependent. Load-induced joint modeling occurs from 12 weeks of age [7]. From 12 months onwards, no age-related or sex-specific changes are observed.

In addition to its role in steering during turning movements, the tail contributes to behavioral expression in dogs. Surprisingly, the direction of tail wagging is significant in this regard [72]. Wagging to the right indicates positive emotion, whereas left-sided tail wagging leads to expression of fear and elevated heart rate. In addition, it has been reported that puppies with longer tails stand 1–2 days earlier. Thus, the tail may also serve to maintain balance in puppies, a function that would be of considerable evolutionary significance.

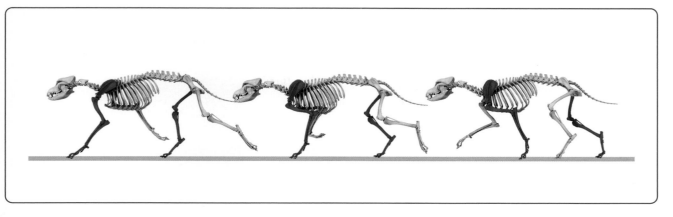

▶ **Fig. 1.35** Movement of functionally analogous limb segments (femur and scapula, brachium and crus, front and hind foot) in diagonal unison, illustrated by three snapshots of the trot cycle. (source: Martin S. Fischer, Jonas Lauströer, Amir Andikfar)

> ⚡ **Practical Application**
> The greatest range of movement of the lumbar vertebral column occurs at L7/S1 and L7/L6. The degree of movement of the lumbar vertebral column, and the demonstrated increase in mobility towards its caudal end, are reflected in the structure of the intervertebral discs, which increase in thickness towards the caudal end of the lumbar spine.

Limbs

The locomotor system of all terrestrial animals is constantly working against gravity. Particularly on uneven terrain, energy expenditure during locomotion (p. 12)increases when there is vertical displacement of the body's center of gravity, i.e. when the body moves up and down. This can be ameliorated or prevented by connecting the joints between the ground and the trunk in a way that allows changes in height to be counterbalanced. The double-angled construction of mammalian legs fulfils this spring and shock absorber function, though it is also inherently energetically expensive.

The three-segment limb of mammals, including the dog, leads to a functional analogy between the femur and scapula (i.e. as opposed to the thigh and brachium), brachium and crus, and front and hindfoot (▶ Fig. 1.35). Particularly in the trot, these functional pairs move in diagonal unison. The pivot points of the forelimb (upper third of the scapula) and hindlimb (hip joint) are optimally positioned at the same vertical height (▶ Fig. 1.5).

However, as the serially homologous segments (brachium/thigh, antebrachium/crus and front foot/hind foot) develop from the same embryological origins, a conflict has arisen between function (in this case biomechanical requirements) and development. This conflict can be reduced to a simple denominator: the hindlimb of mammals corresponds to the leg of non-mammalian tetrapods, but the mammalian forelimb comprises the arm and scapula. Arms and legs have the same developmental program, whereas forelimbs and hindlimbs do not. It has been established that the scapula has a different embryonic origin, arising from multiple somites, not from the limb buds.

The three-segment limbs of dogs are angled not only in the sagittal plan, but also in the transverse plane. The scapula is abducted (its dorsal border is tilted inward) by the serratus ventralis, which attaches to its dorsal border. When the animal is standing, this tilting counteracts the scapular and acromial parts of the deltoid. As described in the chapter Limb Kinematics (p. 18), abduction torque is observed in the shoulder joint throughout the stance phase.

> ⚡ **Practical Application**
> The locomotor system of all terrestrial animals is constantly working against gravity. The primary action of numerous muscles is to work against gravity and to maintain the angulation and matched motion of the (p. 18)limbs through sustained, isometric contraction. The pivot points of the forelimb (upper third of the scapula) and hindlimb (hip joint) are optimally positioned at the same vertical height.

Scapula

The scapula is a flat bone consisting predominantly of cortical osseous tissue. It has a thin cranial border and a caudal border that is considerably thickened, due to the attachment of (primarily) the teres major and the long head of the triceps brachii at this location. The dorsal border is slightly enlarged by a layer of cartilage, which serves as the site of attachment of the serratus and rhomboid muscles. During embryological development, the spine of the scapula grows into the laterally adjacent myoblast mass, dividing this into the supraspinatus and infraspinatus (this occurs in other mammals, and presumably also in the dog). Mechanically, the spine of the scapula acts to reduce bending stress on the flat portion of the bone. Distally, the spine expands to form the acromion and hamate process. The spine of the scapula is the site of insertion of the trapezius and, distally, the omotransversarius (syn. levator scapulae ventralis) and, together with the acromion, forms the origin of the deltoid. The cranial border merges with the supraglenoid tubercle, from which the biceps brachii arises. The weak coracobrachialis arises from a medial thickening, the poorly developed coracoid process.

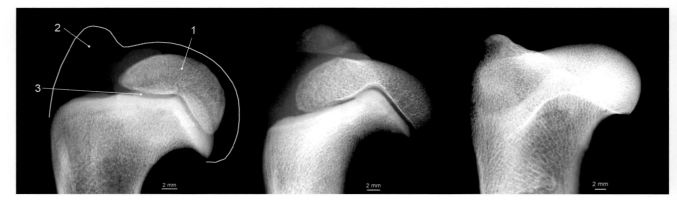

▶ **Fig. 1.36** Micro-focus radiograph of the proximal humerus of a 6-week old, 13-week old and adult dog. 1 caput humeri, 2 tuberculum majus, 3 proximal epiphyseal plate; after [65] (source: PD Dr. Anke Schnapper, Tierärztliche Stiftung Hannover)

Except for the ventral angle and a strip of cartilage at the dorsal border, the scapula is completely ossified at birth. Growth of the scapula occurs primarily at the cranial and caudal borders and at the spine of the scapula, through periosteal ossification. Only the supraglenoid tubercle has a separate ossification center that appears in the sixth week post partum, is fully formed at 13 weeks and fuses with the scapula from 5 months of age [65]. The growth plate of the glenoid cavity runs along the entire cartilage-bone boundary.

> ⚡ **Practical Application**
> Growth of the scapula occurs primarily at the cranial and caudal borders and at the spine of the scapula, through periosteal ossification. Only the supraglenoid tubercle has a separate ossification center.

Humerus

Based on experimental assessment of breaking strength, the humerus is the strongest long bone. It is divided into the humeral head, body and condyle; the articular portion of the condyle is subdivided into the capitulum and the trochlea (▶ Fig. 5.38). Proximally, prominent muscle attachment sites include the greater tubercle, lesser tubercle, tricipital line, deltoid tuberosity and the medially located crest of the lesser tubercle. Their formation can be explained, in part, in terms of function.

The very strong supraspinatus, which attaches at the greater tubercle, is the anti-gravity muscle of the shoulder joint. In all gaits, and during the stance phase, it exerts a tensile force on the proximal humerus. The primary function of the infraspinatus, a similarly strong muscle that also inserts at the greater tubercle, is to exert a weak abduction force when the dorsal scapula is tilted, and to slow the extension of the swinging forelimb.

The marked prominence of the deltoid tuberosity is not explained by the magnitude of the combined force generated by the scapular and acromial parts of the deltoid; this reaches a maximum 283 N in the Greyhound, making the deltoid one of the medium strength muscles of the forelimb (compared with: extensor capri radialis 292 N, infraspinatus 823 N, biceps brachii 853 N [84], [85]). Nor is it a consequence of the power of these muscular components (1 W and 3 W respectively). Instead, it results from their constant activity. The deltoid is the main muscle tasked with meeting the aforementioned need to ensure that the scapula and humerus remain in the same plane; refer also to Limb Kinematics (p. 18).

At birth, there is partial ossification of the diaphysis, extending from the middle of the bone. Ossification of the epiphyses occurs during the first year of life. Around 80% of the longitudinal growth of the humerus (▶ Fig. 1.36) occurs proximally. In the 6-week old dog, only one ossification center is evident, in the caudal half of the proximal epiphysis (greater tubercle). The other components of the humeral head are still cartilaginous at this stage. Ossification of the epiphysis is complete by 5 months of age.

An ossification center for the capitulum is present at the distal humeral epiphysis at 2 to 3 weeks after birth. This is followed one week later by the center for the trochlea. The two centers fuse in the sixth week post partum.

The apophyseal ossification center of the medial epicondyle appears in the eighth week and develops until week 13 post partum. All three ossification centers fuse by 5 months of age. During this period, the apophysis of the medial epicondyle also closes. This chronology exhibits individual and breed-specific variation. Closure of the proximal epiphysis commences at the humeral head from 10 months of age. The distal epiphyseal growth plate closes between 5 and 8 months.

Antebrachium

The radius and ulna are fixed in pronation by the proximal interosseous ligament, a structure measuring up to 2 mm in thickness. The two bones cross over one another, so that the radius lies latero-cranial to the ulna proximally, and medial to the ulna distally. No active movement is possible in the proximal radioulnar joint or the flat distal joint. However, the capacity of these joints for extensive passive rotation is utilized in situations such as sprinting around a bend (p. 16), whereby the front foot and radius act during the stance phase to provide an anchor point around which the ulna and rest of the body can rotate. In the German Shepherd Dog, there is passive internal and external rotation of up to 18° and 50° respectively. The equivalent values for the wire-haired Dachshund are 28° and 48°.

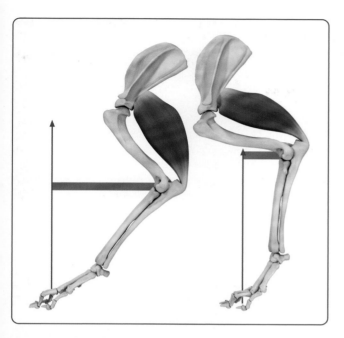

▶ **Fig. 1.37** Relationship between the muscle moment arm and resistive moment arm at the elbow joint. The resistive moment arm, represented by a red bar, shortens during the stance phase. The muscle moment arm is the perpendicular distance between the line of action of the triceps brachii and the center of rotation of the elbow joint. (source: Martin S. Fischer, Jonas Lauströer, Amir Andikfar)

The four-headed triceps brachii is the strongest muscle in the forelimb, generating immense forces of around 2000 N, 1500 N of which are produced by the long head alone (values given are for Greyhounds [84], [85]). Moment arm relationships are significant in this regard. In the forelimb, these are unfavorable: the resistive moment arm (antebrachium + front foot) is long, compared with the short muscle moment arm (olecranon), particularly at the beginning of the stance phase (▶ Fig. 1.37).

The triceps brachii must be strong enough to produce sufficient extensor torque at the elbow joint to counterbalance gravity-induced bending of the heavy front end of the body. All heads of the triceps brachii are active from the end of the swing phase to about two thirds into the stance phase, with maximum activity in the first half. Throughout its active phase, the muscle only shortens by 5% (walk), 7% (trot) and 8% (gallop), mainly due to flexion of the shoulder joint. The angle of the elbow largely remains constant. Were it not for the olecranon, the triceps brachii would need to be much stronger. The function of the olecranon as a lever arm corresponds to that of the calcaneal tuberosity, except that the moment arm relationships in the hindlimb are more favorable for producing strong movements of the hind foot, because the hind foot is much shorter than the antebrachium and front foot (▶ Fig. 1.38). Accordingly. the gastrocnemius muscles generate only two thirds as much force as the triceps brachii.

In the standing position, the antebrachium is almost vertical, to minimise torque, whereas the hind foot is angled. The perpendicular of the forelimb extends from the pivot point of the scapula through the axis of rotation of the elbow and along the antebrachium to a point behind the contact area of the front feet.

The coronoid process of the ulna consists of the prominent medial coronoid process and the smaller lateral coronoid process. The medial coronoid process is an important weight bearing component of the elbow joint (p. 64) during locomotion. It is also adjacent to the main site of insertion of the biceps brachii. In giant breed dogs, the medial coronoid process is broader and aligned more horizontally, which is associated with greater load bearing in these breeds. In large breeds, the articular surface is proportionally smaller. This, together with high body weight, results in increased load. In contrast, the surface area of the articular facet of the radial head increases with body weight, except in chondrodystrophic breeds.

In short-legged breeds (e.g. Dachshund, Welsh Corgi, Bassett Hound, Scottish Terrier) and also in the Chihuahua and French Bulldog, the antebrachium is shortened, compared to other segments of the limb, due to earlier closure of the growth plates. In all breeds examined to date, this achondroplasia is caused by the mutation of a single gene (FGF4). On this basis, it is assumed that all modern short-legged breeds have a common origin [52].

Longitudinal growth occurs at two epiphyses in the radius, and predominantly at the distal epiphysis in the ulna. The proximal growth plate of the radius contributes about 30–40% of longitudinal growth; the distal growth plate correspondingly accounts for 60–70%. The apophyseal growth plate of the olecranon tuber contributes a maximum of 15% to the total longitudinal growth of the ulna. The two osseous components of the antebrachium grow at the same rate, because the distal epiphysis of the ulna is conical while the radial growth plate is flat. This increases the area over which growth takes place in the ulna by a factor of 1.5.

The two ossification centers of the radius are evident in the second to fifth week post partum. The distal ulnar epiphysis appears in weeks 6–8. The radial and ulnar growth plates close at approximately the same time, at 7–11 months of age (for more precise values, see Flinsbach [26]). The ossification center for the olecranon appears in weeks 7–10; the growth plate closes at 6–10 months. In several breeds, the anconeal process has a separate ossification center that becomes apparent at 12–14 weeks. Closure of the growth plate exhibits breed-related and individual variation, occurring between 14 and 20 weeks. The coronoid processes do not have separate ossification centers. Ossification of the medial coronoid process proceeds from the base to the apex and is completed by 20–22 weeks.

- The radius and ulna are fixed in pronation; there is no active movement in the joints between these bones. However, the capacity of these joints for extensive passive rotation is used in movements such as sprinting around a bend (p. 16), whereby the front foot and radius act during the stance phase to provide an anchor point around which the ulna and rest of the body can rotate.
- The function of the olecranon as a lever arm corresponds to that of the calcaneal tuberosity, except that the moment arm relationships in the hindlimb are more favorable for producing strong movements of the hind foot, because the hindfoot is much shorter than the antebrachium and front foot.
- The medial coronoid process is an important load bearing component of the elbow joint (p. 64) during locomotion and is adjacent to the main insertion site of the biceps brachii.
- Longitudinal growth occurs at two epiphyses in the radius, and predominantly at the distal epiphysis in the ulna. These components of the antebrachium grow at the same rate because the distal epiphysis of the ulna is conical (in contrast to the flat radial epiphyses), resulting in an increase in the area over which growth takes place.
- In several breeds, the anconeal process has a separate ossification center that becomes apparent at 12–14 weeks. Closure of the growth plate exhibits breed-related and individual variation, occurring between 14 and 20 weeks. The coronoid processes do not have separate centers of ossification.

Femur

The femur is the second-strongest long bone in the body. The shape of the femoral head varies with breed, as does the angle between the neck and the shaft of the femur. The average neck-shaft angle is 147°. In the dog, the greater trochanter usually reaches the same height as the head of the femur, except in the German Shepherd Dog, Boxer and Poodle. In the Dachshund, it extends beyond the femoral head. The greater trochanter serves as the prominent attachment site for the medial and deep gluteals and the piriformis. Yet the femur represents a striking example of how powerful retraction of the hindlimb is achieved by various muscles that act together, while leaving highly variable traces of their presence on the bone. Whereas the biceps femoris does not leave so much as a line, the greater trochanter develops under the tensile forces exerted by the gluteals. Due to the insertion of the adductors on the facies aspera, the action of these muscles includes both adduction and internal rotation of the femur, as seen in the first half of the stance phase.

Proximal ossification centers are found in the head of the femur, the greater trochanter and the lesser trochanter. The first of these appears in weeks 3 to 4, the others in week 5 post partum. The distal femoral epiphysis forms in week 3. Closure of the apophyseal and epiphyseal growth plates occurs as follows: head of the femur (6–9 months), greater trochanter (8–13 months) and distal epiphysis (6–12 months).

Whereas the biceps femoris does not leave so much as line on the femur, the greater trochanter forms under the tensile forces exerted by the gluteals.

Crus

The skeleton of the crus consists of the closely associated long bones, the tibia and fibula. As the middle segment of the three-segment limb, the crus has the important function of transmitting the propulsion generated by the proximal segment (femur) to the distal hindfoot. The smaller the degree of flexion of the stifle joint or dorsiflexion of the tarsus, the more effective is the propulsion. The biarticular gastrocnemius muscles form a longitudinal tensioning system that passes along the caudal aspect of the limb and contributes substantially to the stability of the entire hindlimb. Except for the gastrocnemius muscles, the muscles of the foot arise from the tibia and the fibula. The tibial plateau and the lateral and medial malleolus are described in the section on the stifle joint (p. 67).

There are four centers of ossification in the tibia and two in the fibula (proximal and distal epiphysis). Fusion of the apophyseal and epiphyseal growth plates of the tibia occurs at the following times: tibial tuberosity (8–10 months), proximal epiphysis (6–15 months), distal epiphysis (5–11 months) and medial malleolus (4–5 months). The proximal and distal epiphyses of the fibula close at 6–12 months and 5–13 months, respectively.

As the middle segment of the three-segment limb, the crus has the important function of transmitting the propulsion generated by the proximal segment (femur) to the distal hindfoot.

Hindfoot

The calcaneal tuberosity is functionally equivalent to the olecranon, though the associated resistive moment arm is much shorter. Since the foot is retracted as a consequence of retraction of the whole limb, the gastrocnemius muscles only need to generate half as much force after 70% of the stance phase as during the first 30%, because the altered leg position results in disproportionate shortening of the resistive moment arm, compared to the muscle moment arm (▶ Fig. 1.38).

The calcaneal tuberosity is functionally equivalent to the olecranon, though the associated resistive moment arm is much shorter.

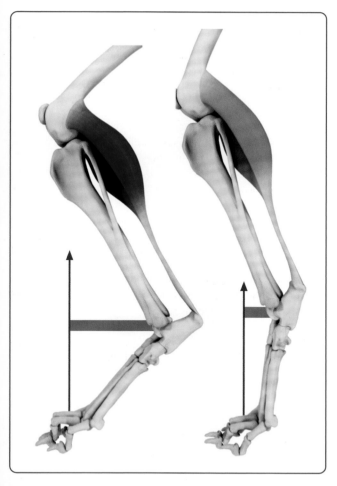

► **Fig. 1.38** Relationship between the muscle moment arm and resistive moment arm at the tarsal joint. The resistive moment arm, represented by a red bar, shortens during the stance phase. The muscle moment arm of the gastrocnemius muscles is the perpendicular distance between the line of action of the gastrocnemius muscles and the center of rotation of the tarsal joint. (source: Martin S. Fischer, Jonas Lauströer, Amir Andikfar)

1.5.2 Functional Myology

The descriptions of muscle activity in this chapter are based on electromyographic studies of various functional muscle groups (► Fig. 1.41, ► Fig. 1.42). Electromyography measures changes in electrical activity of muscle; muscle activity at the measurement site is recorded in the form of an electromyogram (EMG). In early electromyography techniques, the electrical signal was transmitted from individual needle electrodes inserted into the muscle at different depths. More recent studies using multi-electrodes have shown that a muscle is rarely activated as a whole. In some cases, waves of activation are observed in individual muscles, exemplified by the sequential activation of different regions of the triceps brachii during cyclic locomotion. Regional activation patterns are particularly pronounced in the large, flat muscles that connect the forelimb to the trunk. Alternatively, the EMG may reveal only very small regions of activation when, in the course of cyclic locomotion, small regions of muscle rich in type I fibres (p.37) are active, while regions dominated by type II fibres are inactive (ordered recruitment).

It is important to be aware that an electromechanical delay, measuring 5–20 ms depending on the muscle, occurs at the beginning and end of muscle contraction. Thus, the production of force within the muscle commences later, and continues for longer, than indicated in the EMG trace. This explains observations such as the onset of muscle activation just before touch down, ensuring timely delivery of force.

While the EMG provides information about muscle activity (► Fig. 1.41, ► Fig. 1.42), it des not indicate whether this activity contributes to, or inhibits, movement, i.e. it does not distinguish between isotonic, isometric and auxotonic contraction. The direction of force exerted by a muscle changes when the geometry of the leg is altered kinematically. With the aid of modeling, an approximation of the degree of force generated by the muscle can be determined from amplitudes measured by the EMG or from joint torque calculations (► Fig. 1.39, ► Fig. 1.40).

Retractors

The scapula is retracted by the cervical part of the serratus, which is active from the middle of the swing phase to midstance. It may be that this is supported by the action of the trapezius and rhomboid muscles. The thoracic part of the serratus ventralis probably acts exclusively to suspend the trunk and all of the extrinsic shoulder muscles serve to stabilize the pivot point of the scapula. It is striking that the main action of the forelimb, i.e. rotation and translation of the scapula, requires so little muscular work. During steady movement on even ground, the limb (p.17)acts as a strut. This transfers the work from the extrinsic muscles of the shoulder to the muscles of the distal joints, which in turn make extensive use of opportunities to recover energy (p.38) from structures that are passively stretched under load [12],[13].

A new perspective has emerged on the function of some muscles, such as the latissimus dorsi. During cyclic locomotion on a level surface, activity of this muscle only occurs consistently in the second half of the swing phase. Like the deep pectoral, the latissimus dorsi only serves to retract the limb when moving on an incline. Otherwise, its action is to brake the swinging limb and to retract it until the point of touch down, when its activity ceases.

Retraction of the hindlimb, and thereby forward movement of the body, is brought about mainly by the cranial part of the biceps femoris, the gluteals, the semimembranosus and the adductor magnus. The caudal part of the biceps femoris initially brakes the swinging limb and remains active until the point at which the stifle joint passes the point of touch down. Until this time, it acts as a retractor, since the vastus muscles compensate for its flexor components. Immediately after passing the point of touchdown, the flexor action predominates over the retractor function. The activity of the cranial part of the biceps femoris and the gluteus medius begins at the end of the swing phase and continues until the moment in the stance phase when the hip joint passes over the point of touch down. The activity of the retractors can increase severalfold during running on an incline; at a grade of just 10%, the increase is already 20-fold. Any

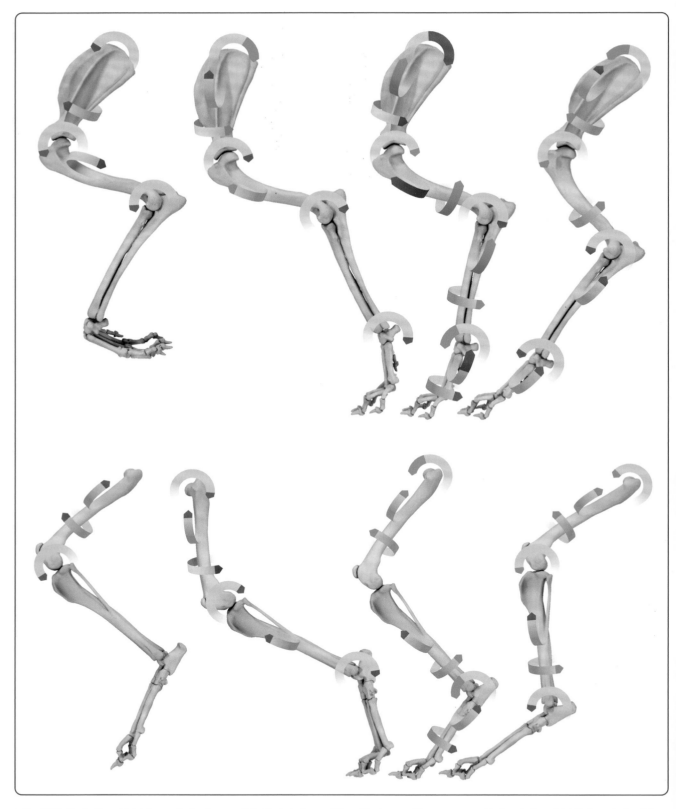

▶ **Fig. 1.39** Illustration of joint torque in the fore- and hindlimb during **walking**. The four positions correspond to touch down (right), the middle of the stance phase, lift off and the middle of the swing phase. The arrows indicate the direction and magnitude of joint torque. The larger the coloured area of the arrow, the greater is the net torque. Three levels of magnitude are represented: 0–0.15 N m/kg, >0.15–0.3 N m/kg and >0.3 N m/kg. Green indicates positive joint work; red represents negative joint work. Dark grey indicates that the joint is static. The number of red arrows is markedly higher in the forelimb than in the hindlimb. In the forelimb, braking takes place over a longer period, while the hindlimb generates propulsion, with storage of energy in the tarsus. The femur undergoes marked internal rotation while the crus rotates externally. The appearance of the clockwise arrow on the scapula at the middle of the stance phase indicates a joint torque action opposing the direction of movement. This signifies slowing of the retraction of the scapula. At lift off, protraction of the scapula (green arrow) has already commenced. (source: Martin S. Fischer, Emanuel Andrada, Jonas Lauströer, Amir Andikfar)

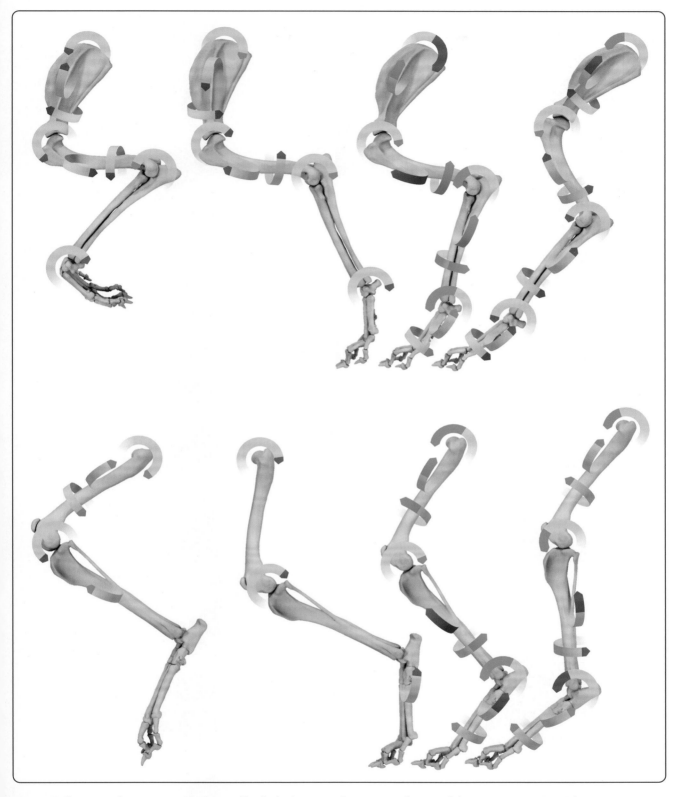

▶**Fig. 1.40** Illustration of joint torque in the fore- and hindlimbs during **trotting**. For an explanation of the arrows, see ▶**Fig. 1.39**. (source: Martin S. Fischer, Emanuel Andrada, Jonas Lauströer, Amir Andikfar)

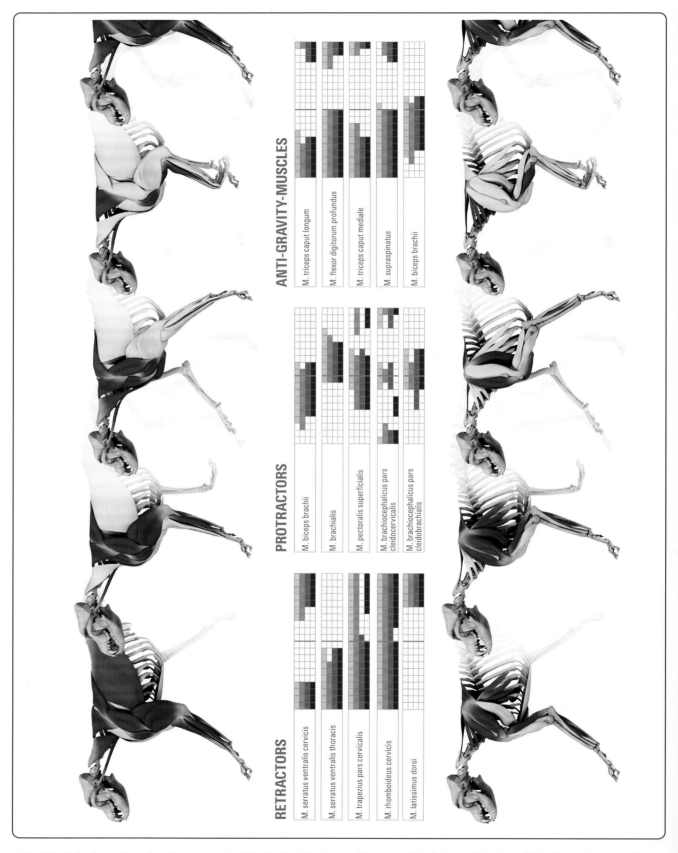

▶ **Fig. 1.41** Activation patterns for selected muscles of the forelimb. The images illustrate activity during walking. The table indicates, from top to bottom for each muscle, normalized activity during walking, trotting and galloping (trailing limb followed by leading limb) from touch down to subsequent touch down. The vertical line bisecting the table indicates the point of lift off (after [12], [13], [29], [76], [77], [78]). (source: Martin S. Fischer, Jonas Lauströer, Amir Andikfar)

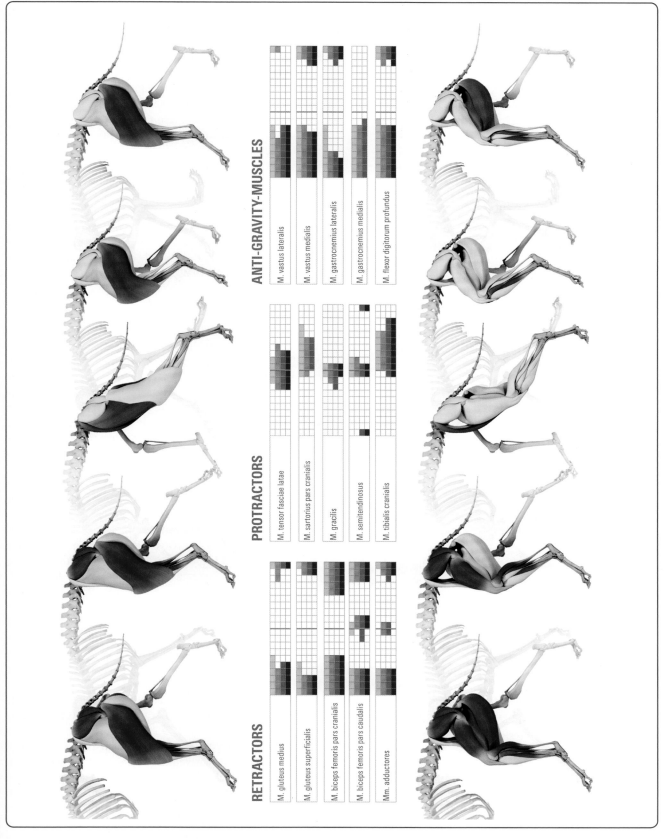

▶ **Fig. 1.42** Activation patterns for selected muscles of the hindlimb. The images illustrate activity during walking. The table indicates, from top to bottom for each muscle, normalized activity during walking, trotting and galloping (trailing limb followed by leading limb) from touch down to subsequent touch down. The vertical line bisecting the table indicates the point of lift off (after [13], [76], [77], [78], [82], [83]). (source: Martin S. Fischer, Jonas Lauströer, Amir Andikfar)

extension in the hip joint and tarsal joint at the end of the stance phase is due to the effect of gravity.

> **🔧 Practical Application**
> - It is striking that the main action of the forelimb, i.e. rotation and translation of the scapula, requires little muscular work.
> - Retraction of the hindlimb, and thereby forward movement of the body, is brought about mainly by the cranial part of the biceps femoris, the gluteals, the semimembranosus and the adductor magnus.

Muscles Acting as Protractors to Advance the Limb During the Swing Phase

Contraction of the biceps brachii and brachialis results in lifting of the forelimb and, together with the action of the superficial pectoral, initiates forelimb protraction; the latter is facilitated by the catapult effect produced by rapid flexion of the carpal joint (p. 18). Protraction is continued by the omotransversarius and brachiocephalicus. The activity of the flexors, particularly the brachialis and biceps brachii, is greater during trotting and galloping than during walking, as the limbs are lifted higher from a usually lower starting position against the trunk. As described earlier, contraction of the latissimus dorsi – and concurrent contraction of the deep and superficial pectorals – results in braking of the swinging forelimb and initiates its retraction.

The following muscles are active from towards end of the stance phase and until early in the swing phase and are thus responsible for lifting and subsequent protraction of the hindlimb. The tensor fasciae latae, pectineus and sartorius initiate flexion of the hip joint and limb protraction. The caudal part of the biceps femoris and the semitendinosus and gracilis flex the stifle joint. Flexion of the tarsal joint at lift off results from the action of the cranial tibial and peroneus longus. In situations where more force is required to drive the body forward, such as running uphill or pulling on a lead, these muscles are activated early and serve as retractors. From the middle of the swing phase, protraction is continued by the action of the iliopsoas, sartorius, extensor digitorum longus, and by the rectus femoris, which exhibits biphasic activity in the symmetrical gaits.

Muscles Acting Against Gravity-induced Flexion

Understandably, the activity of the muscles that counteract gravity-induced flexion on landing is greater during trotting and galloping than during walking. Few muscles are active for the duration of the stance phase (supraspinatus, flexor digitorum profundus). The supraspinatus prevents flexion of the shoulder joint, while the flexor digitorum profundus, supported by the extensor carpi ulnaris and flexor carpi ulnaris, prevents dorsiflexion of the carpal joints. The heads of the triceps brachii are active from the end of the swing phase to the point in the stance phase at which the point of touch down passes the elbow joint during the stance phase. The biceps brachii becomes active shortly thereafter, initially serving to counteract passive, gravity-induced extension of the elbow joint. Only hereafter does the activity of the biceps brachii lead to lifting and protraction of the forelimb.

The gluteals initially act against flexion of the hip joint at the commencement of the stance phase. Retraction of the femur by these muscles occurs subsequently. The stifle joint, which exhibits only limited effective angular movement during the stance phase, is stabilized against gravity-induced flexion by the vastus muscles and, from midstance, also by the rectus femoris. For the tarsal joint, the same function is performed by the gastrocnemius muscles and also the flexor digitorum superficialis and flexor digitorum profundus; the activity of these muscles, like that of the muscles mentioned above, extends from the end of the swing phase into the last third of the stance phase. Their contraction is essentially isometric. The vastus and gastrocnemius muscles act as extensors to control the degree of bending of the hindlimb. As the gastrocnemius muscles are also flexors of the stifle joint when the tarsal joint is fixed, the vastus muscles must also counteract this effect. Together, the vastus muscles are more powerful (25 W combined) than the gastrocnemius muscles (9 W combined).

Muscles of the Back

As in other mammals, the back muscles of the dog consist of three longitudinal systems: the transversospinalis, longissimus and iliocostalis systems. The muscle segments of the longissimus and iliocostalis systems span several vertebrae, while the transversospinalis system consists of long and short muscle segments. Adjacent vertebrae are connected primarily by deep muscles lying close to the bone (e.g. the rotatores). For a long time, the action of the back muscles during locomotion remained unclear. To date, EMG recordings have been made for just three of the canine back muscles: the multifidus lumborum, longissimus thoracis et lumborum and iliocostalis thoracis et lumborum [57], [62]. The first quantitative evaluation of the epaxial muscles of the dog was published only recently [81].

During walking and trotting, these three muscles exhibit two phases of activity per gait cycle (▶ Fig. 1.43, ▶ Fig. 1.44). These occur in the second half of the stance phase and in the swing phase. Activation of the same muscle produces two different effects. During the swing phase, muscle contraction results, as expected, in lateral flexion of the trunk. This does not occur in the stance phase; here, the muscles stabilize the trunk against torsion. The back muscles thus establish a static base for the work performed by the extrinsic limb muscles (arising from the trunk) and compensate for the torques that pass into the trunk. In the walk and gallop, the cranial portions are activated earlier than those located caudally; activation occurs sequentially along the back. In contrast, all portions are activated concurrently in the trot.

Muscle activity recorded during galloping can be reconciled readily with observed movement of the vertebral column. On both sides of the body, the muscles exhibit a concurrent phase of activity per gait cycle. This commences in the suspension phase, shortly before touch down of the trailing hindlimb (first hindlimb to strike the ground), and results in extension of the back. The activity of the back muscles and extension of the back ceases when the trailing hindlimb lifts off.

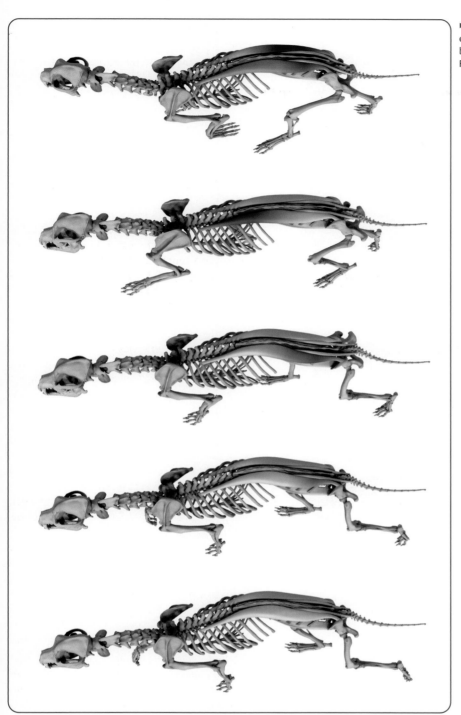

▶ **Fig. 1.43** Activity of the longissimus thoracis et lumborum and iliocostalis thoracis et lumborum during walking. (source: Martin S. Fischer, Jonas Lauströer, Amir Andikfar)

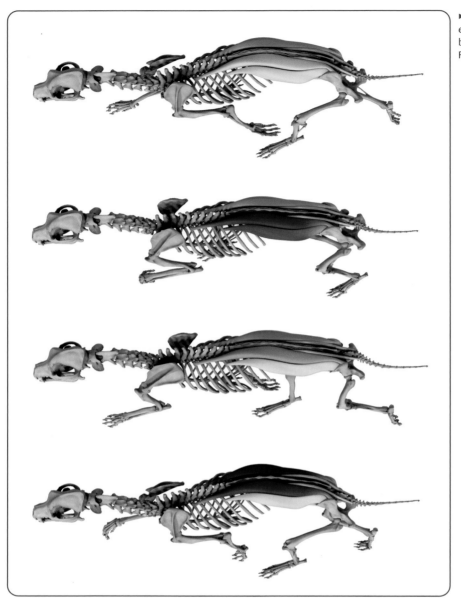

▶ **Fig. 1.44** Activity of the longissimus thoracis et lumborum and iliocostalis thoracis et lumborum during trotting. (source: Martin S. Fischer, Jonas Lauströer, Amir Andikfar)

⚙ Practical Application

The trunk does not flex during the stance phase; here, the muscles stabilize the trunk against torsion. The back muscles thus establish a static base for the work performed by the extrinsic limb muscles (arising from the trunk) and compensate for the torques that pass into the trunk

1.5.3 Functional Arthrology

As described in detail in previous sections, movement in all joints of the fore- and hindlimbs comprises a combination of retraction/protraction (in the sagittal plane), abduction/adduction (in the frontal plane) and internal and external rotation. Functional consideration of the loading of these joints can now be addressed, underpinned by an understanding of dynamic, three-dimensional kinematics, associated torques and action of

the muscles of the limbs. Joint topography, joint capsules, ligaments etc. are covered under Diagnostic Procedure (p. 78).

Considerable differences exist between proximally and distally located joints. Without question, the greatest tolerance is exhibited by the force driven „joint" at the pivot point of the scapula; its impressive cushioning effect is obvious during landing after a jump. The wide range of joint movement observed in the shoulder and hip joints becomes increasingly limited more distally. The shoulder and hip joints are held in place by an adhesion-cohesion mechanism, while the elbow and tarsal joints are largely mechanically controlled. Ligamentous stabilization becomes increasingly prominent from the proximal to the distal end of the limb. The shoulder and hip joints have no extracapsular ligaments. External support consists, at most, of thickenings of the joint capsule wall, with additional stabilization provided by muscular cuffs. Distribution of muscular work and energy recovery across the joints is highly uneven. As a rule, positive work is performed at the proximal joints, for which energy must be expended. At the distal joints, muscle contraction often only serves to inhibit movement, to compensate for the effects of gravity.

At the Ludwig Maximilians University Munich, a method has been developed in recent years - first in human, then in veterinary anatomy - for determining long-term load transmission in joints based on analysis of the thickness of the articular cartilage and the underlying subchondral bone layer [15], [17], [18], [32], [41], [43], [44], [47], [56], [86]. This technique includes assessment of the distribution of cartilage thickness, as a reflection of compressive load, and evaluation of osseous and cartilaginous split-line patterns that indicate the predominant direction of collagen fibers and, thus, the main lines of tension. These joint characteristics reflect long-term distribution of strain on the joint. The above studies have greatly expanded current understanding of loading of individual joints and have elucidated the function of incongruent joints. The following descriptions are based on this research.

Shoulder Joint

The anatomically incongruent shoulder joint is formed by the head of the humerus and the concave articular surface of the scapula; the latter is almost three times smaller than the former. The shoulder has the greatest range of movement of all joints in the dog. In the presence of an intact joint capsule, the joint surfaces are drawn towards one another, like two sheets of glass separated by a fluid layer (adhesion-cohesion mechanism). This is a consequence of the finite volume of synovial fluid in the shoulder joint – comprising just 1 ml of free fluid – and its cohesive properties. Even slight separation of the joint surfaces reduces the pressure within the capsule, drawing the walls of the capsule inwards. In the shoulder joint, as in the hip joint, this mechanism may explain why joint capsule thickenings, intracapsular ligaments and radiation of tendons into the joint capsule („shoulder cuff") are an adequate alternative to extracapsular ligaments.

At the concave articular surface, the glenoid cavity, the subchondral bone layer is 6–7 times thicker than in the humeral head. As is characteristic of incongruent joints, subchondral bone density and cartilage thickness is lower at the center of the glenoid cavity than at the periphery (▶ Fig. 1.45). Under a load equivalent to 50% body weight, only 30% of the articular surface of the glenoid cavity and barely 15% of that of the humeral head are in contact; even at 4 times body weight, the corresponding values are just 65% and 30% (all values from [18], [61]).

Based on evaluation of various breeds of dog, maximum shoulder extension is generally 140–150°, though in Dachshunds it is just 115°. Values reported for total range of movement are highly variable and are mostly between 90° und 110°. Considerable breed-related variation (up to 40°) is evident in values for abduction and adduction, and for rotation around the longitudinal brachial axis. The 90° standing shoulder angle specified in several breed standards is hardly ever observed.

During the stance phase, the head of the humerus slides caudally within the glenoid cavity from a cranial position. Maxi-

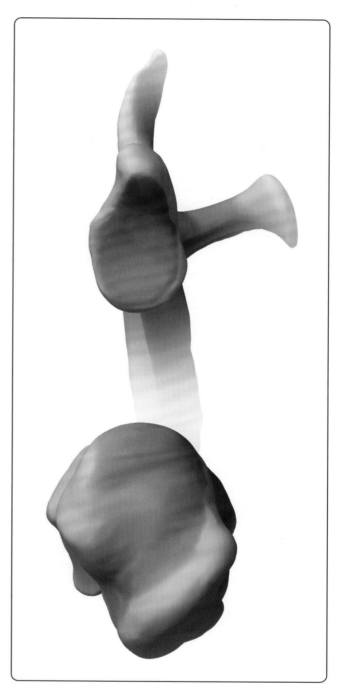

▶ **Fig. 1.45** Subchondral bone density at the shoulder joint. The more intense the red coloring, the denser the bone layer and the greater the long-term loading at this location (after [18]). (source: Martin S. Fischer, Jonas Lauströer, Amir Andikfar)

mum range of movement during the stance phase is less than 30° while the effective angular movement is below 20°; the extent of abduction/adduction and rotation is less than 10°. Furthermore, small loads are unevenly distributed over the joint surface; there are usually two differently sized contact areas, one in the cranial region of the glenoid cavity and one located caudolaterally on its medial rim. As the load increases, pressure is distributed over a larger area.

- Even slight separation of the joint surfaces reduces pressure within the capsule, drawing the walls of the capsule inwards. In the shoulder joint, as in the hip joint, this mechanism may explain why joint capsule thickenings, intracapsular ligaments and radiation of tendons into the joint capsule („shoulder cuff") are an adequate alternative to extracapsular ligaments.
- Based on evaluation of various breeds of dog, maximum shoulder extension is generally 140–150°. Values reported for total range of movement are highly variable and are mostly between 90° und 110°.

Elbow Joint

The elbow joint has three components: the articulation between the humerus and the radius (head of humerus with articular facet of the head of the radius), the articulation between the humerus and the ulna (trochlea of the humerus with the trochlear notch of the ulna) and the proximal radioulnar joint (articular circumference of the radius with the radial notch of the ulna, ▶ Fig. 5.38). The first two form a physiologically incongruent hinge joint; the radioulnar articulation is a pivot joint. Particularly with respect to the elbow, it is important to note the distinction between physiological incongruity (p. 34) and use of the term incongruity in a clinical veterinary context. The latter refers to the presence of a step within the joint, caused by excessive growth-related projection of the ulna above the radius. For reasons that are unclear, the Nomina Anatomica Veterinaria (NAV 2012) only includes the humeroulnar and humeroradial articulations in the elbow joint, thus deviating from the human Terminologia Anatomica (1998) and the conventional, equivalent veterinary interpretation.

While the total range of movement of the elbow joint is about 130° (based on a maximum angle of extension of up to about 165° in most breeds [140° in Dachshunds] and a maximum flexion angle of 20–35°), the effective angular movement during locomotion is usually less than 20°, irrespective of gait. The elbow joint is actively stabilized.

Maierl reports that, during locomotion, the antebrachium rotates around a central pivot point located medially in the elbow joint, causing the anconeal process to be pressed against the lateral epicondyle, and the medial coronoid process to be pressed against the humeral trochlea [43]. In addition to axial forces, this generates considerable transverse forces that act especially on the medial coronoid process, a structure that is relevant in the context of elbow dysplasia (ED).

Contrary to the contemporary view that the radius is the load-bearing element, recent work by Maierl suggests that load is mostly borne by the ulna. In terms of the total articular contact area between the humerus and the radius/ulna, the contact area of the ulna is considerably larger than that of the radius. This is clearly also dependent on joint angle: with increasing flexion, the ulnar component increases further.

The load on the ulna is greatest on the medial side of the trochlear notch, between the anconeal process and the medial coronoid process. At the medial coronoid process, subchondral bone mineralization and articular cartilage thickness are great-

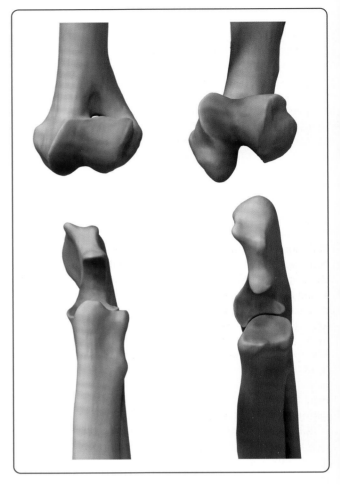

▶ **Fig. 1.46** Subchondral bone density at the elbow joint, from [43]. (source: Martin S. Fischer, Jonas Lauströer, Amir Andikfar)

er than anywhere else in the elbow (▶ Fig. 1.46). In contrast, subchondral bone density at the lateral coronoid process is minimal. On the head of the radius, maximum bone denisty is also observed medially, in a clearly circumscribed area, indicating that this part of the articular surface bears more load over extended periods than the lateral and caudal regions.

Under small loads of up to 100 N, there is limited contact between the joint surfaces at the inner aspect of the two epicondyles, occurring particularly near the anconeal process and the medial coronoid process. At higher loads, these punctate contact areas expand and merge. The width of the joint space is 0.6 mm under limited load, decreasing to 0.1 mm under heavy load.

- While the total range of movement of the elbow joint is about 130°, the effective angular movement during locomotion is usually less than 20°, irrespective of gait.
- Maierl reports that, during locomotion, the antebrachium rotates around a central pivot point located medially in the elbow joint, causing the anconeal process to be pressed against the lateral epicondyle and the and medial coronoid process to be pressed against the humeral trochlea [43].
- In terms of the total articular contact area between the humerus and the radius/ulna, the contact area of the ulna is considerably larger than that of the radius.

Joints of the Front Foot

The carpal joint consists of 15 individual bones plus sesamoid bones and 33 discrete joints with a total of 68 articular surfaces. To a large extent, the bones of each carpal row form a functional unit (▸ Fig. 5.32). A distinction is made between the distal radioulnar joint, the antebrachiocarpal joint, the middle carpal joint and the carpometacarpal joint. In addition, intercarpal joints are present between individual carpal bones within each row and a joint is formed by the accessory carpal bone and the ulnar carpal bone. Tension arising in the flexor carpi ulnaris under heavy load causes the accessory bone to be pressed into the joint formed with the ulnar carpal bone; this has a stabilizing effect on the carpal joint.

The distal radioulnar joint and the antebrachiocarpal joint have a common joint cavity. Like its proximal equivalent, the distal radioulnar joint exhibits only passive movement. Distal to the joint, a fibrocartilaginous ligament forms an additional connection between the radius and ulna.

In the antebrachiocarpal joint, the intermedioradial carpal bone articulates with the radius and the ulnar carpal bone forms a joint with the ulna. Fusion of three carpal bones to form the intermedioradial carpal bone is typical of Carnivora and occurs in the first months post partum. The concave radial articular surface is approximately three times larger than the weakly concave ulnar surface. Under high loads, there is up to 50% contact of the joint surfaces [32]. Greatest long-term loading in the antebrachiocarpal joint is observed at the proximo-dorsal edge of the intermedioradial carpal bone (▸ Fig. 1.47). Thus, transmission of ground reaction forces into the antebrachium occurs largely via the radius. Within the antebrachium, this function transfers to the ulna, which transmits the bulk of the load to the humerus.

The middle carpal joint connects the proximal and distal rows of carpal bones. The intermedioradial carpal bone contacts all four distal bones. The articulation with the third carpal bone is arranged in such a way that a small osseous protuberance on the intermedioradial carpal bone prevents hyperextension of the joint. In contrast, the ulnar carpal bone only forms a joint with the fourth carpal bone and the fifth metacarpal bone. Under heavy load, contact between the articular surfaces reaches a maximum of 40% [32]. The middle carpal joint represents the functional boundary of the carpal joint, situated between a proximal and a distal (second row of carpal bones and metacarpus) entity.

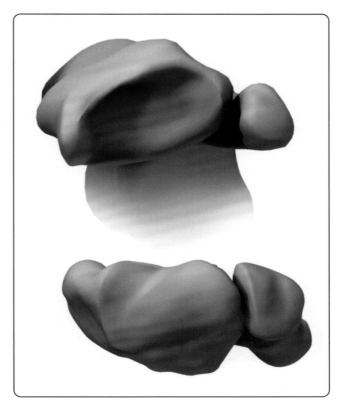

▸ **Fig. 1.47** Subchondral bone density at the antebrachiocarpal joint, after [32]. (source: Martin S. Fischer, Jonas Lauströer, Amir Andikfar)

The carpometacarpal joint is formed by the distal, mildly concave articular surfaces of carpal bones I to IV and the corresponding slightly convex surfaces of the metacarpal bones. These joints are capable of only very limited movement.

Movement of the carpal joints (p. 102), with their complex ligamentous apparatus and taut fascial coverings, is limited mainly to flexion and extension. The range of movement exceeds 180°, of which 70% occurs in the antebrachiocarpal joint, 25% in the middle carpal joint and 5% in the carpometacarpal joint. Varus/valgus angulation is 5–20°/15–30°, occurring predominantly in the antebrachiocarpal joint. Carpal mobility facilitates sure-footedness, even when maneuvering.

The individually variable normal hyperextension of the front foot is around 25° ± 10°, with valgus of up to 15°. In measuring the angle of the carpal joint in the standing position in 50 dogs over 15 kg body weight, Kaiser observed a highly significant correlation between age and the magnitude of the carpal joint angle [32]. According to these findings, the degree of hyperextension increases with advancing age. No association was detected between hyperextension and body weight or breed.

The density of the subchondral bone in the front foot increases throughout life, though the location of maximum density is generally constant [32]. Bone density increases more rapidly in the distal joints and is high, compared to other joints.

Hip Joint

The hip joint is formed by the hemispherical head of the femur and the acetabulum. The lunate surface of the acetabulum is Ω-shaped. The pelvic joint surface is enlarged by the fibrocartilaginous acetabular labrum, and the adhesion-cohesion mechanism is optimized by the hermetic seal produced by the joint capsule. The head of the femur is almost completely covered by a layer of articular cartilage (a few millimeters thick) and is considerably larger than the acetabulum. Breed-related variation is evident in the hip joint (▶ Fig. 1.48) [55].

Although the surface of the femoral head is spherical, only a belt-shaped zone is subjected to load during locomotion. With increasing load, the contact area more than doubles (▶ Fig. 1.48). Even at four times body weight, only 55% of the articular surface of the femoral head is under load. As is characteristic of incongruent joints, transmission of load occurs primarily at the joint periphery. As load increases, the head of the femur spreads out and forces the acetabulum apart. The internal margin of the joint surface is only incorporated into the contact area under very large loads [41]. The load impacts differently on the inner and outer sides of the femur. Compressive forces occur on the medial side, while tensile forces arise on the outside, as reflected by the orientation of bone trabeculae. The

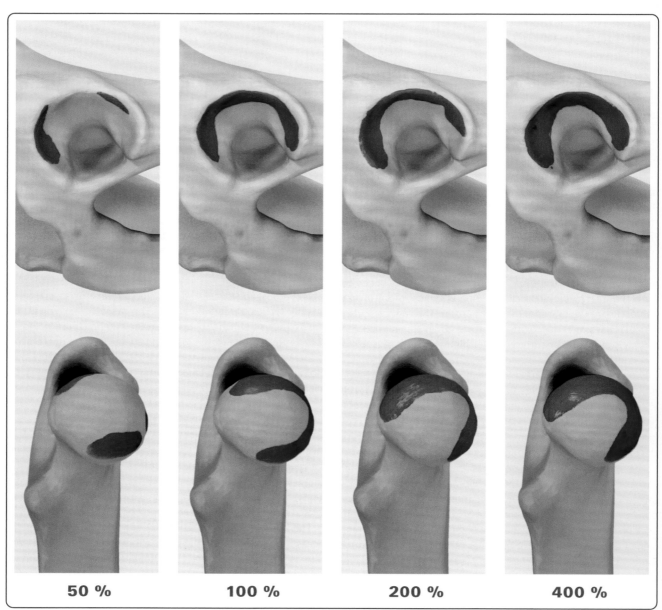

50 %   **100 %**   **200 %**   **400 %**

▶ **Fig. 1.48** Size of the contact area in the hip joint, depending on the degree of load (expressed as a percentage of body weight) [41]. (source: Martin S. Fischer, Jonas Lauströer, Amir Andikfar)

density of the subchondral bone also corresponds to long-term loading (▶ Fig. 1.49).

The maximum ranges of movement of the hip joint are as follows: 70–80° flexion, 80–90° extension, 70–80° abduction, 30–40° adduction, 50–60° internal rotation and 80–90° external rotation. Breed-specific patterns of abduction and adduction, and also internal and external rotation, are evident during locomotion. Particularly extensive rotational movement (p. 13) is observed during idiomotor (non-locomotor) movements.

The hip joint has no mechanically active ligaments. The intra-articular, extrasynovial ligament of the head of the femur, which attaches at the notch of the acetabular „Ω", is the remnant of a developmental supply system and has little mechanical function. During the growth of the femur, the femoral head is supplied by the epiphyseal artery, that passes through the ligament, rather than by vessels of the limb.

> **ℹ Practical Application**
> - Although the surface of the femoral head is spherical, only a belt-shaped zone is subjected to load during locomotion.
> - In incongruent joints, load transmission occurs mainly at the joint periphery.
> - The maximum ranges of movement of the hip joint are as follows: 70–80° flexion, 80–90° extension, 70–80° abduction, 30–40° adduction, 50–60° internal rotation and 80–90° external rotation.

Stifle Joint

The stifle joint is a multi-chambered joint consisting of the mechanically coupled femorotibial and femoropatellar articulations, and the proximal tibiofibular joint. Fibrocartilaginous menisci are located between the articular surfaces of the femur and tibia. These structures compensate for the incongruity between the convex femoral condyles and the weakly concave condyles of the tibial plateau.

The femoropatellar joint is a sliding joint between the patella and the femoral trochlea. The medial and lateral fascia lata and the often insubstantial femoropatellar ligaments hold the patella in place within the proximal trochlear groove. The articular surface of the trochlea is expanded by the presence of fibrocartilage at the edges of the patella. The section of the tendon of insertion of the quadriceps femoris that passes from the patella to the tibia is referred to as the patellar ligament. It is separated from the joint capsule by a large fat pad. The patella alters the direction of pull of the quadriceps femoris. By increasing the distance to the center of rotation of the stifle joint, it enhances the lever action of the quadriceps femoris, or reduces the force needed for the same amount of leverage. According to recent findings, the patella is not a sesamoid bone in the traditional sense that mechanical forces induce ossification within the quadriceps femoris tendons. Instead, it develops as a bony process and subsequently forms a joint with the femur [20].

The large joint capsule incorporates three communicating cavities, 2 between the femur and tibia and one beneath the patella. The first two correspond to the originally separate joints between the femur and tibia/fibula. Numerous sensory structures including free nerve endings (nociceptors) and Ruffini's

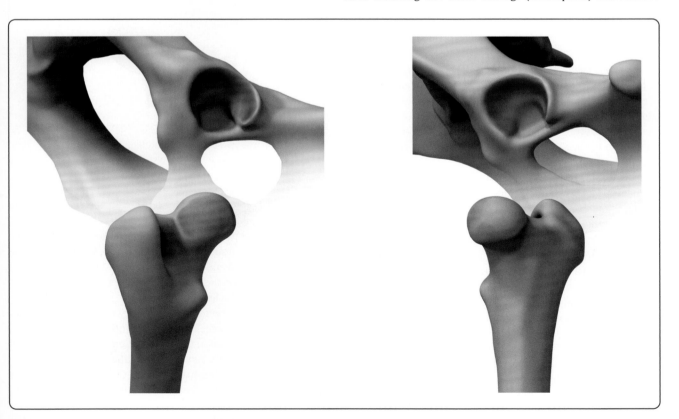

▶ **Fig. 1.49** Subchondral bone density in the hip joint, after [41]. (source: Martin S. Fischer, Jonas Lauströer, Amir Andikfar)

corpuscles (stretch receptors) are located in the joint capsule. The normal stifle joint contains just 0.2–2 ml of watery synovial fluid. In the stifle joint, the synovial fluid serves the additional purpose of nourishing the avascular menisci.

The biconcave menisci consist of about two thirds water, allowing them to function effectively as shock absorbers. The remaining third is composed of collagen, proteoglycans and glycosaminoglycans. Menisci also serve to reduce the synovial fluid layer between the condyles and the tibial plateau to a thin film, thus regulating its lubricating function (moistening of the hyaline cartilage with joint fluid). The lateral meniscus is larger and thicker than its medial counterpart. Both menisci are thick abaxially, becoming thinner towards their axial margin. The menisci (▶ Fig. 5.14) have an elaborate support system composed of 6 ligaments.

During extension and flexion of the stifle joint, the menisci are forced to undergo a sliding, rolling movement. Movement of the medial meniscus is more limited, due to its firm attachment to the medial collateral ligament and the joint capsule. The lateral collateral ligament permits greater movement of the lateral femoral condyle and thereby the lateral meniscus. Moreover, the tendons of origin of the popliteus and extensor digitorum longus preclude an attachment between the lateral meniscus and the joint capsule. Since the contact area of the femur and tibia lies in front of the functional axis of the tibia and the rotational axis of the stifle joint, the tibia slides cranially when the stifle is under load (cranial tibial thrust). This is counteracted by the cranial cruciate ligament.

The stifle joint moves through a maximum of 130°; its maximum angle of extension is 150°. Posture-dependent varus/valgus angulation is also observed. When the stifle joint is extended, only minimal rotation is possible as both collateral ligaments (particularly the lateral ligament) oppose this movement. However, while the lateral collateral ligament is completely lax when the joint is flexed, only the caudal portion of the medial collateral ligament is slack; the cranial component remains taut. Together with the greater mobility of the lateral meniscus and the more caudal position of the lateral condyle, this results in passive internal rotation of the tibia during flexion of the stifle joint, as seen during the swing phase. During extension, this is „automatically" reversed by the increasing tension in the lateral collateral ligament („screw home mechanism"). This rotation under extension is limited by the collateral and cruciate ligaments. During the stance phase, the stifle is flexed; in this position, laxity of the lateral collateral ligament permits internal rotation of the femur. Thus, the femur may rotate internally at the same time as the tibia rotates externally. The degree of internal femoral rotation is limited by the caudal cruciate ligament.

The cruciate ligaments are remnants of the capsular septum that originally separated the femorotibial and femorofibular joints in tetrapods. Consequently, they are intra-articular, yet extrasynovial, as also reflected in their arterial vascular supply. From a functional perspective, both cruciate ligaments have two components that exhibit different degrees of tension. The caudolateral portion of the cranial cruciate ligament (CrCL), which arises most distally and inserts most caudally, is taut during extension and lax when the joint is flexed. The cranio-

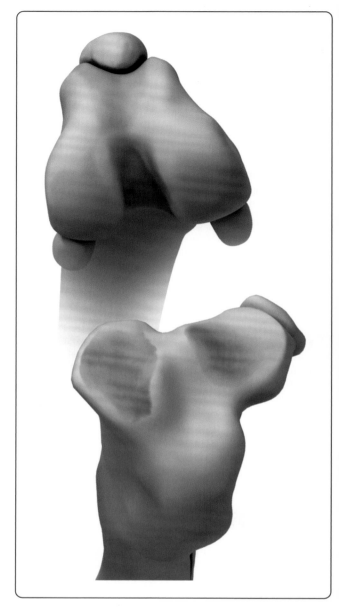

▶ **Fig. 1.50** Subchondral bone density at the stifle joint, after [56]. (source: Martin S. Fischer, Jonas Lauströer, Amir Andikfar)

medial part is constantly under tension. In the caudal cruciate ligament (CdCL), the cranial part is only taut during flexion, while the caudal part is only taut during extension. The cranial cruciate ligament limits cranial movement of the tibia, internal rotation of the tibia and hyperextension of the joint; the caudal cruciate ligament restricts caudal movement of the tibia and internal rotation of the femur.

In the femur, subchondral bone density is greatest at the center of the femoral trochlea (▶ Fig. 1.50) [56]. A further, less pronounced peak is found in the proximal portion of the curve of the intercondylar fossa. Substantially higher bone density is observed in the tibial plateau, though in the lateral condyle this decreases concentrically from the center towards the periphery. The region of greatest density is approximately twice as large in the medial condyle. Distribution of bone density in the patella has been found to vary considerably [56]. While density was greatest at the apex in some specimens, this region was least dense in other dogs.

> ⚡ **Practical Application**
> - During extension and flexion of the stifle joint, the menisci are forced to undergo a sliding, rolling movement.
> - Since the contact area of the femur and tibia lies in front of the functional axis of the tibia and the rotational axis of the stifle joint, the tibia slides forward when the stifle is under load (cranial tibial thrust). This is counteracted by the cranial cruciate ligament.
> - The cranial cruciate ligament limits cranial movement of the tibia, internal rotation of the tibia or external rotation of the femur and hyperextension of the joint; the caudal cruciate ligament restricts caudal movement of the tibia and internal rotation of the femur.

Joints of the Hindfoot

The tarsal joint (p. 87) is composed of 14 individual bones bearing a total of usually 66 articular surfaces, thirty of which are associated with the 4 transverse levels of the joint.

The distal tibiofibular joint, which exhibits only limited, exclusively passive movement, is incorporated into a common joint capsule with the talocrural joint. The talocrural joint is the only significant joint of the foot in terms of active limb movement, as all the other joints are close-fitting and relatively immovable. The talocrural articulation is formed by the tibial cochlea and the prominently ridged trochlea of the talus. The ridges are slanted craniolaterally; the angle of inclination (up to 25°) exhibits individual and breed-related variation. Laterally, the trochlea of the talus articulates with the malleolus of the fibula. On its medial side, the trochlea forms an articulation with the tibial malleolus. Together, the malleoli form a tight, pincer-like guide for the proximal tarsal joint. On the caudal aspect of the talus, two separate joint surfaces meet with the calcaneus to form the talocalcaneal joint. The articulation with the second row of tarsal bones is formed between the distal end of the talus and the navicular (central tarsal) bone, offset relative to the position of the trochlea, and between the calcaneus and the cuboid (fourth tarsal) bone. The compact distal intertarsal joints connect the navicular (central) tarsal bone with cuneiform bones (tarsal bones I–III). In the tarsometatarsal joints, articulations are formed between the cuboid (fourth tarsal) bone and metatarsals IV and V, the lateral cuneiform (third tarsal) bone and metatarsal III, and the intermediate cuneiform (second tarsal) bone with metatarsal II. The small medial cuneiform (first tarsal) bone may articulate or fuse with metatarsal I. If present, the first digit is usually rudimentary. Dew claws are usually present in some breeds and may contain two phalanges. However, the presence of a dew claw is not necessarily indicative of the degree of development of metatarsal I. A claw-bearing phalanx may be connected with the tarsus purely by connective tissue.

1.6

Anatomy and Physiology of the Nervous System

Daniel Koch, Martin S. Fischer

1.6.1 Anatomy

Spinal Cord

The spinal cord lies in the vertebral canal. In the thoracolumbar region, the cord occupies a slightly greater proportion of the canal than in the cervical region. The gap between the cord and the vertebral column is filled with epidural fat. The spinal cord begins at the end of the brain stem and, in most dogs, ends approximately at the level of the sixth lumbar vertebra. The spinal cord is divided into the following segments (▶ Fig. 1.51): cervical (C1–C8; though there are only 7 cervical vertebrae), thoracic (Th1–Th13), lumbar (L1–L7), sacral (S1–S3) and coccygeal (variable). At the cervical (C6–Th2) and lumbar (L4–S3) intumescence, the spinal cord is somewhat broader, as these regions give origin to the lower motor neurons (LMN) supplying the fore- and hindlimbs. The spinal cord consists of central grey matter and peripheral white matter. The spinal nerve roots arise from the dorsal and ventral horns of the spinal cord. In the cervical region, the nerve roots exit the vertebral column cranial to the vertebral body of the same number; C8 exits caudal to cervical vertebra 7. From the thoracic region onwards, the roots leave the vertebral column caudal to the equivalently numbered vertebra. Due to the shortening of the spinal cord relative to the length of the vertebral column, the spinal nerves arising from the caudal portions travel extended distances within the vertebral canal, before exiting through the intervertebral foramina. The thus formed cauda equina is protected within the vertebral canal, where it is generously accommodated within the epidural space.

Meninges

The meninges enclose the CNS and are composed of three layers. The innermost layer, the pia mater, lies directly upon the spinal cord. The space between the pia mater and the arachnoid membrane contains the cerebrospinal fluid. Located outermost is the fibrous dura mater. The meningeal sac usually ends at the sacrum.

Cerebrospinal Fluid (liquor cerebrospinalis)

The cerebrospinal fluid is produced mainly by the choroid plexuses of the brain. It leaves the brain, passing caudad, and fills the subarachnoid space. A small amount also enters the central canal of the spinal cord. In the brain and spinal cord, the cerebrospinal fluid is reabsorbed into veins, via arachnoid projections. Cerebrospinal fluid is usually colourless and contains little protein and few cells. It protects the brain and spinal cord by absorbing shock, evens out differences in pressure, nourishes the CNS and serves as a cerebral transport medium for disposal of waste (glymphatic system).

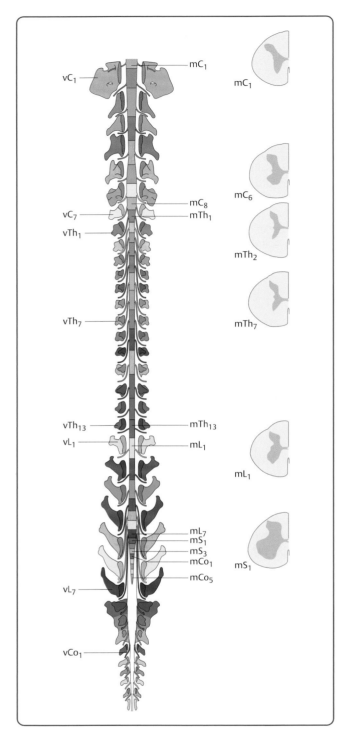

► **Fig. 1.51** Illustration of the division of the spinal cord into cervical (C1–C8), thoracic (Th1–Th13), lumbar (L1–L7), sacral (S1–S3) and coccygeal (Co1–Co5) segments. The spinal cord segments are identified by the letter „m" (medullary) and the vertebrae by the letter „v". The corresponding bony and medullary portions are shown in the same colour, illustrating the topographic staggering of the spinal cord and vertebral column (ascensus medullae). (source: Stoffel MH, Geiger D, Guldimann C, Kocher M. Funktionelle Neuroanatomie für die Tiermedizin. Enke 2010)

Peripheral Nerves

The spinal nerves, together with the 12 cranial nerves, constitute the peripheral nerves. In the dog, there are 8 cervical-, 13 thoracic, 7 lumbar 3 sacral and around 5 coccygeal pairs of spinal nerves. The spinal nerve roots arise from the spinal cord: the dorsal root contains afferent fibers, while efferent fibers are found in the ventral root. The roots combine to form the spinal nerve trunk, which leaves the vertebral canal through the intervertebral foramen (► Fig. 1.52). At the fore- and hindlimbs, the ventral branches of the spinal nerves form nerve plexuses, the brachial plexus (► Fig. 1.53) and the lumbosacral plexus (► Fig. 1.54). The brachial plexus incorporates cervical nerves 6, 7 and 8 and the first two thoracic nerves, the lumbosacral plexus is formed by lumbar nerves 4 to 7 and sacral nerves 1 to 3. The afferent fibers innervate a specific cutaneous region known as a dermatome. The efferent equivalent is the myotome. Rather than resulting in clearly defined neural deficits, injuries affecting the plexuses usually lead to complex abnormalities of movement and coordination. This is consistent with the observation that nerves located within the limb contain fibers originating from various spinal nerves.

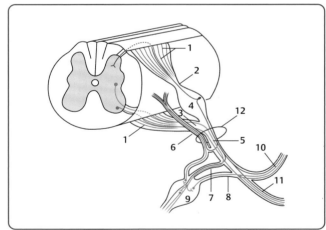

► **Fig. 1.52** Schematic illustration of the components of a spinal nerve in the thoracolumbar region of the spinal cord. 1 fila radicularia, 2 radix dorsalis, 3 radix ventralis, 4 ganglion spinale, 5 truncus nervi spinalis, 6 ramus meningeus, 7 ramus communicans albus, 8 ramus communicans griseus, 9 sympathetic ganglion, 10 ramus dorsalis, 11 ramus ventralis, 12 foramen intervertebrale; afferent fibers = blue; motor fibers = red; sympathetic fibers = green. (source: Salomon F-V, Geyer H, Gille U. Anatomie für die Tiermedizin. 3. Auflage. Stuttgart. Enke 2015)

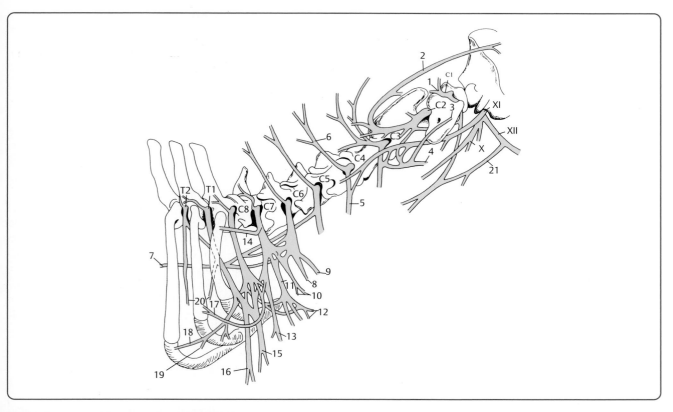

▶ **Fig. 1.53** Simplified illustration of the cervical nerves and brachial plexus of the dog. 1 n. suboccipitalis, 2 n. occipitalis major, 3 n. auricularis magnus, 4 n. transversus colli, 5 r. ventralis, 6 r. dorsalis, 7 n. phrenicus, 8 n. suprascapularis, 9 branch to m. brachiocephalicus, 10 nn. subscapulares, 11 n. musculocutaneus, 12 nn. pectorales craniales, 13 n. axillaris, 14 n. thoracicus longus, 15 n. radialis, 16 nn. medianus and ulnaris, 17 n. thoracodorsalis, 18 n. thoracicus lateralis, 19 nn. pectorales caudales, 20 intercostal nerves, 21 ansa cervicalis, C1–C8 = cervical nerves 1–8, T1–T2 = thoracic nerves 1–2, X n. vagus, XI n. accessorius, XII n. hypoglossus (after Evans, 1993). (source: Salomon F-V, Geyer H, Gille U. Anatomie für die Tiermedizin. 3. Auflage. Stuttgart. Enke 2015)

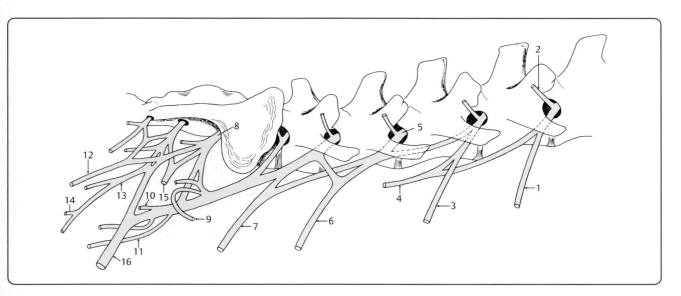

▶ **Fig. 1.54** Simplified illustration of the lumbosacral plexus of the dog. 1 n. ilioinguinalis, 2 r. dorsalis of lumbar nerve 3, 3 n. cutaneus femoris lateralis, 4 n. genitofemoralis, 5 lumbar nerve 5, 6 n. femoralis, 7 n. obturatorius, 8 sacral nerve 1, 9 n. gluteus cranialis, 10 n. gluteus caudalis, 11 branch to m. obturatorius internus, 12 n. cutaneus femoris caudalis, 13 n. pudendus, 14 n. rectalis caudalis, 15 nn. pelvini, 16 n. ischiadicus (after Evans, 1993). (source: Salomon F-V, Geyer H, Gille U. Anatomie für die Tiermedizin. 3. Auflage. Stuttgart. Enke 2015)

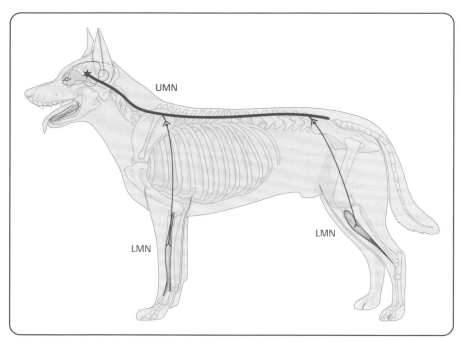

▶ **Fig. 1.55** Lower motor neurons (LMN) include all peripheral descending nerves. Upper motor neurons (UMN) initiate voluntary movement, maintain muscle activity and generally have a slight inhibitory effect on LMN activity. (source: Karin Baum)

1.6.2 Divisions

The nervous system is divided into the central (CNS) and peripheral (PNS) nervous systems. The brain and spinal cord belong to the CNS, the ganglia, plexuses and spinal nerves are components of the PNS. Nerves are composed of a cell nucleus as well as information-receiving processes (dendrites) and a single, long process, the axon, that transmits information to other nerves or muscles via synapses and neurotransmitters, such as acetylcholine or catecholamines. Glial cells form the supportive, ensheathing and nourishing tissue of the nervous system.

From a functional perspective, the nervous system can be divided into somatic and visceral components. The somatic or animalistic nervous system is responsible for communication between an organism and the environment. The visceral nervous system controls vegetative body functions, such as digestion, thermoregulation, cardiac function and breathing. It is of lesser importance for the diagnosis of locomotor abnormalities.

The terms afferent and efferent have come to be used conventionally to describe the direction of impulse transmission. Afferent pathways arise at a receptor and continue within peripheral nerves. Afferent signals generally comprise sensory inputs such as proprioception, pain etc. In the spinal ganglion, the stimulus is transferred to the axon component that enters the CNS, for subsequent transmission to the brain. Efferent neurons transmit information to an effector organ and are thus considered descending pathways; their functions include control of muscle activity.

1.6.3 Upper and Lower Motor Neurons, Reflex Arcs

Efferent neurons are divided into two motor neuron systems. Upper motor neurons (UMN) include regulatory neurons in the brain and connecting pathways that course to the intumescences. The cell body is located in the brain. Upper motor neurons are responsible for conscious triggering of voluntary movement. Switching between upper motor neurons and lower motor neurons (LMN) occurs in the ventral horn of the grey matter of the spinal cord (▶ Fig. 1.55). In functional terms, the lower motor neuron system includes the peripheral nerve and the muscle. Lower motor neurons exhibit baseline involuntary activity, in response to impulses originating from the periphery. This activity may become apparent in the presence of deep spinal cord lesions where the hindlimbs exhibit autonomous movement that is asynchronous with that of the rest of the body („spinal walker").

In a reflex arc, a peripheral sensory neuron sends a signal through the brachial or lumbosacral plexus to the ventral horn of the spinal cord, where it is passed directly on to a lower motor neuron, giving rise to muscle activity (▶ Fig. 1.56). There is no voluntary input from the brain. However, in a normally functioning nervous system, the brain exerts a dampening influence on lower motor neuron activity. This relationship is utilized when examining reflexes. An increased reflex response and limb spasticity indicate that the upper motor neurons have been damaged, for example by protrusion of an intervertebral disc. If only the hindlimbs are affected, the lesion is located between Th3 and L3. Involvement of all four limbs indicates a lesion between C1 und C5. A special case is presented by the Schiff-Sherrington phenomenon, involving a deep lesion of the thoracolumbar spinal cord. This results in loss of inhibitory pathways that regulate forelimb movement, leading to spasticity of these limbs. Reduced to absent reflex responses and

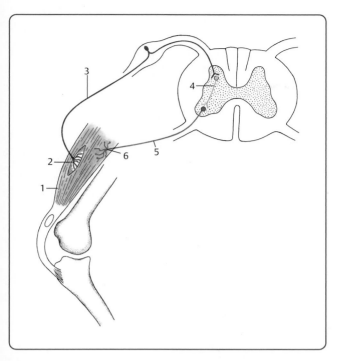

▶ **Fig. 1.56** Schematic illustration of the intrinsic or monosynaptic reflex arc of the patellar reflex. 1 m. rectus femoris, 2 muscle spindle, 3 afferent neuron, 4 interneuron, 5 efferent neuron, 6 motor end plate. (source: Salomon F-V, Geyer H, Gille U. Anatomie für die Tiermedizin. 3. Auflage. Stuttgart. Enke 2015)

flaccid limbs signify a LMN lesion. Typical examples include degenerative lumbosacral stenosis or radial nerve trauma following a motor vehicle accident. Compression of the spinal cord at C6–Th2 and L4–S3 result in LMN deficits in the corresponding limbs.

1.7
Bibliography

[1] Andersson LS et al. Mutations in DMRT3 affect locomotion in horses and spinal circuit function in mice. Nature 2012; 488:642–646

[2] Andrada E, Reinhardt L, Lucas K, Fischer MS. 3D- inverse dynamics of beagles' forelimbs during walk and trot. AJVR 2017; 78: 804–817

[3] Armstrong R, Saubert IV C, Seeherman H et al. Distribution of fiber types in locomotory muscles of dogs. Am J Anat 1982; 163(1):87–98

[4] Benninger MI, Seiler GS, Robinson LE et al. Effects of anatomic conformation on three-dimensional motion of the caudal lumbar and lumbosacral portions of the vertebral column of dogs. Am J Vet Res 2006; 67(1):43–50

[5] Blickhan R. The spring-mass model for running and hopping. J Biomech 1989; 22(11–12):1217–1227

[6] Blickhan R, Seyfarth A, Geyer H et al. Intelligence by mechanics. Phil Trans R Soc A 2007; 365:199–220

[7] Breit S, Kunzel W. On biomechanical properties of the sacroiliac joint in purebred dogs. Ann Anat 2001; 183(2):145–150

[8] Budsberg SC, Verstraete MC. Canine center of pressure patterns during a trotting gait. Vet Surg 1993; 22(5):373–374 (Meeting Abstracts)

[9] Bürger R, Lang J. Kinetische Studie über die Lendenwirbelsäule und den lumbosakralen Übergang beim Deutschen Schäferhund. Schweizer Arch Tierheilk 1993; 135(2):35–43

[10] Caicoya AG, Illert M, Jämkie R. Monosynaptic Ia pathways at the cat shoulder. J Physiol 1999; 518:825–841

[11] Carrier D, Chase K, Lark K. Genetics of canid skeletal variation: Size and shape of the pelvis. Genome Res 2005; 15(12):1825–1830

[12] Carrier DR, Deban SM, Fischbein T. Locomotor function of the pectoral girdle 'muscular sling' in trotting dogs. J Exp Biol 2008; 209:2224–2237

[13] Carrier DR, Deban SM, Fischbein T. Locomotor function of forelimb protractor and retractor muscles of dogs: evidence of strut–like behavior at the shoulder. J Exp Biol 2008; 211(1):150–162

[14] Cetinkaya MA, Yardimci C, Sağlam M. Carpal laxity syndrome in forty-three puppies. Vet Comp Orthop Traumatol 2007; 2(02):126–130

[15] Dickomeit MJ. Anatomische und biomechanische Untersuchungen am Ellbogengelenk des Hundes (Canis familiaris) [Dissertation]. München: Ludwig-Maximilians-Universität; 2002

[16] Dobenecker B, Endres V, Kienzle E. Energy requirements of puppies of two different breeds for ideal growth from weaning to 28 weeks of age. Journal of animal physiology and animal nutrition 2013; 97 (1):190–196

[17] Eckstein F, Steinlechner M, Müller-Gerbl M et al. Mechanische Beanspruchung und subchondrale Mineralisierung des menschlichen Ellbogengelenks. Unfallchirurg 1993; 96:99–104

[18] Eller D. Anatomische und biomechanische Untersuchungen am Schultergelenk (Articulatio humeri) des Hundes (Canis familiaris) [Dissertation]. München: Ludwig-Maximilians-Universität; 2003

[19] Evans HE. Miller's Anatomy of the Dog. Philadelphia: WB Saunders; 2013

[20] Eyal S, Blitz E, Shwartz Y et al. On the development of the patella. Development 2015; 142:1831–1839

[21] Fish FE, Dinenno NK. The 'dog paddle': Stereotypic swimming gait pattern in different dog breeds. SICB Meeting; 2014

[22] Fischer MS. Kinematics, EMG, and inverse dynamics of the therian forelimb – a synthetical approach. Ann Anat 1999; 238:41–54

[23] Fischer MS, Blickhan R. The tri-segmented limbs of therian mammals: kinematics, dynamics, and self-stabilization A review. J exp Zool 2006; 305A:935–952

[24] Fischer MS, Lehmann S, Andrada E. Three-dimensional kinematics of canine hind limbs: in vivo, biplanar, high-frequency fluoroscopic analysis of four breeds during walking and trotting. Scientific Rep. 2018; 8:1–22. doi:10.1038/s41598–018–34310–0

[25] Fischer MS, Lilje KE. Hunde in Bewegung. Stuttgart: Franckh-Kosmos; 2011

[26] Flinsbach S. Röntgenologische und sonographische Überprüfung ausgewählter Parameter des Knochenwachstums an mit Kalzium, Phosphor oder Vitamin A fehlversorgten Beagles und Foxhound-Boxer-Labrador- Mischlingen [Dissertation]. München: Ludwig-Maximilians-Universität; 2003

[27] German AJ. Promoting healthy growth in pets. Abstract International Nutritional Sciences Symposium 2016, Atlanta, USA

[28] Geyer H, Seyfarth A, Blickhan R. Compliant leg behaviour explains basic dynamics of walking and running. Proceedings of the Royal Society of London B: Biological Sciences 2006; 273(1603): 2861–2867

[29] Goslow G, Seeherman H, Taylor C et al. Electrical activity and relative length changes of dog limb muscles as a function of speed and gait. J Exp Biol 1981; 94(1):15–42

[30] Gregersen C, Silverton N, Carrier D. External work and potential for elastic storage at the limb joints of running dogs. J Exp Biol 1998; 201(23):3197–3210

[31] Hedhammar A, Wu FM, Krook L. Overnutrition and skeletal disease: an experimental study in growing Great Dane dogs. X. Discussion, Cornell veterinarian

[32] Kaiser A. Morphologische und biomechanische Eigenschaften des Karpalgelenks (Articulatio carpi) des Hundes (Canis familiaris) [Dissertation]. München: Ludwig-Maximilians-Universität; 2006

[33] Kempt T. Functional trade-offs in the limb bones of dogs selected for running versus fighting. J Exp Biol 2005; 208(18):3475–3482

[34] Kiefer-Hecker B, Kienzle E, Dobenecker B. Effects of low phosphorus supply on the availability of calcium and phosphorus, and musculoskeletal development of growing dogs of two different breeds. Journal of animal physiology and animal nutrition 2018; 102(3): 789–798

[35] Kienzle E, Brenten T, Dobenecker B. Impact of faecal DM excretion on faecal calcium losses in dogs eating complete moist and dry pet foods–food digestibility is a major determinant of calcium requirements. Journal of nutritional science 2017; 6

[36] Kienzle E, Dobenecker B. Effect of dietary cation-anion balance on faecal calcium excretion in dogs. Abstract ESVCN Congress 2017 Cirencester, UK

[37] Klein C, Thes M, Böswald LF et al. Metabolisable energy intake and growth of privately-owned growing dogs in comparison with official recommendations on the growth curve and energy supply. J Anim Physiol Anim Nutr 2019; 103: 1952–1958

[38] Kubein-Meesenburg D, Nägerl H, Fanghänel J. Elements of a general theory of joints. 1. Basic kinematic and static function of diarthrosis. Anat Anz 1990; 170:301–308

[39] LaFlamme DP. Development and Validation of a Body Condition Score System for Cats. A Clinical Tool. Feline Practice 1997; 25:13–17

[40] LaFlamme DP, Hume E, Harrison J. Evaluation of Zoometric Measures as an Assessment of Body Composition of Dogs and Cats. Compendium 2001; 23 [Suppl gA]:88

[41] Lieser B. Morphologische und biomechanische Eigenschaften des Hüftgelenks (Articulatio coxae) des Hundes (Canis familiaris) [Dissertation]. München: Ludwig-Maximilians-Universität; 2003

[42] Mack JK, Alexander LG, Morris PJ et al. Demonstration of uniformity of calcium absorption in adult dogs and cats. J Anim Physiol Nutr (Berl.) 2015; doi: 10.1111/jpn.12294

[43] Maierl J. Zur funktionellen Anatomie und Biomechanik des Ellbogengelenks (Articulatio cubiti) des Hundes (Canis familiaris) [Habilitationsschrift]. München: Ludwig-Maximilians-Universität; 2003

[44] Maierl J, Böttcher P. Dreidimensionale Visualisierung der subchondralen Knochendichte entlang der Oberflächennormalen am Schulter- und Ellbogengelenk des Hundes. Ann Anat (Suppl) 1999; 181:288

[45] Meyer H, Zentek J. Ernährung des Hundes. Stuttgart: Enke; 2013

[46] Morris PJ, Salt C, Raila J et al. Safety evaluation of vitamin A in growing dogs. Br J Nutr 2012; 108:1800–1809

[47] Müller-Gerbl M. CT-Osteoabsorptiometrie (CT-OAM) und ihr Einsatz zur Analyse der Langzeitbeanspruchung der großen Gelenke in vivo [Habilitationsschrift]. München: Ludwig-Maximilians-Universität; 1991

[48] Nanua P, Waldron KJ. Energy comparison between trot, bound, and gallop using a simple model. J Biomech 1995; 117(4):466–473

[49] Nap RC, Hazewinkel HAW, Voorhout G et al. The influence of the Dietary Protein Content on Growth in Giant Breed Dogs. Vet Comp Orthop Traumatol 1993; 6(1):5–12

[50] Nap RC, Mol JA, Hazewinkel HAW. Age-related plasma concentrations of growth hormone (GH) and insulin-like growth factor I (IGF-I) in Grat Dane pubs fed different dietary levels of protein. Domest Anim Endocrin 1993; 10(3):237–247

[51] Oury F, Sumara G und O et al. Endocrine regulation of male fertility by the skeleton. Cell 201; 144(5):796–809

[52] Parker HG, Vonholdt BM, Quignon P et al. An expressed Fgf4 retrogene is associated with breed-defining chondrodysplasia in domestic dogs. Science 2009; 325:995–998

[53] Pasi BM, Carrier DR. Functional trade-offs n the limb muscles of dogs selected for running vs. fighting. J Evol Biol 2003; 16:324–332

[54] Pauwels F. Die Druckverteilung im Ellenbogengelenk, nebst grundsätzlichen Bemerkungen über den Gelenkdruck. 11. Beitrag zur funktionellen Anatomie und kausalen Morphologie des Stützapparates. Z Anat Entw-Gesch 1963; 123:643–667

[55] Richter V, Löffler K. Rassespezifische Merkmale am Becken des Hundes. Dtsch Tierärztl Wschr 1976; 83:455–461

[56] Riegert S. Anatomische und biomechanische Untersuchungen am Kniegelenk (Articulatio genus) des Hundes (Canis familiaris) [Dissertation]. München: Ludwig-Maximilians-Universität; 2004

[57] Ritter D, Nassar P, Fife M et al. Epaxial muscle function in trotting dogs. J Exp Biol 2001; 204(17):3053–3064

[58] Rode C, Siebert T, Blickhan R. Titin induced force enhancement and force depression: A 'sticky spring' mechanism in muscle contractions? J Theor Biol 2009; 259: 350–360

[59] Rode C, Tomalka A, Blickhan R, Siebert T. Myosin filament sliding through the Z-disc relates striated muscle fibre structure to function. Proc Roy Soc B 2016; 283: 20153030

[60] Salomon F-V, Geyer H, Gille U. Anatomie für die Tiermedizin. 3. Auflage. Stuttgart. Enke 2015

[61] Scherrer PK, Hillberry BM, Sickle DV. Determining the in-vivo areas of contact in the canine schoulder. J Biomech 1979; 101:271–278

[62] Schilling N, Carrier D. Function of the epaxial muscles during trotting. J Exp Biol 2009; 212(7):1053–1063

[63] Schilling N, Carrier DR. Function of the epaxial muscles in walking, trotting, and galloping dogs: Implications for the evolution of epaxial muscle funtion in tetrapods. J Exp Biol 2010; 213:1490–1502

[64] Schleip R, Findley TW, Chaitow L, Huijing PA. Lehrbuch Faszien. München: Urban & Fischer; 2014

[65] Schnapper A. Direkte Zell-Zell-Interaktionen während der Wachstums- und funktionell-adaptiven Reifungsvorgänge im Skelett des Hundes [Habilitationsschrift]. Hannover: Stiftung Tierärztliche Hochschule; 2007

[66] Seyfarth A, Geyer H, Günther M et al. A movement criterion for running. J Biomech 2002; 35(5):649–655

[67] Shahar R, Milgram J. Morphometric and anatomic study of the hind limb of a dog. Am J Vet Res 2001; 62(6):928–933

[68] Shahar R, Milgram J. Morphometric and anatomic study of the forelimb of the dog. J Morph 2005; 263(1):107–117

[69] Sharp NJ, Wheeler SJ. Small animal spinal disorders: diagnosis and surgery. Philadelphia: Elsevier Mosby; 2005

[70] Siebert T, Stutzig N, Rode C. A hill-type muscle model expansion accounting for effects of varying transverse muscle load. J Biomech 2018; 66: 57–62

[71] Siedler S, Dobenecker B. The source of phosphorus influences serum PTH, apparent digestibility and blood levels of calcium and phosphorus in dogs fed high phosphorus diets with balanced Ca/P ratio. In Proc. Waltham International Nutritional Sciences Symposium 2016, p. 21

[72] Siniscalchi M et al. Seeing Left- or Right-Asymmetric Tail Wagging Produces Different Emotional Responses in Dogs. Curr Biol 2013; 23:1–4

[73] Snow D, Billeter R, Mascarello F et al. No classical type IIB fibres in dog skeletal muscle. Histochem Cell Biol 1982; 75(1):53–65

[74] Stoffel MH. Funktionelle Neuroanatomie für die Tiermedizin. Stuttgart: Enke; 2010

[75] Thes M, Köber N, Fritz J et al. Metabolizable energy intake of client owned adult dogs. Proceedings of the WALTHAM International Nutritional Sciences Symposium 2013, October 2013, Portland, USA; P107

[76] Tokuriki M. Electromyographic and joint-mechanical studies in quadrupedal locomotion. I. Walk. Nippon Juigaku Zasshi. Japan J Vet Sci 1973; 35(5):433–436

[77] Tokuriki M. Electromyographic and joint-mechanical studies in quadrupedal locomotion. II. Trot. Nippon Juigaku Zasshi. Japan. J Vet Sci 1973; 35(6):525–533

[78] Tokuriki M. Electromyographic and joint-mechanical studies in quadrupedal locomotion. III. Gallop. Nippon Juigaku Zasshi. Japan. J Vet Sci 1974; 36(2):121–132

[79] Usherwood JR, Wilson AM. Biomechanics: no force limit on greyhound sprint speed. Nature 2005; 438(7069):753–754

[80] Wachs K. Kinematische Analyse von 3D-rekonstruierten Bewegungen der Lendenwirbelsäule und des Beckens beim Beagle in Schritt und Trab [Dissertation]. Hannover: Stiftung Tierärztliche Hochschule; 2015

[81] Webster EL, Hudson PE, Channon SB. Comparative functional anatomy of the epaxial musculature of dogs (Canis familiaris) bred for sprinting vs. fighting. J Anat 2014; 225(3): 317–327

[82] Wentink G. The action of the hind limb musculature of the dog in walking. Acta anat 1976; 96:70–80

[83] Wentink G. Biokinetical analysis of hind limb movements of the dog. Anat Embryol 1977; 151:171–181

[84] Williams SB, Wilson AM, Rhodes L et al. Functional anatomy and muscle moment arms of the pelvic limb of an elite sprinting athlete: the racing greyhound (Canis familiaris). J Anat 2008; 213(4):361–372

[85] Williams SB, Wilson AM, Daynes J et al. Functional anatomy and muscle moment arms of the thoracic limb of an elite sprinting athlete: the racing greyhound (Canis familiaris). J Anat 2008; 213 (4):373–382

[86] Winhard FE. Anatomische und computertomographische Untersuchungen am gesunden und degenerativ veränderten Schulter- und Ellbogengelenk des Hundes (Canis familiaris) [Dissertation]. München: Ludwig-Maximilians-Universität; 2007

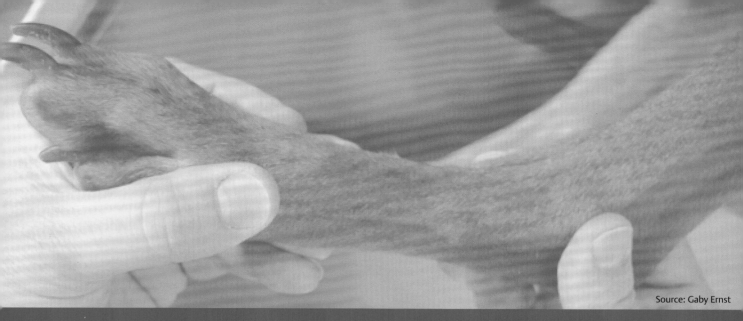

Source: Gaby Ernst

Part 2
Diagnostic Procedure

2 Introduction

Daniel Koch, Martin S. Fischer

2.1
General

The requirements for conducting a lameness examination include a sufficiently large room, an examination table with a non-slip surface, appropriate lighting, an assistant and an outside area for gait analysis.

The lameness examination is divided into 4 main components:
1. Anamnesis (signalment and history)
2. Visual assessment and gait analysis
3. Examination of the dog in a standing position
4. Examination of the dog in recumbency

Gait analysis is used to **identify the affected limb**. Examination of the dog in a standing position permits identification of the relevant **region or joint**. After the dog has been examined in recumbency, it should be possible to establish a provisional **clinical diagnosis**.

The examination always commences distally and proceeds proximally. **All** limbs are assessed. The limb identified during gait analysis as the source of lameness is examined last. This allows the dog to become accustomed to the procedure and permits the examiner to familiarize themselves with the normal characteristics of the individual animal. It also ensures that tests that may elicit pain are conducted at the end of the examination. It is important to gain the dog's trust, as pain responses are generally not exhibited in the presence of fear.

The orthopedic examination can be integrated with other relevant forms of appraisal, such as general and neurological examination. Additional investigative methods, such as radiography, ultrasound, blood testing and computed tomography, should only be conducted after the orthopedic examination has been completed.

For examination in a standing position, the dog is held at the head by an assistant. During examination in recumbency, the assistant holds the dog against the table by its two ventrally positioned limbs.

The methods used for examination can be divided into inspection, palpation and manipulation:

- Inspection: observation of angular deformities, abnormal surface contours and pain responses.
- Palpation: detection of increases in temperature, abnormal surface contours, fluctuating swelling and pain responses.
- Manipulation: identification of angular deformities, crepitation, hypermobility and hypomobility, and possible elicitation of pain responses.

The validity of a test can be confirmed by comparing one side with the other and by conducting the test several times [87], [88], [89], [90], [91].

> **Examination Guidelines**
> - investigation sequence:
>   - which limb is affected?
>   - which region/joint is affected?
>   - provisional clinical diagnosis
> - examination should proceed from distal to proximal; all limbs, affected limb last
> - tests should be conducted on both sides and repeated several times

2.2
Bibliography

[87] Hazewinkel HAW, Meutstege FJ. Locomotieaparaat. In: Rijnberk A, De Vries H. Anamnese en lichamelijk onderzoek bij gezelschapsdieren. Houten, Bohn, Stafleu, Van Loghum, 1990: 175–200

[88] Krämer M. Der klinisch-orthopädische Untersuchungsgang der Gliedmasse, demonstriert am gesunden Hund. Ein Videofilm [Dissertation]. Zürich: Universität; 1998

[89] Scharvogel S. Klinisch-orthopädischer Untersuchungsgang. In: Kramer M, Hrsg. Kompendium der Allgemeinen Veterinärchirurgie. Hannover: Schlütersche; 2004: 20–36

[90] Piermattei DL, Flo GL, DeCamp CE. Brinker, Piermattei and Flo's Handbook of Small Animal Orthopedics and Fracture Repair. Philadelphia: WB Saunders; 2006

[91] Brunnberg L, Waibl H, Lehmann J. Lahmheit beim Hund. Kleinmachnow: Procane Claudo; 2015

3 Anamnesis

Daniel Koch, Martin S. Fischer

3.1
Signalment

A lame dog is initially encountered via the telephone, when an appointment is made. Based on the signalment, the examiner can organize their thoughts and identify clinically suspicious factors. Orthopedically relevant characteristics include breed, age and sex.

> ### 🔲 Interpretation of Signalment
> **General Breed Predispositions**
> - large breeds:
>   - elbow dysplasia (p. 224)
>   - hip dysplasia (p. 212)
>   - panosteitis (p. 188)
>   - cruciate ligament rupture (p. 201)
> - small breeds:
>   - patellar luxation (p. 204)
>   - aseptic necrosis of the femoral head
> - Molosser, fighting dogs:
>   - cruciate ligament rupture (p. 201)
> - chondrodystrophic breeds:
>   - spinal disorders
>   - disorders of growth in the forelimbs
>
> **General Age Predispositions**
> - puppies and dogs under one year of age:
>   - patellar luxation (p. 204)
>   - elbow dysplasia (p. 224)
>   - hip dysplasia (p. 212)
>   - disorders of growth (panosteitis (p. 188), hypertrophic osteodystrophy (p. 189))
>   - malalignment following growth plate trauma
> - Dogs over one year of age:
>   - neoplasia
>   - cruciate ligament rupture (p. 201)
>   - diseases resulting in osteoarthritis
>
> **General Sex Predispositions**
> Disorders of growth and all forms of dysplasia are more common in males due to their greater size and rate of weight gain, compared to females.

3.2
History

The history provides important information about lameness. It gives the client an opportunity to describe the problem from their perspective and the examiner should listen to their account without interrupting. Questioning by the examiner forms the second phase of history-taking. Open questions are followed by closed questions.

The following represents a sample history-taking sequence:
1. How would you describe the problem?
2. What do you observe when the dog gets up/jumps into the car/climbs stairs/goes down stairs?
3. Has there been any prior treatment and what were the outcomes?
4. What do you feed the dog?
5. Do you have any information about litter-mates?
6. Is the dog used for a particular purpose?
7. Does the dog have any other diseases?
8. Does the dog drag its toes on the ground when walking?
9. Is lameness worse at the beginning of a walk than at the end?
10. Does the dog have more difficulty moving over uneven ground?
11. Is there anything else that you consider worth mentioning?
12. Additional questions

> ### 🔲 Interpretation of Anamnesis
> - lameness improves as the dog warms up (temporary lameness after rest)
>   - joint disorder
> - lameness does not improve as the dog warms up
>   - muscle disorder
>   - neurological disorder
> - difficulty climbing hills/stairs
>   - hindlimbs affected
> - difficulty descending hills/stairs
>   - forelimbs affected
> - performance dog
>   - muscle disorder
>   - disorder of the cervical vertebrae
> - toe-dragging
>   - neurological disorder
>   - hip disorder
>   - fatigue due to a medical disorder
> - shifting lameness
>   - panosteitis (p. 188)
>   - polyarthritis (p. 191)
> - lameness increases on uneven ground
>   - disorder localized to the distal limb

4 Visual Assessment and Gait Analysis

Daniel Koch, Martin S. Fischer

4.1 Visual Assessment at Rest

The dog is observed in standing and sitting positions. Particular attention is given to the distribution of weight over the joints (back – front, left – right), the angle of the joints (internal rotation, external rotation, valgus, varus), the relationship between individual body parts, and body shape.

> **Interpretation of Posture**
> - head in extended position
>   - relief of pressure on the hindlimbs
> - back hunched
>   - intervertebral disc disease, abdominal pain
> - stifle joint positioned under the body
>   - pain on extension of the stifle joint(s)
> - external rotation of the forelimbs
>   - elbow or shoulder disorder
>   - premature growth plate closure
>   - asynchronous growth of the radius and ulna
> - plantigrade/palmigrade stance
>   - rupture of the plantar or palmar ligaments
>   - collagen defect
> - completely plantigrade stance
>   - ruptured common calcaneal tendon
>   - tarsal trauma
>   - avulsion of the gastrocnemius
> - abduction of the entire forelimb
>   - pressure-relieving stance, indicative of elbow or carpus disorder
> - hyperextension of the talocrural joint
>   - excessive muscle mass in the hindlimbs
>   - growth disorder
> - lateral deviation of the body center
>   - disorder affecting other body side
> - low tail carriage
>   - cauda equina compression syndrome
> - back disorder

4.2 Gait Analysis

Gait analysis is used to check the information provided in the history, to identify the affected limb and to gain insight into the nature of the disorder from the gait pattern. Ideally, gait analysis is conducted in the open, both on even and uneven ground, and on stairs. It should be performed away from distracting influences such as other dogs, cars and pedestrians.

4.2.1 Evaluation during Rising

An initial impression of locomotor function is obtained when the patient is required to rise. Good opportunities to watch the dog stand up include the greeting in the waiting room and the end of the history-taking process. In both situations, it is likely that the dog will have been lying down for several minutes. Any temporary lameness after rest will be more obvious during these first few steps than when the dog subsequently rises during one of the phases of gait analysis.

4.2.2 Evaluation from the Back, Front, and Side

To obtain as much information as possible from gait analysis, the dog should be observed from the back, front and side as it moves over even ground (▶ Fig. 4.1). A triangular area with sides approximately 20 m long is suitable for this purpose. If this is not available, the examiner should move to a different position to observe the dog from the side. The dog is led on a leash by the client or an assistant.

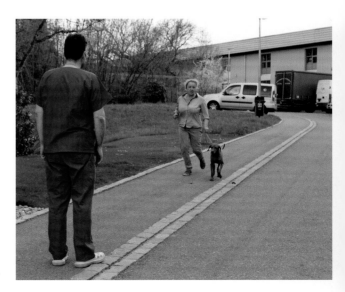

▶ **Fig. 4.1** Gait analysis in an outdoor environment. The dog is led by an assistant or by the client over various types of ground. All gaits are observed from the front, back and side.

Lameness is most apparent during trotting. In order to detect even very subtle temporary lameness, gait analysis thus commences with the trot. The hindlimbs are observed from behind the trotting dog, stride length is examined from the side and the forelimbs are observed as the dog trots towards the examiner. The process is repeated at the walk and gallop.

If pain or functional derangements are present, the affected limb bears less weight, or spends less time in contact with the ground, than the contralateral limb. This results in transfer of weight to the unaffected side. The healthy limb is recognized by its noticeably longer stance phase and, in the case of forelimb disorders, by displacement of the head towards the unaffected limb. This is referred to as a weight-bearing (supporting limb) lameness. Non-weight bearing (swinging limb) lameness is relatively rare, but easy to identify as touch down is intermittent or impossible. Lameness is classified into different grades (p.81). As a rule, distally located abnormalities result in marked, potentially non-weight bearing lameness, while clinical signs resulting from proximal lesions tend to be less pronounced. The well-developed muscle mass surrounding the proximal joints has an inherently stabilizing effect. Exceptions include strong pain (e.g. osteosarcoma) and neurological deficits.

The gallop is of relatively limited use in gait analysis. However, in the presence of forelimb lameness, the trailing, more heavily loaded limb may indicate the unaffected side, and back or hip pain may manifest as concurrent, rather than staggered, touch-down of the hindlimbs.

4.2.3 Evaluation on Uneven Terrain

Lameness arising from structures of the distal limb, including the digits, pads or metacarpals/metatarsals, becomes more pronounced on uneven terrain, such as gravel or a dirt track. Gait analysis should thus be conducted on these surfaces, as well as on grass (▶ Fig. 4.2). A similar grade of lameness on different types of ground suggests a lesion in the proximal half of the limb, from the stifle or elbow onwards.

4.2.4 Evaluation on Stairs

Assessment of the dog's ability to negotiate stairs begins with questioning during history-taking. This is because of the likelihood that the dog will warm up during gait analysis and no longer exhibit signs of lameness when moving up and down stairs. The dog should be led on a short leash. Weight is transferred to the front when descending stairs, and to the back during stair ascent. Thus, lameness that may be barely detectable on even ground may become apparent on stairs, in the form of delayed touch down or evidence of pain on grounding. Ramps and hills may produce similar effects; this can be determined from the history.

4.2.5 Evaluation of Jumping

The ability to jump over obstacles or into a car depends on the presence of normally functioning orthopedic and neurological pathways between the foot and the caudal vertebrae. Dogs can generally compensate very effectively for orthopedic disorders distal to the stifle joint by transferring weight to the contralateral side. Reluctance to jump or inability to jump sufficiently high thus suggests that the abnormality more likely involves the hip, pelvis or vertebral column and the corresponding neuromuscular environment. It is useful to watch the dog jump into the client's car. When the dog jumps out again, the forelimbs can also be observed during touch down. As this form of assessment is strenuous, it should clearly be avoided if the problem is obvious or the dog is in pain, so that further tissue damage is prevented.

4.2.6 Grading of Lameness

Grading of lameness according to Brunnberg:
- Grade 1: barely affected
- Grade 2: affected, but consistently weight-bearing
- Grade 3: affected, inconsistently weight-bearing
- Grade 4: affected, non-weight bearing

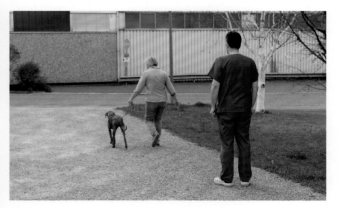

▶ **Fig. 4.2** Abnormalities of the distal limbs are more apparent when gait analysis is conducted on uneven terrain, compared with a soft surface.

⚡ Interpretation of Gait Analysis

- difficulty rising
  - hindlimb disorder
  - back disorder
  - cervical spondylopathy
- lameness improves as dog warms up (temporary lameness after rest)
  - joint disorder
- buckled limb
  - disorder of the contralateral limb
- short stride length in the hindlimbs
  - joint disorder
  - involvement of the hip joint
- hindlimb hopping
  - patellar luxation (p. 204)
- intermittent non-weight bearing lameness
  - patellar luxation (p. 204)
- non-use of limb
  - trauma
  - panosteitis (p. 188)
  - neoplasia
  - cruciate ligament rupture (p. 201) with meniscal damage
- toe-touching in the hindlimbs
  - cruciate ligament rupture (p. 201)
- internal rotation of the stifle with concurrent external rotation of the tarsus during the swing phase
  - fibrosis of the gracilis
- difficulty moving over uneven terrain
  - distal limb disorder

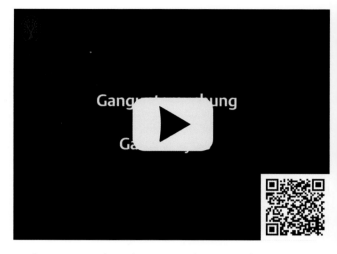

▶ **Video 4.1** Gait analysis. This sequence shows a complete gait examination in a healthy dog: walking, trotting and galloping, evaluation from all sides, movement over different surfaces, jumping in and out of a car, ascending and descending stairs. (source: Tele D, Diessenhofen, Switzerland)

Refer to ▶ **Video 4.1** for a video showing gait analysis.

5 Examination of the Dog in a Standing Position

Daniel Koch, Martin S. Fischer

5.1
Preliminary Examination

5.1.1 General Examination

Before proceeding further with the orthopedic examination, a general examination is conducted (▶ **Video 5.1**). This includes:

- breathing
- pulse
- temperature
- capillary refill time
- mucous membrane color
- lymph nodes
- cardiac auscultation
- skin
- overall body shape

> 🔧 **Interpretation of General Examination**
> - elevated body temperature
>   - hypertrophic osteodystrophy (p. 189)
>   - panosteitis (p. 188)
>   - acute episode of polyarthritis (p. 191)
> - barely perceptible femoral pulse
>   - thrombus
> - regional lymph node enlargement
>   - neoplasia (p. 194)
>   - injury
>   - infection

5.1.2 Brief Neurological Examination

Lameness cannot automatically be attributed to an orthopedic disorder. To exclude a neural etiology, a brief neurological examination should be conducted as part of an orthopedic evaluation (▶ **Video 5.2**).

This includes:

- deep palpation of the entire vertebral column
- turning the head in all directions
- testing for proprioceptive deficits
- brief evaluation of cranial nerve function
- testing of the main limb reflexes

If this brief examination reveals deviations from the norm, a full neurological examination must be conducted. For a detailed description and demonstration, see Neurological Examination (p. 159).

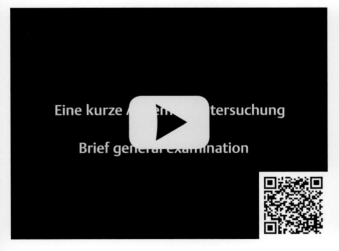

▶ **Video 5.1** Brief general examination. This sequence includes standing symmetry, pulse evaluation, examination of the cardiovascular system including capillary refill time, and assessment of body temperature. (source: Tele D, Diessenhofen, Switzerland)

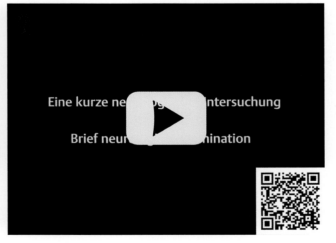

▶ **Video 5.2** Brief neurological examination. This sequence includes assessment of positioning reflexes, palpation of the vertebral column and testing for pain. (source: Tele D, Diessenhofen, Switzerland)

5.2

Orthopedic Examination of the Dog in a Standing Position

The dog is examined on a table with a non-slip surface. An assistant restrains the dog as required. The degree of restraint should allow the dog to move its head and limbs as an indication of pain experienced during the examination.

When examining the dog in a standing position, both hands are used to assess the left and right limb simultaneously and in the same sequence, allowing differences between the two sides to be identified. Positioning of the feet on the tabletop should be similar on both sides. The hindlimbs are examined from behind, the forelimbs from the front.

The following features should be noted:
- symmetry (bone, muscle and joint contours)
- heat
- joint effusion
- presence and nature of masses
- pain

The examination proceeds from distal to proximal. All structures should be examined (bones, joints, tendons, ligaments, muscles, skin, subcutis).

5.3
Hindlimb

5.3.1   Digits, Metatarsus and Tarsus
Standing Symmetry

Standing behind the dog, the examiner grasps the metatarsals of both limbs. Standing symmetry is assessed by pulling the metatarsals caudally, ideally with bilaterally equivalent force. During this procedure, the digits should remain on the surface of the examination table (▶ **Fig. 5.1**).

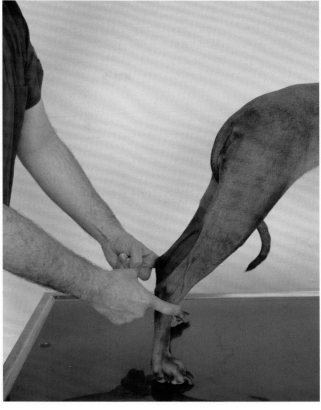

> ⚡ **Findings and Differential Diagnosis**
> * one limb is more easily retracted
>   – general weakness of the more easily retracted limb

▶ **Fig. 5.1** Examination of hindlimb symmetry and stability. The examiner draws both legs backwards with their hands. (source: Gaby Ernst, Saland, Switzerland)

Anatomy

* The muscle mass of the dog constitutes approximately 60% of its total body weight. The musculature is concentrated proximally, with little muscle present in the distal limbs. Thus, the examination should include assessment of mobility and possible muscular abnormalities, as well as evaluation of the bones and joints.
* The following anatomical descriptions and illustrations relate to structures that are relevant to the orthopedic examination. These perspectives do not represent conventional topographical anatomy. They deviate from classical representations in that they have been selected to provide the best view of the selected structures (▶ **Fig. 5.2**).

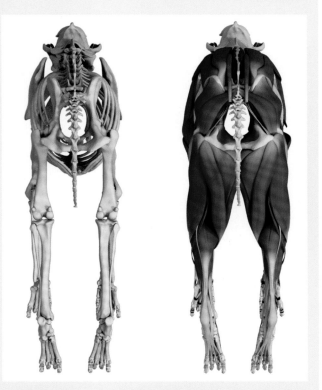

▶ **Fig. 5.2** Skeleton and musculature of a dog. Caudal view. (source: Martin S. Fischer, Jonas Lauströer, Amir Andikfar)

Testing for Pain in the Distal Limb

Standing behind the dog, the examiner grasps the metatarsals firmly and presses the hindlimbs onto the surface of the examination table, checking for a pain response (▶ Fig. 5.3).

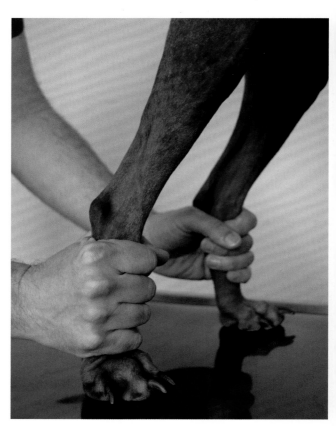

> **⚡ Findings and Differential Diagnosis**
> - pain response and/or lifting of the paw after application of pressure suggests an abnormality in the distal limb, e.g.
>   - swelling of the digital joints
>   - digital fracture
>   - metatarsal fracture
>   - tarsal disorder
> - dorsoflexion of the digits
>   - rupture of the digital flexors (rare in the hindlimbs)

▶ **Fig. 5.3** Pain testing in the distal hindlimbs: the examiner grasps the metatarsals and applies downward pressure. (source: Gaby Ernst, Saland, Switzerland)

Anatomy

- Dogs have a digitigrade posture. The hindfoot is held in tension by the long tendons of the digital flexor muscles. The flexor digitorum superficialis forms a cap as it passes over the calcaneal tuberosity. The deep flexor tendon is formed by the union of the tendons of the flexor digitorum medialis (syn. flexor digitorum longus) and the flexor digitorum lateralis (▶ Fig. 5.4).

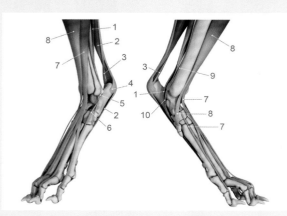

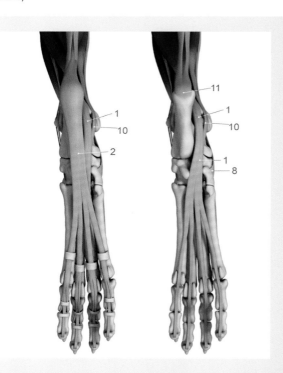

▶ **Fig. 5.4** Tarsus and associated muscles of the crus.
1 mm. flexores digitorum profundi, 2 m. flexor digitorum superficialis, 3 m. biceps femoris (caudal portion), 4 calcaneal cap, 5 m. peroneus longus, 6 m. extensor digitorum lateralis, 7 m. extensor digitorum longus, 8 m. tibialis cranialis, 9 m. tibialis caudalis, 10 m. flexor digitorum longus, 11 common calcaneal tendon. (source: Martin S. Fischer, Jonas Lauströer, Amir Andikfar)

Tarsus

Standing behind the dog, the examiner performs a comparative palpation of the bones of the metatarsus and tarsus (▶ Fig. 5.5). The virtually immobile tarsometatarsal and intertarsal joints cannot be palpated as these joints produce very little synovial fluid, even in the presence of injury.

> **Findings and Differential Diagnosis**
> - angular deformity
>   - fracture of tarsal bones, intertarsal or tarsometatarsal ligament injury/abnormality
>   - calcaneal fracture (p. 198)
> - abnormal plantar surface contour (swelling)
>   - old injury
>   - pathological calcaneal fracture (p. 198) or spontaneous rupture of intertarsal ligaments in old dogs, Collies and related breeds

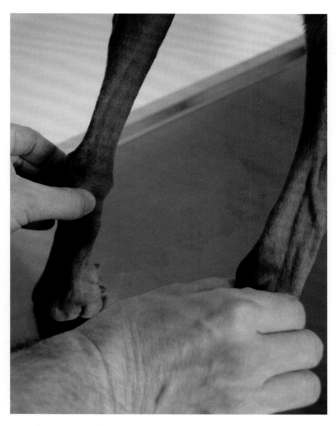

▶ **Fig. 5.5** Comparative palpation of the left and right tarsus. (source: Gaby Ernst, Saland, Switzerland)

Anatomy

- long and short collateral ligaments (▶ Fig. 5.6)
- long collateral ligaments: pass from the lateral or medial malleolus to the metatarsal bones, with attachments to the tarsal bones
- short collateral ligaments: pass from the lateral or medial malleolus to the talus, calcaneus and thence to the metatarsal bones

- fan-shaped dorsal tarsal ligament: passes from the talus to the third and fourth tarsal bones
- internal tarsal ligaments: pass between the central tarsal, third tarsal and fourth tarsal bones
- long plantar ligament: passes from the calcaneus to the metatarsus
- short tarsometatarsal ligaments: pass from the distal tarsal bones to the metatarsal bones

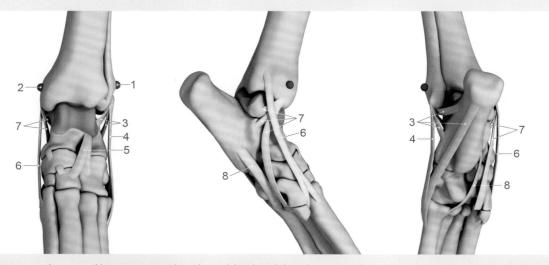

▶ **Fig. 5.6** Tarsus and associated ligaments. Cranial, mediocaudal and caudolateral view. 1 malleolus lateralis (palpable feature), 2 malleolus medialis (palpable feature), 3 lig. collaterale tarsi laterale breve, 4 lig. collaterale tarsi laterale longum, 5 lig. tarsi dorsale, 6 lig. collaterale tarsi mediale longum, 7 lig. collaterale tarsi mediale breve, 8 lig. plantare longum. (source: Martin S. Fischer, Jonas Lauströer, Amir Andikfar)

5.3.2   Tarsal Joint

Joint Palpation

The examiner stands behind the dog. The medial and lateral malleoli serve as reference points. The thumb and index finger are used to palpate the cranial, distal and caudal aspects of the joint along a sickle-shaped line. The medial and lateral collateral ligaments each have two components and are palpable as taut structures extending cranially and caudally from the malleolus (▶ **Fig. 5.7**).

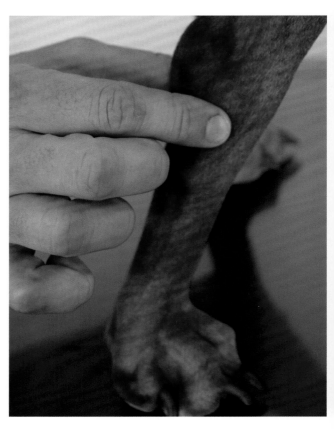

> ☑ **Findings and Differential Diagnosis**
> • Effusion, heat and/or pain in the tarsal joint
>   – talus fracture
>   – osteochondrosis
>   – polyarthritis (p. 191)
>   – collateral ligament rupture
>   – malleolus fracture
> • lateral or medial axial deviation
>   – collateral ligament rupture
>   – tibial malalignment

▶ **Fig. 5.7** Palpation of the talocrural joint, following a semicircular course around the medial and lateral malleoli. The normal joint is palpable as a narrow seam. (source: Gaby Ernst, Saland, Switzerland)

Anatomy

• The tarsal joint has 4 levels in the transverse plane (▶ **Fig. 5.8**):
  – talocrural joint (tarsocrural joint, orange)
  – proximal intertarsal joints (blue)
  – distal intertarsal joints (red)
  – tarsometatarsal joints (yellow)

• The distal tibiofibular joint and the talocrural joint have a common joint capsule.
• The medial and lateral malleoli form a pincer-like guide for the talocrural joint. On the caudal aspect of the talus, two separate joint surfaces articulate with the calcaneus (talocalcaneal joint).
• Palpable features: lateral malleolus and medial malleolus.

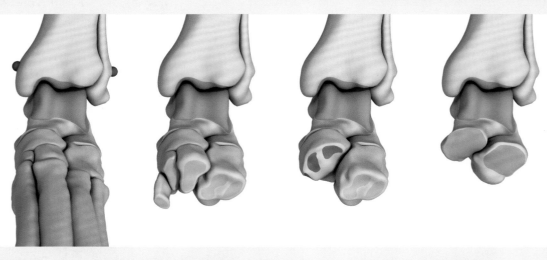

▶ **Fig. 5.8** The levels of the tarsal joint in the transverse plane. (source: Martin S. Fischer, Jonas Lauströer, Amir Andikfar)

Common Calcaneal Tendon

Standing behind the dog, the examiner first palpates the distal portion of the common calcaneal tendon. The tendon inserts on the calcaneus and is normally under considerable tension when the dog is standing. The calcaneal cap (flexor digitorum superficialis) on the caudal aspect of the calcaneal tuberosity is subsequently inspected (▶ Fig. 5.9).

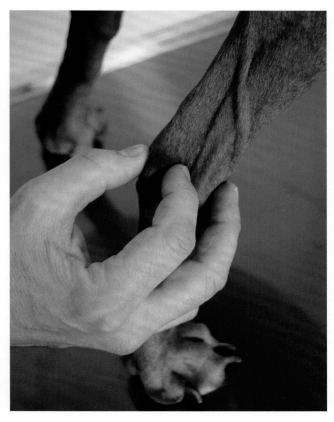

▶ **Fig. 5.9** The common calcaneal tendon is clearly visible and palpable proximal to the calcaneus. (source: Gaby Ernst, Saland, Switzerland)

🗐 Findings and Differential Diagnosis

- calcaneus in contact with the surface of the table
  - common calcaneal tendon rupture
  - avulsion of the medial or lateral head of the gastrocnemius from the femur
  - calcaneal fracture
- firm swelling at the insertion of the common calcaneal tendon
  - partial common calcaneal tendon rupture
- hypermobility of the calcaneal cap
  - lateral luxation of the calcaneal cap (p. 200) (less commonly medial luxation) in Shelties

Anatomy

- The common calcaneal tendon is not equivalent to the Achilles tendon in humans, which is formed by the tendon of the gastrocnemius and soleus muscles. The soleus is absent in the dog.
- In the dog, the common calcaneal tendon is formed by the following muscles: gastrocnemius (main portion), biceps femoris (caudal portion), semitendinosus, gracilis (reinforcing strand). The muscles insert at different locations (▶ Fig. 5.10 and ▶ Fig. 1.29).
- Rather than attaching to the dorsal aspect of the calcaneal tuberosity, the tendon of insertion of the gastrocnemius muscles

is redirected towards the distal edge of the tuberosity by the bursa of the common calcaneal tendon.

- The portion of the common calcaneal tendon arising from the biceps femoris attaches separately at the dorsomedial edge of the calcaneal tuberosity.
- The flexor digitorum superficialis forms the calcaneal cap that is attached by connective tissue to the calcaneal tuberosity. Short tendons arising from the sides of the muscle attach to the calcaneal tuberosity dorsally.

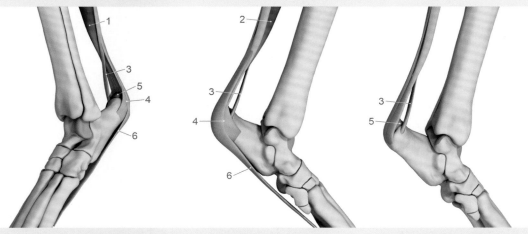

▶ **Fig. 5.10** Insertion sites of the components of the common calcaneal tendon. 1 m. gastrocnemius lateralis, 2 m. gastrocnemius medialis, 3 m. biceps femoris (caudal portion), 4 calcaneal cap, 5 bursa tendinis calcanei, 6 m. flexor digitorum superficialis. (source: Martin S. Fischer, Jonas Lauströer, Amir Andikfar)

5.3.3 Crural region

The tibia and fibula are palpated from distal to proximal. The palpable features of the fibula are the lateral malleolus, distally, and the head of the fibula, proximally. The medial aspect of the body of the tibia (planum cutaneum) is palpable along its length. The muscles of the crus are tested for swelling and pain on digital pressure. Swelling due to trauma occurs particularly in the lateral compartment, where the large tibialis cranialis is located (▶ Fig. 5.11).

> 🔾 **Findings and Differential Diagnosis**
> * swelling
>   – neoplasia (p. 194)
>   – hematoma
>   – compartment syndrome
> * crepitation
>   – fracture
> * axial deviation
>   – fracture
>   – malalignment
> * pain
>   – fracture
>   – neoplasia (p. 194)
>   – panosteitis (p. 188)
>   – compartment syndrome

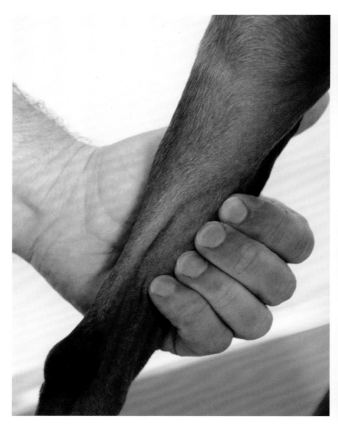

▶ **Fig. 5.11** Assessment of the medial surface of the body of the tibia (planum cutaneum) for abnormal surface contours and pain on digital pressure. (source: Gaby Ernst, Saland, Switzerland)

Anatomy
* The tibial planum cutaneum separates the extensors and flexors. For the most part, the muscles continue as long tendons in the lower half of the crus (▶ Fig. 5.12).

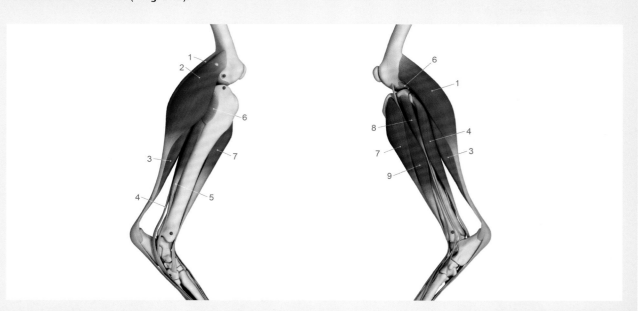

▶ **Fig. 5.12** Muscles of the crus. Medial and lateral view. 1 m. gastrocnemius lateralis, 2 m. gastrocnemius medialis, 3 m. flexor digitorum superficialis, 4 mm. flexores digitorum profundi, 5 m. flexor digitorum longus, 6 m. popliteus, 7 m. tibialis cranialis, 8 m. peroneus longus, 9 m. extensor digitorum lateralis. (source: Martin S. Fischer, Jonas Lauströer, Amir Andikfar)

5.3.4 **Stifle Region**

Joint Palpation

Positioned behind the patient, the examiner uses their left and right hand to examine both stifle joints simultaneously (► **Fig. 5.13**). The thumb and index finger are used to assess the region between the patella and the tibial plateau, just caudal to the patellar ligament, for joint effusion, pain on palpation and heat. In the healthy dog, the patellar ligament can be distinguished clearly from the caudally located joint.

⚡ Findings and Differential Diagnosis

- swelling, heat and/or pain
  - cruciate ligament rupture/partial cruciate ligament rupture
  - meniscal injury
  - avulsion of the extensor digitorum lateralis
  - neoplasia (p. 194)
  - patellar luxation (p. 204)
  - osteochondrosis (p. 185)
- fluctuating swelling
  - acute trauma
  - joint fracture

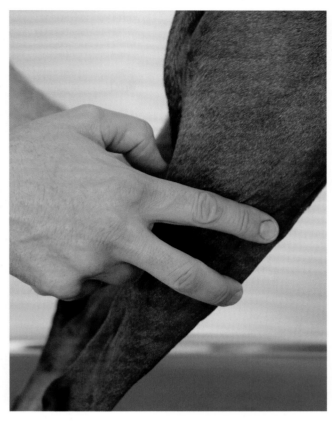

► **Fig. 5.13** Reference points for identification of the stifle joint: patella, tibial crest and femoral condyles. (source: Gaby Ernst, Saland, Switzerland)

Anatomy

- The stifle joint consists of 3 articular components (► **Fig. 5.14**):
  - femorotibial joint
  - femoropatellar joint
  - proximal tibiofibular joint
- The lateral meniscus is larger and thicker than its medial counterpart, both are thick abaxially and taper towards their axial border. Extension and flexion of the stifle joint forces the menisci to undergo a rolling, sliding movement. The medial meniscus is less mobile due to its attachments to surrounding structures.
- The menisci are stabilized by 6 ligaments. A single ligament attaches the lateral meniscus to the femur.
- Up to 3 additional sesamoid bones are associated with the stifle joint. These are located in the tendon of origin of the gastrocnemius lateralis and gastrocnemius medialis (fabellae) and the popliteus. According to recent findings, the patella is not a sesamoid bone in the traditional sense that mechanical forces induce ossification within the quadriceps femoris tendons. Instead, it develops as a bony process and subsequently forms a joint with the femur [20].

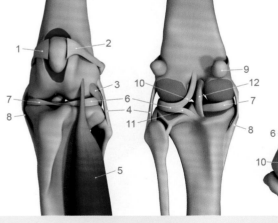

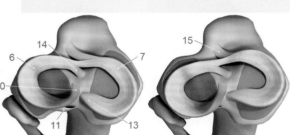

► **Fig. 5.14** The stifle joint with ligaments and menisci. Cranial and caudal view and illustration of the menisci in the extended and flexed joint. 1 lig. femoropatellaris medialis, 2 lig. femoropatellaris lateralis, 3 m. popliteus, 4 lig. collaterale laterale, 5 m. extensor digitorum longus, 6 meniscus lateralis, 7 meniscus medialis, 8 lig. collaterale mediale, 9 fabella, 10 lig. meniscofemorale, 11 lig. tibiale caudale menisci lateralis, 12 lig. cruciatum caudale, 13 lig. tibiale caudale menisci medialis, 14 lig. tibiale craniale menisci lateralis, 15 lig. tibiale craniale menisci medialis. (source: Martin S. Fischer, Jonas Lauströer, Amir Andikfar)

Bone Contours

The tibia, patella and distal femur are assessed along the joint margins for pain on palpation and the presence of osteophytes (▶ Fig. 5.15).

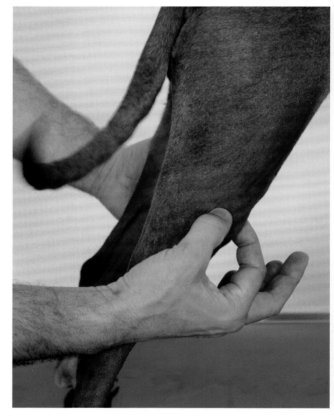

▶ **Fig. 5.15** Osteophytes occur at the joint margins. They may be palpable, particularly on the femur. (source: Gaby Ernst, Saland, Switzerland)

⚡ Findings and Differential Diagnosis
- abnormal bone contours
  - osteosarcoma (p. 194) of the distal femur or proximal tibia
  - severe osteoarthritis

Anatomy
- The large joint capsule forms 3 communicating cavities between the femur and tibia, and beneath the patella (▶ Fig. 5.16).
- The stifle joint has 15 ligaments, 6 of which are attached to the menisci. The meniscal ligaments attach the menisci to the tibia and also attach the lateral meniscus to the femur. These are conventionally referred to as the cranial and caudal ligaments of the medial and lateral meniscus, the meniscofemoral ligament and the transverse ligament.
- Lateral collateral ligament (LCL): passes from the lateral epicondyle, immediately proximal to the origin of the popliteus, to the head of the fibula; loosely connected to the joint capsule.
- Medial collateral ligament (MCL): passes from the medial epicondyle to a broad area of attachment on the proximal tibia. A bursa is located near the site of attachment. The MCL is approximately one third longer than the LCL.
- During extension, the tensed ligaments prevent rotational joint movement; during flexion, internal rotation is permitted by the laxity of the lateral collateral ligament, though this is counteracted by the cruciate ligaments. External rotation is prevented only by the lateral collateral ligament.

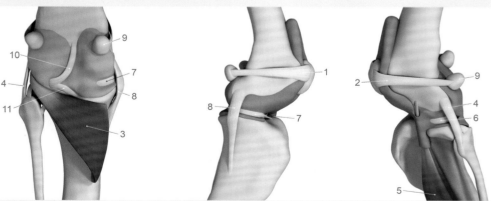

▶ **Fig. 5.16** Stifle joint with ligaments and joint capsule (green). Caudal, medial and lateral view. 1 lig. femoropatellaris medialis, 2 lig. femoropatellaris lateralis, 3 m. popliteus, 4 lig. collaterale laterale, 5 m. extensor digitorum longus, 6 meniscus lateralis, 7 meniscus medialis, 8 lig. collaterale mediale, 9 fabella, 10 lig. meniscofemorale, 11 lig. tibiale caudale menisci lateralis. (source: Martin S. Fischer, Jonas Lauströer, Amir Andikfar)

Position of the Patella

The position of the patella is assessed. It should be located in the middle of the distal femur, positioned firmly in its sulcus. The thumb and index finger are used to attempt to luxate the patella medially and laterally (▶ Fig. 5.17). This can be facilitated by reducing the tension in the quadriceps femoris to some degree. To achieve this, the examiner places their knee under the dog's thigh, allowing the dog to take weight off the limb.

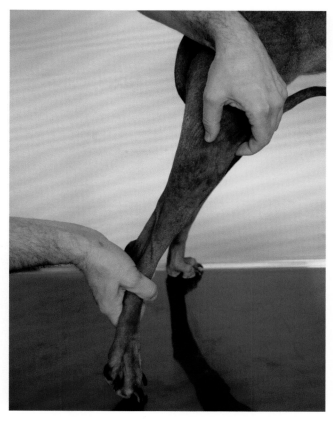

> **Findings and Differential Diagnosis**
> - hypermobility of the patella
>   - medial or lateral patellar luxation
> - hypomobility of the patella
>   - contracture of the quadriceps femoris
> - pain on palpation of the patella and patellar ligament
>   - cartilage wear
>   - polyarthritis (p. 191)
>   - traction osteochondritis at the insertion of the patellar ligament

▶ **Fig. 5.17** Assessment of the position of the patella relative to the femur and preliminary testing for patellar luxation. (source: Gaby Ernst, Saland, Switzerland)

Anatomy

- The patella is held in the proximal portion of the trochlear groove by the lateral and medial fascia lata and by the femoro-patellar ligaments (▶ Fig. 5.18).
- Patellar ligament: component of the tendon of insertion of the quadriceps femoris that passes from the patella to the tibia, separated from the joint capsule by a fat pad.
- The cruciate ligaments are intra-articular but extrasynovial.
- Cranial cruciate ligament (CrCL): passes from the caudomedial region of the lateral condyle to the cranial intercondyloid area of the tibia, twisting on itself along its course; restricts cranial movement and internal rotation of the tibia.
- Caudal cruciate ligament (CdCL): passes from the lateral side of the medial condyle (medial to the CrCL) to the popliteal notch; counteracts internal rotation of the femur and external rotation of the tibia.
- Each cruciate ligament has 2 functional components that exhibit varying states of tension.

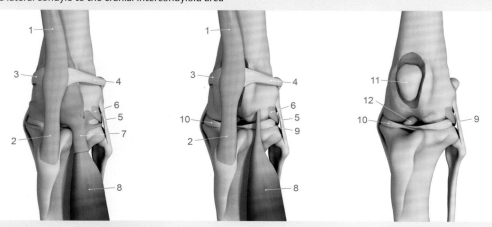

▶ **Fig. 5.18** Stifle joint and patella, cranial view.
1 tendon of insertion of m. quadriceps femoris, 2 lig. patellae, 3 lig. femoropatellaris medialis, 4 lig. femoropatellaris lateralis, 5 lig. collaterale laterale, 6 m. popliteus, 7 vagina synovialis m. extensoris digitorum longus, 8 m. extensor digitorum longus, 9 meniscus lateralis, 10 meniscus medialis, 11 patella, 12 lig. cruciatum craniale. (source: Martin S. Fischer, Jonas Lauströer, Amir Andikfar)

5.3.5 Thigh

The muscles of the thigh are palpated from distal to proximal, noting their position, course and dimensions, and the presence of any pain. The total circumference of the musculature of the thigh is determined using a measuring tape, a piece of cord or the examiner's hands. To achieve reliable results, the circumference should be measured proximally, with the hands or measuring tape positioned at the level of the inguinal region (▶ Fig. 5.19).

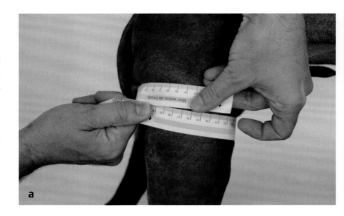

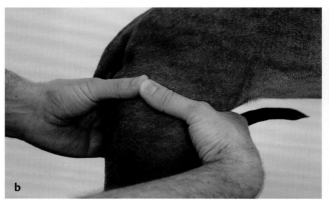

> 🔍 **Findings and Differential Diagnosis**
> - painful or hypomobile muscles in the caudal thigh
>   - fibrosis of the ischiocrural („hamstring") muscles
> - reduced thigh muscle circumference, compared with the contralateral limb
>   - chronic reduction of limb loading, disorder located within the limb or laterally in the region of the vertebral column
> - painful or swollen quadriceps femoris
>   - contracture of the quadriceps femoris
> - painful pectineus
>   - hip dysplasia (p. 212) or coxofemoral osteoarthritis (p. 212)

▶ **Fig. 5.19** Assessment of thigh muscle circumference.
a Using a measuring tape. (source: Gaby Ernst, Saland, Switzerland)
b Using the hands. (source: Gaby Ernst, Saland, Switzerland)

Anatomy
- The ischiocrural („hamstring") muscles are comprised of the biceps femoris, semitendinosus and semimembranosus (▶ Fig. 5.20).

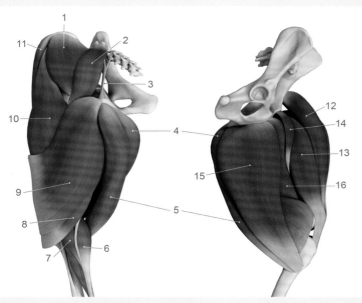

▶ **Fig. 5.20** Proximal hindlimb with palpable features. Muscles of the thigh. 1 m. glutaeus medius, 2 m. glutaeus superficialis, 3 lig. sacrotuberale, 4 m. semimembranosus, 5 m. semitendinosus, 6 m. gastrocnemius medialis, 7 m. gastrocnemius lateralis, 8 m. biceps femoris pars caudalis, 9 m. biceps femoris pars cranialis, 10 m. tensor fasciae latae, 11 m. sartorius pars cranialis, 12 m. rectus femoris, 13 m. vastus medialis, 14 m. pectineus, 15 m. gracilis, 16 mm. adductores. (source: Martin S. Fischer, Jonas Lauströer, Amir Andikfar)

5.3.6 Hip Region

Hip Joint Position

The relative positions of the ischial tuberosity, greater trochanter and iliac crest are palpated using the thumb, index finger and middle finger (▶ Fig. 5.21). These points should form similarly shaped triangles on the left and right sides.

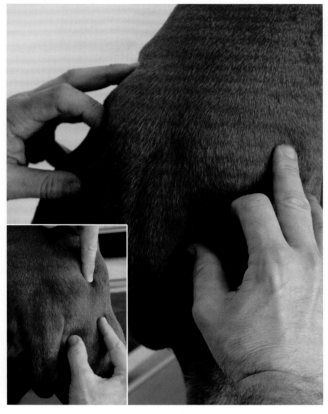

> **🗹 Findings and Differential Diagnosis**
> - greater trochanter abnormally positioned or not palpable
>   - luxation of the hip joint (p. 218) in a craniodorsal, caudoventral or cranioventral direction

▶ **Fig. 5.21** Palpation of the three bony prominences (ischial tuberosity, greater trochanter and iliac crest) used in the diagnosis of femoral head luxation. (source: Gaby Ernst, Saland, Switzerland)

Anatomy

- Forces generated in the hindlimbs are transmitted through the pelvis and sacrum into the lumbar vertebral column and thereby into the trunk. Movement of the lower vertebral column results from movement of the limbs. This is reflected in the frame-like construction of the pelvis. The sacroiliac joint acts largely as a buffer designed to absorb peaks of load (▶ Fig. 5.22). Loading of the sacroiliac joint by compressive and tensile forces is disproportionately higher in large breeds.

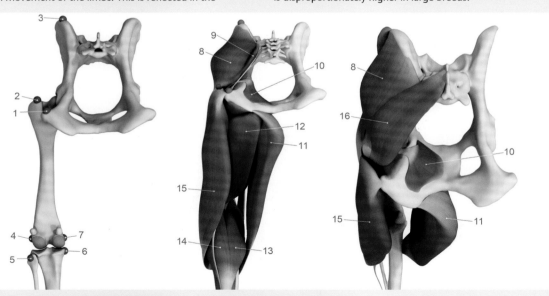

▶ **Fig. 5.22** Proximal hindlimb with palpable features. Deep ischiocrural and croup muscles.
1 tuber ischiadicum, 2 trochanter major, 3 crista iliaca, 4 epicondylus lateralis, 5 caput fibulae, 6 condylus medialis, 7 epicondylus medialis, 8 m. glutaeus medius, 9 m. piriformis, 10 m. obturator internus, 11. m. gracilis, 12 mm. adductores, 13 m. gastrocnemius medialis, 14 m. gastrocnemius lateralis, 15 m. biceps femoris, 16 m. glutaeus superficialis. (source: Martin S. Fischer, Jonas Lauströer, Amir Andikfar)

Manipulation of the Hip Joint

With one hand on the distal femur and the other over the greater trochanter, the hip joint is extended, flexed and abducted on the left and right side. During this procedure, the dog stands only on the contralateral leg. In all of these maneuvres, it should be possible to move the femur into a horizontal position (▶ Fig. 5.23).

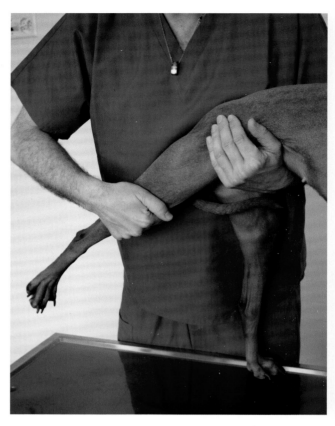

> **Fig. 5.23** Maximum extension of the hip joint. This manipulation places pressure on the hip joint, iliopsoas and the lumbar vertebrae and may elicit a pain response. (source: Gaby Ernst, Saland, Switzerland)

> **Findings and Differential Diagnosis**
> - general reduction in range of movement of the hip joint
>   - coxofemoral osteoarthritis
>   - hip dysplasia (p. 212)
>   - hip joint luxation (p. 218)
>   - neoplasia (p. 194)
> - pain only on extension of the hip joint
>   - coxofemoral osteoarthritis
>   - hip dysplasia (p. 212)
>   - cauda equina compression
>   - spondylosis
>   - intervertebral disc disease
> - crepitation and pain
>   - coxofemoral osteoarthritis
>   - neoplasia (p. 194)

Anatomy

- In the hip joint, the hemispherical head of the femur articulates with the Ω-shaped lunate surface of the acetabulum. The pelvic side of the articulation is enlarged by the fibrocartilaginous acetabular labrum (▶ Fig. 5.24).
- There are no mechanically functional ligaments in the hip joint. The intra-articular, extrasynovial ligament of the head of the femur passes to the Ω-shaped recess of the acetabulum. The transverse acetabular ligament joins the tips of the lunate sur-

- The spacious joint capsule attaches proximally at the edge of the acetabular labrum and below the head of the femur near the cartilage-lined articular surface. Thickenings of the capsule are present dorsally (zona orbicularis) and in the cranial and caudal capsule walls. The fibers of the articularis coxae muscle radiate into the outer layer of the capsule, to which they can apply tension.

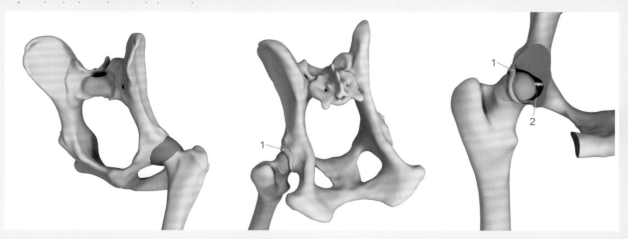

> **Fig. 5.24** Hip joint with joint capsule (green), acetabular labrum and illustration of the ligament of the head of the femur by „removal" of the dorsal acetabulum. 1 labrum acetabulare, 2 lig. capitis femoris. (source: Martin S. Fischer, Jonas Lauströer, Amir Andikfar)

Examination of the Iliopsoas

The femur is rotated inwards at full extension, resulting in maximum stretching of the iliopsoas (▶ Fig. 5.25). Digital pressure can be applied laterally to the cranial and middle portions of the muscle, ventral to the vertebral column. In dogs below approximately 25 kg body weight, the iliopsoas can be palpated rectally, cranial to the ilium.

> ⚡ **Findings and Differential Diagnosis**
> - pain response elicited only when the femur is internally rotated at full extension
>   - iliopsoas strain (p. 220)
>   - coxofemoral osteoarthritis
> - pain elicited by pressure on the iliopsoas
>   - iliopsoas strain (p. 220)

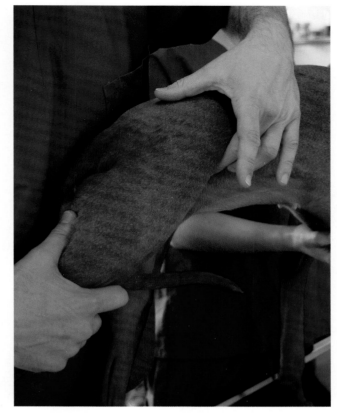

▶ **Fig. 5.25** Maximum lengthening of the iliopsoas via simultaneous extension of the hip joint and internal rotation of the limb. (source: Gaby Ernst, Saland, Switzerland)

Anatomy

- The iliopsoas is formed by the juxtaposition of the psoas major and iliacus (▶ Fig. 5.26). These muscles can easily be separated, as far as their attachment to the lesser trochanter. The psoas major arises from the transverse processes of L2 and L3, by means of an aponeurosis from L3 and L4, and from the ventral surface of L4–L7. The iliacus takes its origin from the caudomedial aspect of the ilium.
- During walking, the iliopsoas is active at the end of the stance phase and in the swing phase. During trotting and galloping, its activity commences earlier, in the first third of the stance phase, thus contributing to stabilization of the limb.

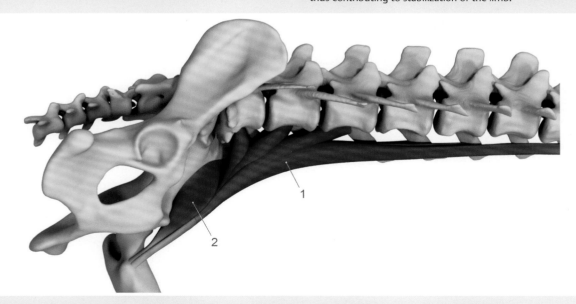

▶ **Fig. 5.26** Medial view of the psoas major (1) and the iliacus (2). (source: Martin S. Fischer, Jonas Lauströer, Amir Andikfar)

5.3.7 Overview of Common Differential Diagnoses and Video of Examination

The following table (▶ **Table 5.1**) provides an overview of the most important differential diagnoses.

▶ **Tab. 5.1** Overview of differential diagnoses.

Region	Key Differential Diagnoses
digits, metatarsus and tarsus	• polyarthritis • fractures • neoplasia
tarsal joint	• instabilities • osteochondrosis of talus • rupture or partial rupture of common calcaneal tendon
crus	• panosteitis • neoplasia
stifle	• cruciate ligament rupture • partial cruciate ligament rupture • patellar luxation
thigh	• neoplasia • panosteitis • muscular induration/fibrosis
hip	• hip dysplasia/osteoarthritis • hip joint luxation • Legg-Perthes-disease

Refer to ▶ **Video 5.3** for a video showing examination of the hindlimb of a dog in a standing position.

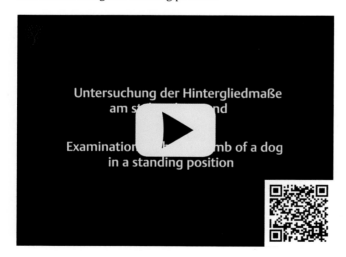

▶ **Video 5.3** Examination of the hindlimb of a dog in a standing position. This sequence includes: standing symmetry, testing for pain in the distal limbs, palpation of the metatarsal and tarsal bones, palpation of the tarsal joint, palpation of the common calcaneal tendon, palpation of the crural region, palpation of the stifle joint and the patella, the cranial drawer test, palpation of the femur and „hamstring" muscles, palpation and examination of the hip joint and examination of the iliopsoas. (source: Tele D, Diessenhofen, Switzerland)

5.4 Forelimb

5.4.1 Digits, Metacarpus and Carpus

Standing Symmetry

Standing in front of the dog, the examiner assesses standing symmetry by placing an index finger around each carpus at the level of the accessory carpal bone and pulling cranially with bilaterally equivalent force (▶ Fig. 5.27).

> 🗐 **Findings and Differential Diagnosis**
> - one leg more easily drawn forward
>   - generalized weakness of the more easily manipulated limb

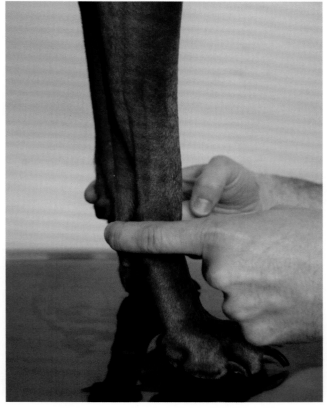

▶ **Fig. 5.27** Assessment of forelimb symmetry and stability by pulling on the forelimbs at the level of the accessory carpal bone. (source: Gaby Ernst, Saland, Switzerland)

Anatomy

- Muscle mass is approximately evenly distributed between the front and hind limbs (▶ Fig. 5.28 and ▶ Fig. 5.2). The total physiological cross-sectional area, which provides a very good approximation of the force that can be generated by the muscles, is also virtually identical. The forelimbs usually carry 60% of the vertical load. Increasing acceleration is accompanied by greater distribution of the vertical body weight force to the hindlimbs. Horizontal forces are higher in the hindlimbs; these generate more propulsion, while the forelimbs exert a longer and stronger braking force.

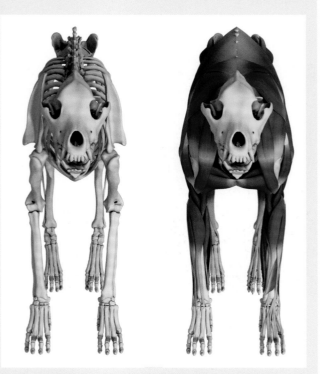

▶ **Fig. 5.28** Skeleton and musculature of the dog. Cranial view. (source: Martin S. Fischer, Jonas Lauströer, Amir Andikfar)

Testing for Pain in the Distal Limb

Both legs are grasped firmly, proximal to the carpus, and pressed onto the surface of the examination table, checking for evidence of pain (▶ Fig. 5.29).

> **✔ Findings and Differential Diagnosis**
> - pain response and/or lifting of paw after testing suggests a disorder of the distal limb, e.g.
>   - swelling of the digital joints
>   - digital fracture
>   - metacarpal fracture
>   - carpal disorder
> - dorsoflexion of the digits
>   - rupture of the digital flexors

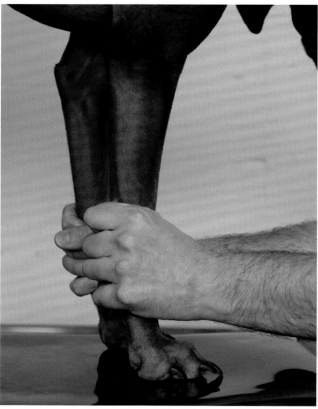

▶ **Fig. 5.29** The procedure used to test for pain in the distal forelimbs is similar to that used in the hindlimbs. The distal antebrachium is grasped firmly and pressed onto the surface of the table. (source: Gaby Ernst, Saland, Switzerland)

Anatomy

- Like the hindfoot, the front foot is held in tension by the tendons of the superficial and deep digital flexors (▶ Fig. 5.30). Storage of elastic energy in these tendons results in a catapult effect when load is removed at lift off.
- The carpal tunnel is formed by the flexor retinaculum, a reinforcement of the deep carpal fascia, and by the palmar portion of the joint capsule. The tunnel is traversed by the tendons of

insertion of the deep digital flexor, arteries, veins and the ulnar and median nerves.

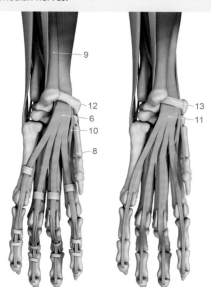

▶ **Fig. 5.30** Carpus with associated muscles of the antebrachium. 1 m. extensor carpi ulnaris, 2 m. extensor digitorum lateralis, 3 m. extensor digitorum communis, 4 m. extensor carpi radialis, 5 m. abductor pollicis longus, 6 m. flexor digitorum superficialis, 7 m. flexor digitorum profundus caput humerale, 8 m. flexor digitorum profundus caput radiale, 9 m. flexor carpi ulnaris, 10 m. flexor carpi radialis, 11 common tendon of insertion of the m. flexor digitorum profundus, 12 carpal fascia (elevated), 13 retinaculum flexorum. (source: Martin S. Fischer, Jonas Lauströer, Amir Andikfar)
a Craniolateral and craniomedial view. (source: Martin S. Fischer, Jonas Lauströer, Amir Andikfar)
b Caudal view with illustration of the superficial and deep flexors. (source: Martin S. Fischer, Jonas Lauströer, Amir Andikfar)

Carpus

The metacarpus and the carpus are assessed by comparative palpation. Palpation is used to determine the position of the accessory carpal bone on the caudolateral aspect of the carpus (▶ Fig. 5.31).

> **Findings and Differential Diagnosis**
> * axial deviation, palmigrade stance
>   - fracture of carpal or metacarpal bones or abnormality of intercarpal or carpal ligaments, particularly on the palmar aspect
>   - accessory carpal bone fracture
>   - rupture of the collateral ligaments of carpus
> * abnormal contours (swelling) in palmar region
>   - old injury
>   - swelling due to acute hyperextension trauma (p. 221)
> * crepitation or displacement of the accessory carpal bone
>   - accessory carpal bone fracture
>   - ligament rupture or carpal flexor tendon tear

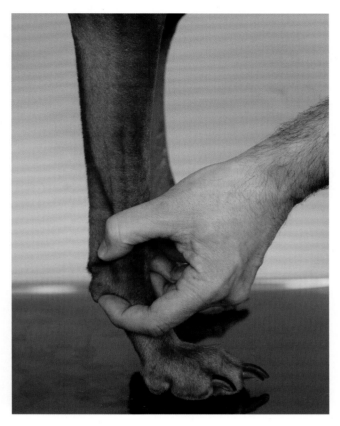

▶ **Fig. 5.31** The accessory carpal bone, on the caudolateral aspect of the main joint, is the most readily identifiable bone in the carpal region. (source: Gaby Ernst, Saland, Switzerland)

Anatomy

15 carpal bones (▶ Fig. 5.32) form 33 individual joints. Each row of carpal bones constitutes a functional unit. The main articulations are as follows:
* distal radioulnar joint (red)
* antebrachiocarpal joint (orange)
* middle carpal joint
* carpometacarpal joint

The distal radioulnar joint and antebrachiocarpal joints have a common joint cavity.

The concave radial articular surface is around 3 times larger than the weakly concave articular surface of the ulna.

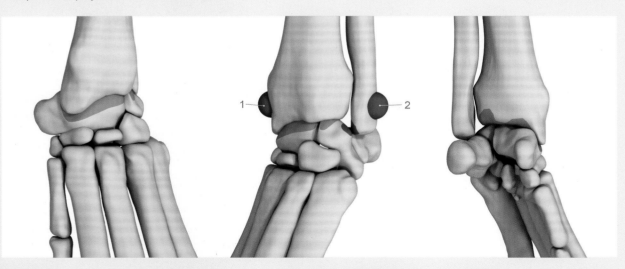

▶ **Fig. 5.32** Palpable features of the carpus. 1 proc. styloideus medialis, 2 proc. styloideus lateralis. (source: Martin S. Fischer, Jonas Lauströer, Amir Andikfar)

5.4.2 Carpal Joint

The cranial part of the antebrachiocarpal joint is palpable between the styloid processes (▶ Fig. 5.33).

> **Findings and Differential Diagnosis**
> * effusion, heat and/or pain
>   – polyarthritis (p. 191)
>   – collateral ligament rupture
>   – joint fracture
>   – neoplasia of the distal radius
> * carpal valgus
>   – medial collateral ligament rupture
>   – asynchronous growth of the radius and ulna
> * abnormal surface contours on medial aspect of joint
>   – chronic ligament damage
>   – tendovaginitis (p. 223) of the abductor pollicis longus

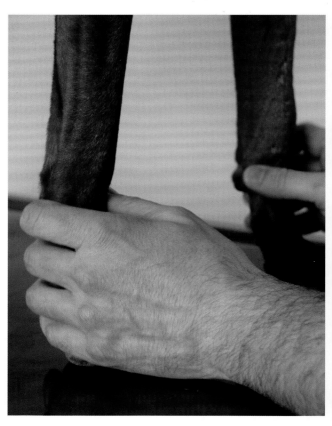

▶ **Fig. 5.33** The normal carpal joint contains little synovial fluid. Any joint swelling is detected in the cranial portion of the joint between the styloid processes. (source: Gaby Ernst, Saland, Switzerland)

Anatomy

* Due to its elaborate ligamentous apparatus and taut fascial coverings, movement of the carpal joint is limited to flexion and extension (▶ Fig. 5.34). In the normal joint, the angle of hyperextension is 25° ± 10°, with valgus of up to 15°.

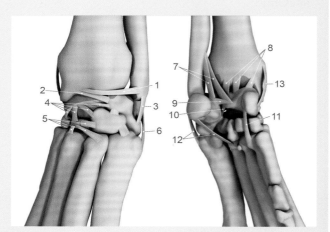

▶ **Fig. 5.34** Ligaments of the carpus.
1 lig. radioulnare, 2 lig. radiocarpeum dorsalis, 3 lig. collaterale carpi laterale, 4 ligg. intercarpea dorsales, 5 ligg. carpometacarpea dorsales, 6 lig. accessoriometacarpeum, 7 lig. ulnocarpeum palmare, 8 lig. radiocarpeum palmare, 9 lig. accessorioulnare, 10 lig. intercarpeum palmare, 11 lig. carpometacarpeum palmare, 12 ligg. accessoriometacarpea, 13 lig. collaterale carpi mediale. (source: Martin S. Fischer, Jonas Lauströer, Amir Andikfar)

5.4.3 Antebrachium

Moving from distal to proximal, the subcutaneously accessible sections of the radius and ulna are palpated and subjected to digital pressure. Particular attention should be given to the styloid processes, the head of the radius and the olecranon (▶ Fig. 5.35).

> **🔲 Findings and Differential Diagnosis**
> - cranial curvature of the radius, valgus and external rotation of the antebrachium (asynchronous growth of the radius and ulna):
>   - premature closure of the growth plate of the distal ulna and possibly the distal radius resulting in malalignment
> - pain in the distal third of the radius
>   - neoplasia of the radius
> - pain along the diaphysis and in the olecranon
>   - panosteitis (p. 188)
>   - fracture
> - swelling of the lateral extensor or medial flexor muscle groups
>   - compartment syndrome
> - swelling, heat and pain throughout the antebrachium
>   - hypertrophic osteodystrophy (p. 189)

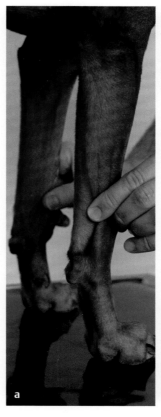
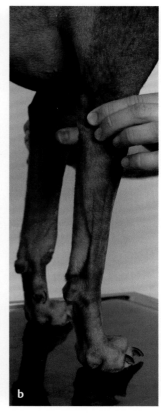

▶ **Fig. 5.35** The radius is palpable distally on the medial side of the limb (a), the ulna can be palpated proximally, on the lateral side, and at olecranon (b). (source: Gaby Ernst, Saland, Switzerland)

Anatomy

- The radius and ulna (▶ Fig. 5.36) cross one another. They are fixed in pronation by the interosseous ligament (up to 2 mm in thickness), though extensive passive rotation occurs during sprinting around a bend.

- Sesamoid cartilage may be present laterally within a connective tissue mesh formed by the tendon of origin of the supinator, lateral collateral ligament and the annular ligament of the radius, particularly in large and giant breed dogs.

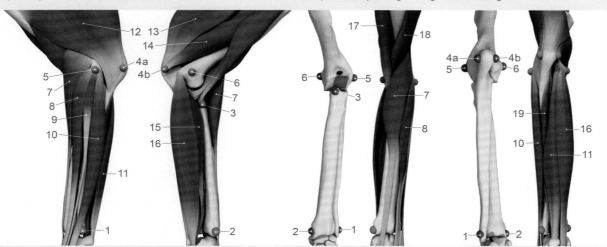

▶ **Fig. 5.36** Antebrachium and associated musculature.
Palpable features of the antebrachium: 1 proc. styloideus lateralis, 2 proc. styloideus medialis, 3 caput radii, 4 a, b olecranon with tuber olecrani, 5 epicondylus lateralis humeri, 6 epicondylus medialis humeri.
Muscles of the antebrachium: 7 m. extensor carpi radialis, 8 m. extensor digitorum communis, 9 m. extensor digitorum lateralis, 10 m. extensor carpi ulnaris, 11 m. flexor carpi ulnaris, 12 m. triceps brachii caput laterale, 13 m. triceps brachii caput longum, 14 m. triceps brachii caput mediale, 15 m. flexor digitorum profundus caput humerale, 16 m. flexor digitorum superficialis, 17 m. biceps brachii, 18 m. brachialis, 19 m. flexor digitorum profundus caput ulnare. (source: Martin S. Fischer, Jonas Lauströer, Amir Andikfar)

5.4.4 Elbow Region

Palpation of the Elbow Joint

The joint capsule of the elbow joint is palpable over a semi-circular area distal to the medial and lateral humeral epicondyle. It extends caudoproximally to the anconeal process (▶ Fig. 5.37).

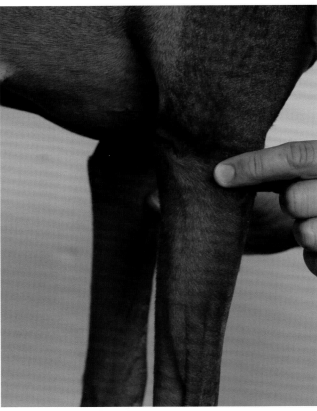

> **Findings and Differential Diagnosis**
> - effusion and heat in the elbow joint
>   - elbow dysplasia (p. 224)
>   - elbow osteoarthritis
> - marked effusion in the lateral compartment of the elbow joint
>   - fracture or ununited anconeal process

▶ **Fig. 5.37** Examination of the elbow joint. Distal to the humeral epicondyles (identified here as reference points), the elbow joint can be palpated over a semi-circular area extending from the anconeal process to the medial and lateral coronoid processes. (source: Gaby Ernst, Saland, Switzerland)

Anatomy

- The humeroulnar joint (yellow/orange) and the humeroradial joint (red) form a physiologically incongruent hinge joint (▶ Fig. 5.38). The humeroulnar joint has the larger joint surface and transmits force into the brachium.
- The joint capsule is reinforced on the flexor aspect by oblique fibers.
- There are 4 pouches under the biceps brachii and the extensor digitorum communis, and 2 pouches on the caudal aspect of the olecranon fossa.
- The radioulnar joint is part of the elbow joint and is incorporated into the joint capsule. It permits passive rotation of the ulna and radius.

- Greatest loading of the ulna occurs on the medial side of the trochlear notch between the anconeal process and the medial coronoid process.
- The trochlear notch articulates with the trochlea of the humerus. In small to medium-sized dogs the joint surface is continuous. In contrast, a reduction in articular cartilage is frequently observed at the deepest point of the trochlear notch in large breeds. In giant breeds, articular cartilage is often found only on the medial part of the joint surface.

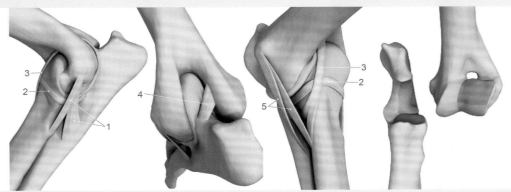

▶ **Fig. 5.38** Joint capsule of the elbow joint with associated ligaments. Illustration of the humeroulnar joint (yellow/orange) and the humeroradial joint (red). 1 Lig. collaterale lateralis, 2 lig. anulare radii, 3 lig. obliquum, 4 lig. olecrani, 5 lig. collaterale medialis. (source: Martin S. Fischer, Jonas Lauströer, Amir Andikfar)

Collateral Ligaments

The medial and lateral collateral ligaments are palpated. They should be tense along their course from the humerus to the head of the radius (laterally) and from the humerus to the ulna (medially). The soundness of the ligaments is tested further by adduction/abduction and by pronation/supination of the antebrachium with the elbow in flexion and extension (▶ Fig. 5.39).

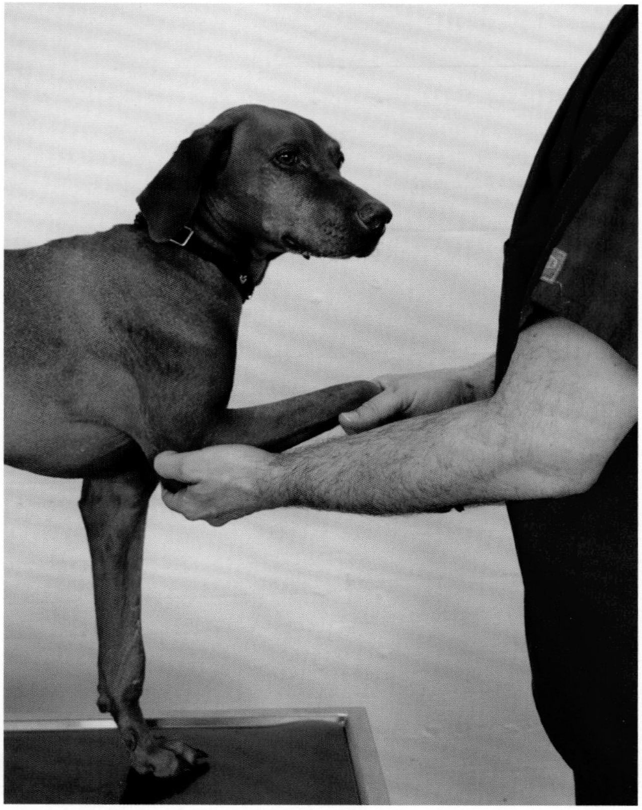

ⓘ Findings and Differential Diagnosis

- abduction of more than 30°
    - medial collateral ligament tear
- head of radius displaced laterally
    - lateral luxation of the antebrachium (lateral elbow luxation)
- increased supination
    - lateral instability
- increased pronation
    - medial instability

▶ **Fig. 5.39** Examination of the collateral ligaments of a dog in a standing position: increased pronation indicates a medial collateral ligament lesion, increased supination a lateral collateral ligament lesion. (source: Gaby Ernst, Saland, Switzerland)

Anatomy

- The lateral and medial collateral ligaments divide at approximately the level of the annular ligament of the radius (▶ Fig. 5.40). Since the attachments of the collateral ligaments are located eccentrically, relative to the axis of rotation of the joint, the joint literally clicks into place from either side of the neutral position (=maximum tension).
- Annular ligament of radius: passes from the medial coronoid process to the LCL and lateral coronoid process.
- Oblique ligament: passes from the lateral edge of the supratrochlear foramen to the medial radius and to the medial collateral ligament.
- Olecranon ligament: passes from the caudal side of the supratrochlear foramen to the anconeal process and the cranial crest of the olecranon.

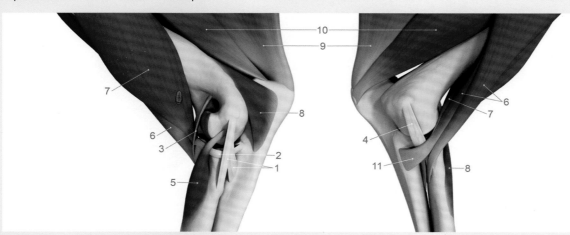

▶ **Fig. 5.40** Elbow joint and associated ligaments and muscles.
1 lig. collaterale lateralis, 2 lig. anulare radii, 3 lig. obliquum, 4 lig. collaterale medialis, 5 m. supinator, 6 m. biceps brachii, 7 m. brachialis, 8 m. anconaeus, 9 m. triceps brachii caput longum, 10 m. triceps brachii caput mediale, 11 common tendon of insertion of m. biceps brachii and m. brachialis. (source: Martin S. Fischer, Jonas Lauströer, Amir Andikfar)

5.4.5 Brachium

The muscle bellies of the brachium are palpated from distal to proximal (▶ Fig. 5.41). The radial insertion of the biceps brachii should be noted and tested for pain by drawing the brachium caudally. The course and humeral attachment of the triceps brachii is palpated. The humerus is only directly palpable in the distal third of the brachium. Proximally, its cranial portion is tested for the presence of pain.

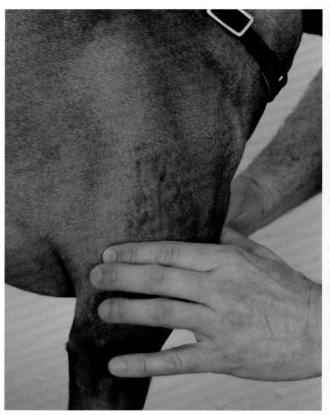

▶ **Fig. 5.41** After coursing over the mediocranial aspect of the shoulder joint, the biceps brachii is held in place between the lesser and greater tubercle by a transverse band before passing distally. Its proximal portion can be palpated. (source: Gaby Ernst, Saland, Switzerland)

> 🛈 **Findings and Differential Diagnosis**
> - pain in biceps brachii
>   - biceps tendinitis (p. 228)
> - swelling at the attachment of the triceps brachii
>   - partial or complete tear of the triceps brachii
>   - olecranon fracture
> - pain in humerus
>   - neoplasia (p. 194)

Anatomy

- From its origin on the supraglenoid tubercle, the biceps brachii winds around the shaft of the humerus and inserts on the radial tuberosity, and at a site distal to the medial coronoid process of the ulna (▶ **Fig. 5.42**).
- The coracobrachialis arises by a tendon from the coracoid process of the scapula. The tendon passes over the medial aspect of the shoulder joint within a tendon sheath. The muscle inserts on the crest of the lesser tubercle.
- The long head of the triceps brachii is the strongest muscle of the limbs.

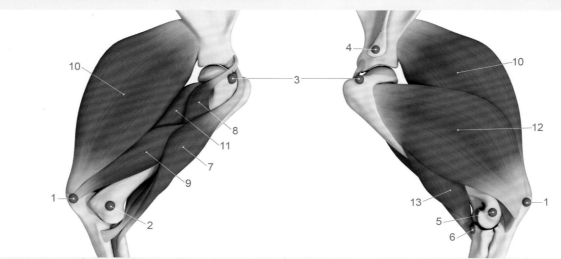

▶ **Fig. 5.42** Brachium with shoulder and elbow joints and associated muscles.
Palpable features: 1 olecranon, 2 epicondylus medialis humeri, 3 tuberculum majus, 4 acromion, 5 epicondylus lateralis humeri, 6 caput radii, 7 m. biceps brachii, 8 m. coracobrachialis, 9 m. triceps brachii caput mediale, 10 m. triceps brachii caput longum, 11 m. triceps brachii caput accessorium, 12 m. triceps brachii caput laterale, 13 m. brachialis. (source: Martin S. Fischer, Jonas Lauströer, Amir Andikfar)

5.4.6 Shoulder Region

Joint Palpation

The shoulder joint is hidden deep beneath the musculature. It can only be palpated directly on its craniomedial aspect, where it is traversed by the biceps brachii (▶ Fig. 5.43). During palpation, the shoulder joint is also manipulated.

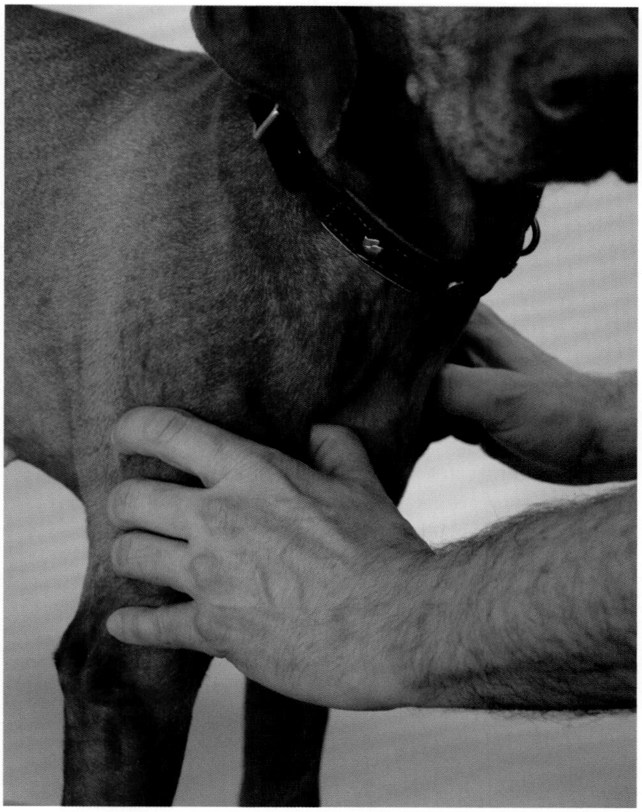

> ⚡ **Findings and Differential Diagnosis**
> - pain and heat
>   - osteochondrosis (p. 185)
>   - biceps tendinitis
>   - shoulder instability (p. 229)
> - crepitation
>   - chronic osteochondrosis
>   - joint fracture
>   - shoulder luxation
>   - neoplasia (p. 194)
>   - avulsion of biceps brachii from supraglenoid tubercle

▶ **Fig. 5.43** The shoulder joint lies deep beneath the muscles of the shoulder and can only be palpated directly on its cranial aspect. (source: Gaby Ernst, Saland, Switzerland)

Anatomy

- Intracapsular ligaments are present; the medial glenohumeral ligament is a discrete ligament, rather than merely a thickening of the capsule (▶ Fig. 5.44).
- The proximal portion of the biceps brachii courses within a tendon sheath. Fibrocartilage is embedded within the gliding portion of the tendon. The head of the humerus moves underneath the tendon; the tendon itself does not move. The tensile strength and loading capacity of the tendon of origin decrease with age. Tensile loading capacity relative to body weight is lower in heavy dogs.

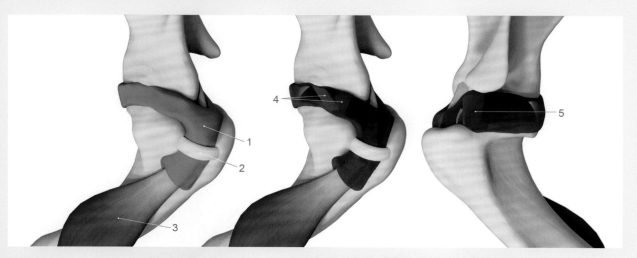

▶ **Fig. 5.44** Joint capsule of the shoulder joint with intracapsular ligaments. The joint capsule is shown as translucent to reveal the course of the tendon of origin of the biceps brachii within the tendon sheath.
1 Vagina synovialis intertubercularis, 2 lig. transversum humeri, 3 m. biceps brachii, 4 lig. glenohumeralis medialis, 5 thickening of the lateral capsule wall. (source: Martin S. Fischer, Jonas Lauströer, Amir Andikfar)

Assessment of Shoulder Stability

With the elbow and shoulder joints fully extended, the limb is abducted and the entire range of motion of the shoulder joint is assessed (▶ Fig. 5.45).

ℹ Findings and Differential Diagnosis
- abduction greater than 20°
  - medial shoulder luxation
  - infraspinatus contracture
- pain on manipulation
  - osteochondrosis (p. 185)
  - biceps tendinitis
  - cranial or caudal luxation
  - contracture of infraspinatus
- increased mobility
  - cranial or lateral luxation
  - shoulder joint dysplasia

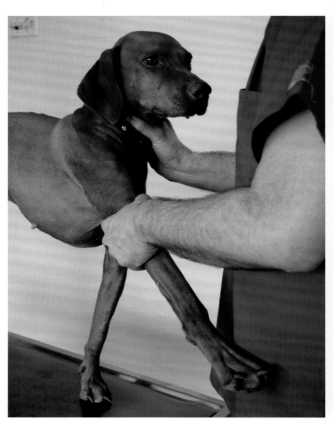

▶ **Fig. 5.45** In a medially stable shoulder joint, the maximum angle of abduction is 20°. (source: Gaby Ernst, Saland, Switzerland)

Anatomy

- The shoulder joint has a large range of movement: extension 140°–150°, abduction/adduction and longitudinal rotation highly breed-specific.
- The shoulder joint is held in place by an adhesion-cohesion mechanism and by the shoulder cuff.

- The joint capsule forms a cuff around the shoulder into which portions of the tendons of insertion of several muscles radiate (subscapularis, medially; infraspinatus, supraspinatus and teres minor, laterally). The term "dynamic ligaments" is also used to describe this type of stabilization (▶ Fig. 5.46).

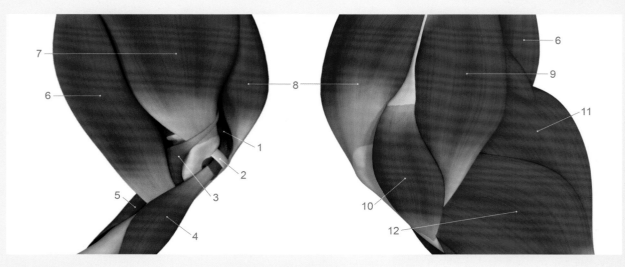

▶ **Fig. 5.46** Lateral and medial view of the shoulder joint with associated muscles.
1 Vagina synovialis intertubercularis, 2 lig. transversum humeri, 3 m. coracobrachialis, 4 m. biceps brachii, 5 m. brachialis, 6 m. teres major, 7 m. subscapularis, 8 m. supraspinatus, 9 m. deltoideus pars scapularis, 10 m. deltoideus pars acromialis, 11 m. triceps caput longum, 12 m. triceps caput laterale. (source: Martin S. Fischer, Jonas Lauströer, Amir Andikfar)

5.4.7 Scapular Region

The scapula is palpated along its cranial and caudal borders. The acromion and scapular spine are assessed with respect to their anatomical location (correct vs incorrect) and the presence of pain. The relative bulk of the muscle groups cranial and caudal to the scapular spine on the left and right side is evaluated (▶ Fig. 5.47).

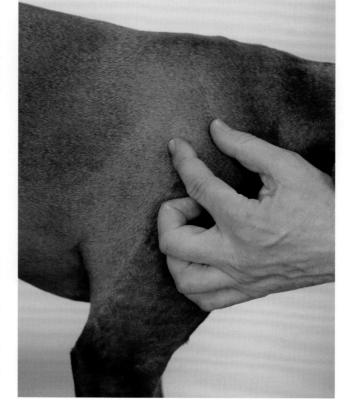

▶ **Fig. 5.47** Comparison of the degree of muscle mass cranial and caudal to the scapula on the left and right sides. This aids in identifying the affected limb. (source: Gaby Ernst, Saland, Switzerland)

> ### ✪ Findings and Differential Diagnosis
>
> - reduced shoulder muscle mass, relative to the contralateral limb
>   - chronic reduction of forelimb loading
>   - disorder located within the limb or in the lateral cervical region
> - pain on palpation of the scapula
>   - fracture
>   - neoplasia (p. 194)

Anatomy

- The scapula is functionally equivalent to the femur and makes the greatest contribution to stride length in the forelimb.
- The pivot point for movement of the entire forelimb is located in the dorsal third of the scapula.
- The articular surface of the glenoid cavity of the scapula is just one third of the size of the joint surface of the head of the humerus (▶ Fig. 5.48). The physiological range of motion of the shoulder joint is regulated by passive and active means, particularly adhesion-cohesion mechanisms and the muscular shoulder cuff.

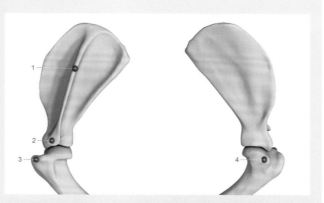

▶ **Fig. 5.48** Articular surfaces of the shoulder joint and palpable features of the humerus and scapula: 1 spina scapulae, 2 acromion, 3 tuberculum majus, 4 tuberculum minus. (source: Martin S. Fischer, Jonas Lauströer, Amir Andikfar)

5.4.8 Overview of Common Differential Diagnoses and Video of Examination

The following table (▶ Table 5.2) provides an overview of the most important differential diagnoses.

▶ **Tab. 5.2** Overview of differential diagnoses.

Region	Key Differential Diagnoses
digits, metacarpus and carpus	• polyarthritis • fractures • sesamoid disease
carpal joint region	• hyperextension trauma • tendovaginitis of abductor pollicis longus • polyarthritis
antebrachium	• neoplasia • panosteitis • asynchronous growth of radius and ulna
elbow	• elbow dysplasia/osteoarthritis • elbow luxation
brachium	• neoplasia • panosteitis • biceps tendovaginitis
shoulder	• osteochondrosis • medial instability • contracture

Refer to ▶ **Video 5.4** for a video showing examination of the forelimb of a dog in a standing position.

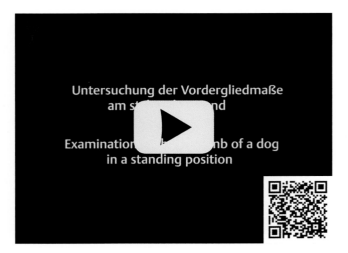

Untersuchung der Vordergliedmaße am s... nd

Examination ... nb of a dog in a standing position

▶ **Video 5.4** Examination of the forelimb of a dog in a standing position. This sequence includes: standing symmetry, testing for pain in the distal limb, palpation of the metacarpal and carpal bones, palpation of the radius and ulna, palpation and examination of the elbow joint, palpation of the humerus and triceps brachii, palpation and examination of the shoulder joint and palpation of the scapula. (source: Tele D, Diessenhofen, Switzerland)

6 Examination of the Dog in Recumbency

Daniel Koch, Martin S. Fischer

6.1
Orthopedic Examination of the Dog in Recumbency

The dog is now placed in lateral recumbency. An assistant restrains the dog by grasping the limbs closest to the table, proximal to the carpus and tarsus, and using the elbow to limit the movement of the dog's head. The degree of restraint should be such that the dog can still express gestures of resistance and pain. It is advisable for the owner to stand near the head of the dog.

The aim of examining the recumbent dog is to establish a provisional clinical diagnosis. While the site of the injury will have been identified from gait analysis and examination of the dog in a standing position, all limbs should be examined with the patient in recumbency, concluding with the affected limb. In this way, subtle abnormalities can be detected by comparison with the contralateral limb. There may also be more than one affected limb; e.g. in cases of panosteitis, polyarthritis, most dysplasias and cruciate ligament rupture.

Any of the following abnormalities should be noted:
- changes in surface contours or swelling
- heat and/or pain
- hypomobility
- hypermobility
- crepitation
- luxation
- instability

6.2

Hindlimb

6.2.1 Digits, Metatarsus and Tarsus

Overall evaluation

The skin of the paw and the interdigital region is inspected and the digital pads are palpated. The digits and metatarsals are then grasped and latero-medially compressed to check for a pain response. The paws, joints and metatarsals are examined for changes in surface contours (▶ Fig. 6.1, ▶ Fig. 6.2).

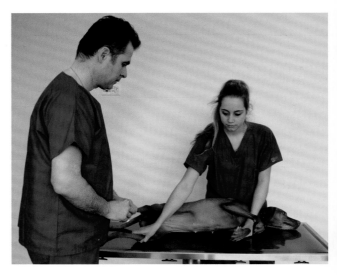

▶ **Fig. 6.1** Examination of the dog in lateral recumbency. An assistant restrains the dog by grasping the limbs closest to the table. (source: Gaby Ernst, Saland, Switzerland)

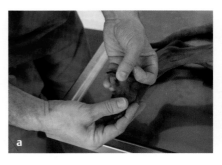 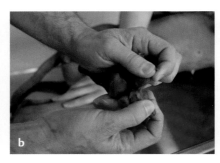 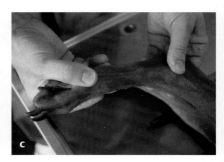

▶ **Fig. 6.2** Paws and Metatarsals.
a Inspection of the interdigital skin for injuries, tumors and foreign bodies. (source: Gaby Ernst, Saland, Switzerland)
b Injuries of the pads result in poorly healing wounds that are highly sensitive to pressure. Foreign bodies may become embedded in the pads. (source: Gaby Ernst, Saland, Switzerland)
c Examination of the structural stability of the metatarsal bones. (source: Gaby Ernst, Saland, Switzerland)

⚡ Findings and Differential Diagnosis

- reddening of the interdigital skin
  - allergy
- abnormal surface contours
  - neoplasia (p. 194)
- pain, heat
  - neoplasia (p. 194)
  - fracture
  - luxation
  - foreign body

Examination of the Digital Joints

The joints are examined for evidence of heat and surface irregularities. Each individual joint is flexed, extended, adducted and abducted (▶ **Fig. 6.3**). While one hand is used to examine joint mobility, the other tests for heat, swelling, crepitation, axial deviation, hypomobility and hypermobility. Any pain responses should be noted. The sesamoid bones of the flexor tendons are examined by hyperextending the metatarsophalangeal joints (▶ **Fig. 6.4**).

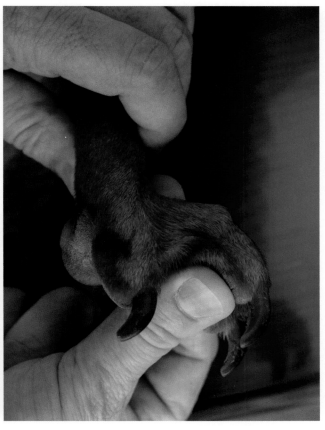

▶ **Fig. 6.4** Examination of the sesamoid bones by hyperextension of the metatarsophalangeal joints: one hand grasps the digits while the other hand is used to test for pain and joint crepitation. Two sesamoid bones are present on the plantar aspect of each metatarsophalangeal joint. (source: Gaby Ernst, Saland, Switzerland)

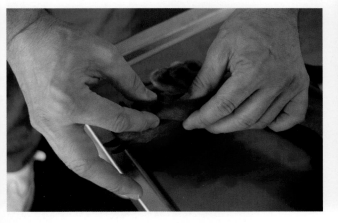

▶ **Fig. 6.3** Examination of individual digital joints. (source: Gaby Ernst, Saland, Switzerland)

Findings and Differential Diagnosis

- crepitation
  - joint fracture
- heat
  - polyarthritis (p. 191)
  - allergy
- axial deviation
  - collateral ligament rupture
  - fracture
- hypomobility
  - sesamoid disease (p. 220)
  - chronic joint disorder
- hypermobility
  - flexor or extensor tendon tear
  - joint capsule tear
  - nerve lesion
- pain
  - joint fracture
  - polyarthritis (p. 191)
  - sesamoid disease
  - joint capsule or ligament trauma

Tarsus

The bones of the tarsus are normally immobile. Each bone is palpated and the short ligaments are tested by extension, flexion abduction and adduction of the joint (▶ Fig. 6.5, ▶ Fig. 6.6).

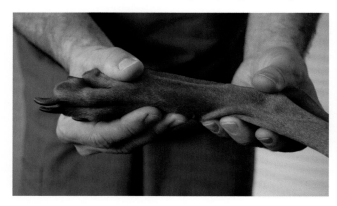

▶ **Fig. 6.5** Assessment of the lateral collateral ligaments of the tarsus. (source: Gaby Ernst, Saland, Switzerland)

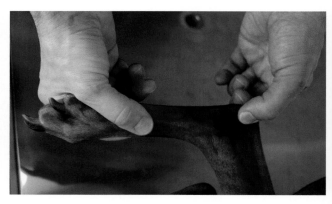

▶ **Fig. 6.6** Assessment of the calcaneus for pain and fractures. (source: Gaby Ernst, Saland, Switzerland)

⚡ Findings and Differential Diagnosis

- hypermobility
  - luxation
  - fracture
- abnormal surface contours on the ventral aspect of the calcaneus
  - pathological calcaneal fracture (p. 198)
- swelling, discharge
  - metatarsal fistula in German Shepherd Dogs

Overview of Common Findings and Video Demonstration

The following table (▶ **Table 6.1**) provides an overview of common findings in this region.

▶ **Tab. 6.1** Overview of findings.

Location/Test	Finding	Interpretation	Frequency
overall evaluation	abnormal contours	• neoplasia	+
	heat and/or pain	• neoplasia	+
		• fracture	+ +
		• luxation	+
		• foreign body	+
interdigital region	skin redness	• allergy	+ +
digital joints	abnormal contours	• fracture	+
	heat and/or pain	• polyarthritis	+ +
		• joint fracture	+ +
		• sesamoid disease	+
		• joint capsule/ligament trauma	+ +
	hypomobility	• sesamoid disease	+
		• chronic arthropathy	+
	hypermobility	• joint capsule tear	+
		• nerve lesion	+
	crepitation	• fracture	+ +
	instability	• collateral ligament rupture	+ +
		• fracture	+ +
tarsus	abnormal contours	• calcaneal fracture	+
	heat and/or pain	• metatarsal fistula (GSD)	+
	hypomobility	• luxation	+ +
		• fracture	+ +

Refer to ▶ **Video 6.1** for a video showing examination of the region from the digits to the tarsus in a dog in recumbency.

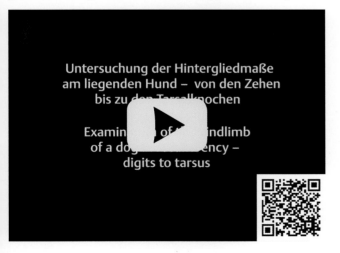

▶ **Video 6.1** Examination of the hindlimb of a dog in recumbency – digits to tarsus. This sequence includes palpation and assessment of the digits and digital joints (including sesamoid bones) and palpation of the metatarsal bones and common calcaneal tendon. (source: Tele D, Diessenhofen, Switzerland)

6.2.2 **Tarsal Joint**

Talocrural Joint

The joint is tested in flexion and extension for crepitation, heat, pain and fluctuating swelling. One hand is rested on the joint, while the other is used to manipulate the tarsus via the metatarsals (▶ Fig. 6.7, ▶ Fig. 6.8, ▶ Fig. 6.9). The talocrural joint is palpable over a semi-lunar shaped area distal to the styloid processes.

The collateral ligaments are examined by abduction and adduction of the joint in extension and flexion. The normal degree of movement is approximately 5–8° in the extended joint and 8–12° when the joint is flexed.

With the talocrural joint in flexion, rotational movements are used to assess the short portions of the collateral ligaments.

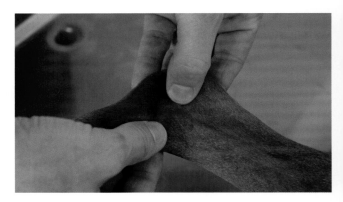

▶ **Fig. 6.7** Palpation of the talocrural joint and testing for crepitation, heat, fluctuating swelling and pain. (source: Gaby Ernst, Saland, Switzerland)

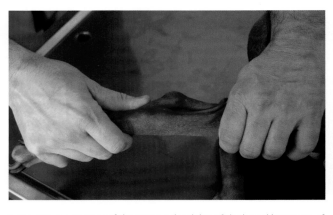

▶ **Fig. 6.8** Assessment of the structural stability of the lateral ligaments of the tarsus in extension. (source: Gaby Ernst, Saland, Switzerland)

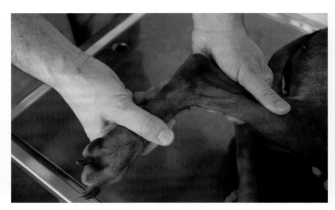

▶ **Fig. 6.9** Assessment of the structural stability of the lateral ligaments of the tarsus in flexion. (source: Gaby Ernst, Saland, Switzerland)

⚡ Findings and Differential Diagnosis

- hypermobility during abduction and adduction
  - collateral ligament rupture
  - luxation
- hypermobility during flexion and extension
  - fracture close to joint
  - luxation
- hypomobility
  - talocrural joint osteoarthritis following fracture
  - luxation or osteochondrosis
  - neoplasia (p. 194)

- instability during rotation of the flexed talocrural joint
  - rupture of the short caudal portions of the lateral collateral ligament or other ligamentous component
- heat, pain and crepitation in the joint
  - joint fracture
  - osteochondrosis (p. 185) of the trochlear ridges of the talus
  - neoplasia (p. 194)

Common Calcaneal Tendon

Moving proximally from its calcaneal attachment, the common calcaneal tendon is assessed for abnormal surface contours or stumps resulting from rupture. The integrity of the tendon is determined with the stifle joint in extension and the talocrural joint in flexion (▶ Fig. 6.10).

The portion of the tendon originating from the flexor digitorum superficialis passes over the calcaneus. In predisposed dogs, this can be luxated, usually in a lateral direction or, after trauma, in either direction. This is assessed by using the thumb to press gently on the calcaneal cap.

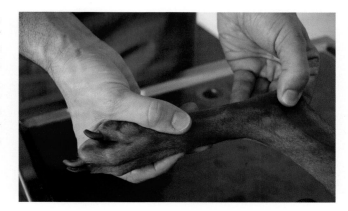

▶ **Fig. 6.10** Assessment of the integrity of the common calcaneal tendon, commencing at the attachment of the tendon to the calcaneus. This is performed at various degrees of flexion and extension. (source: Gaby Ernst, Saland, Switzerland)

⚡ Findings and Differential Diagnosis

- abnormal surface contours of the distal common calcaneal tendon
  - partial rupture of the common calcaneal tendon (p. 199)
- common calcaneal tendon not palpable
  - partial rupture of the common calcaneal tendon (p. 199)
- absence of tension in the common calcaneal tendon
  - partial rupture of the common calcaneal tendon (p. 199)
  - avulsion of the gastrocnemius at the femur
  - calcaneal fracture (p. 198) or intertarsal luxation
  - luxation of talocrural joint
- hypermobility of the calcaneal cap
  - lateral luxation of the calcaneal cap (p. 200), particularly in Shelties

Overview of Common Findings and Video Demonstration

The following table (▶ **Table 6.2**) provides an overview of common findings in this region.

▶ **Tab. 6.2** Overview of findings.

Location/Test	Finding	Interpretation	Frequency
talocrural join	heat and/or pain	• joint fracture	+
		• osteochondrosis of trochlear ridges of talus	+
		• neoplasia	+
	hypomobility	• talocrural joint osteoarthritis following fracture	+
		• luxation or osteochondrosis	+
		• neoplasia	+
	hypermobility during flexion and extension	• fracture near joint	+ +
		• luxation	+ +
	hypermobility during abduction and adduction	• collateral ligament rupture	+
		• luxation	+
	crepitation	• joint fracture	+
		• osteochondrosis of trochlear ridges of talus	+
		• neoplasia	+
	instability during rotation of flexed talocrural joint	• rupture of short caudal portion of lateral collateral ligament or other ligamentous component	+
common calcaneal tendon	abnormal contours	• partial common calcaneal tendon rupture	+ +
	common calcaneal tendon not palpable	• common calcaneal tendon rupture	+
	absence of tension in common calcaneal tendon	• common calcaneal tendon rupture	+
		• avulsion of gastrocnemius from femur	+
		• calcaneal fracture or intertarsal luxation	+
		• luxation of talocrural joint	+
	hypermobility of calcaneal cap	• lateral luxation of calcaneal cap, particularly in Shelties	+

Refer to ▶ **Video 6.2** for a video showing examination of the tarsal joint of a dog in recumbency.

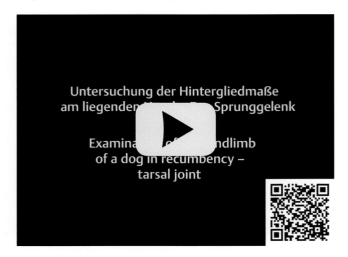

▶ **Video 6.2** Examination of the hindlimb of a dog in recumbency – tarsal joint. This sequence includes palpation and examination of the tarsal joint. (source: Tele D, Diessenhofen, Switzerland)

6.2.3 Crus

The crural region of both limbs is now palpated from distal to proximal. The muscle bellies of the lateral compartment (tibialis cranialis and extensor digitalis lateralis) can be delineated particularly clearly. Palpable features of the fibula include the malleolus and the fibular head. On the tibia, the medial aspect of the body of the tibia (planum cutaneum) is palpable (► Fig. 6.11, ► Fig. 6.12).

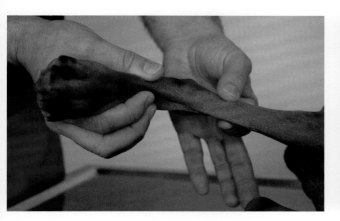

► **Fig. 6.11** Palpation of the distal portion of the tibia and fibula. (source: Gaby Ernst, Saland, Switzerland)

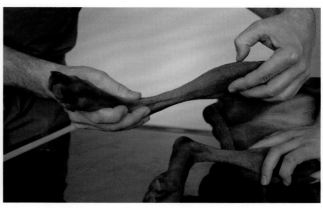

► **Fig. 6.12** Neoplasia may occur in the proximal tibia. (source: Gaby Ernst, Saland, Switzerland)

🗷 Findings and Differential Diagnosis

- swelling
  - neoplasia (p. 194)
  - hematoma
  - compartment syndrome
- crepitation
  - fracture
  - neoplasia (p. 194)
- pain in distal physis
  - malleolus fracture
  - fracture involving growth plate
  - growth disorder e.g. hypertrophic osteodystrophy (p. 189)
- pain in diaphysis
  - fracture
  - neoplasia (p. 194)
  - panosteitis (p. 188)
- pain in proximal physis
  - fracture involving growth plate
  - Osgood-Schlatter disease (p. 209) (large young dogs)
  - neoplasia (p. 194)
  - avulsion fracture of the tibial tuberosity
- pain in muscle belly
  - compartment syndrome

Overview of Common Findings and Video Demonstration

The following table (▶ Table 6.3) provides an overview of common findings in this region.

▶ **Tab. 6.3** Overview of findings.

Location	Finding	Interpretation	Frequency
–	abnormal contours	• neoplasia	+
		• hematoma	+
		• compartment syndrome	+
distal physis	heat and/or pain	• malleolus fracture	+ +
		• fracture involving growth plate	+
		• growth disorder e.g. hypertrophic osteodystrophy	+
diaphysis	heat and/or pain	• fracture	+ +
		• neoplasia	+
		• panosteitis	+
proximal physis	heat and/or pain	• fracture involving growth plate	+
		• Osgood-Schlatter disease (large young dogs)	+
		• neoplasia	+ +
		• avulsion fracture of tibial tuberosity	+
muscle belly	heat and/or pain	• compartment syndrome	+
–	crepitation	• fracture	+ +
		• neoplasia	+

Refer to ▶ **Video 6.3** for a video showing examination of the crural region of a dog in recumbency.

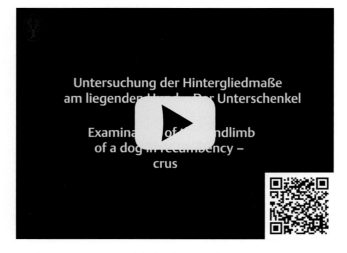

▶ **Video 6.3** Examination of the hindlimb of a dog in recumbency – crus. This sequence includes palpation of the crural region including tibia and fibula, styloid processes, the planum cutaneum and the tibialis cranialis, extensor digitorum lateralis and gastrocnemius. (source: Tele D, Diessenhofen, Switzerland)

6.2.4 Stifle Joint

Extension and Flexion

The tibial tuberosity, patellar ligament and patella are identified (▶ Fig. 6.13) and the stifle joint is flexed and extended. As the joint is manipulated, the thumb and index finger of one hand are used to assess the cranial part of the joint for heat, fluctuation, swelling and crepitation (▶ Fig. 6.14). Where joint pathology is present, pain is most likely to be elicited at maximum extension. Virtually all abnormalities of the stifle joint result in marked swelling. Low grade patellar luxation is a possible exception.

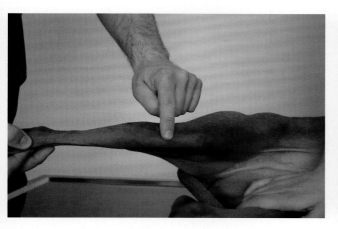

▶ **Fig. 6.13** The reference point for examination of the stifle joint is the cranial border of the tibial tuberosity. (source: Gaby Ernst, Saland, Switzerland)

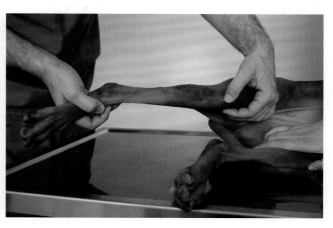

▶ **Fig. 6.14** Examination of the stifle joint: the right hand is rested on the stifle joint to detect crepitation and swelling, while the left hand is used to manipulate the tarsus to flex and extend the stifle joint. (source: Gaby Ernst, Saland, Switzerland)

🔧 Findings and Differential Diagnosis

- swelling of the stifle joint
  - cruciate ligament rupture (p. 201)
  - partial cruciate ligament rupture (p. 201) (pain particularly on internal rotation)
  - meniscal lesion following cruciate ligament rupture
  - joint fracture
  - bite wound
  - avulsion of the extensor digitorum lateralis (p. 209)
  - osteochondritic lesion on the lateral femoral condyle (usually young dogs)
  - insertional patellar tendinitis, so-called Osgood-Schlatter disease (p. 209) (usually affects young dogs)
  - patellar luxation (p. 204)
  - polyarthritis (p. 191)

- crepitation
  - cruciate ligament rupture (p. 201) or chronic partial cruciate ligament rupture
  - poorly healed joint fracture
  - untreated osteochondritic lesion
  - joint erosion in German Shepherd Dogs
  - patellar fracture

Assessment of the Collateral Ligaments

The collateral ligaments are assessed with the stifle joint in extension. The tibia is abducted, adducted and rotated relative to the femur (▶ Fig. 6.15, ▶ Fig. 6.16). In the normal joint, the range of movement is 5–10°.

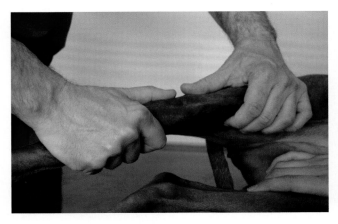

▶ **Fig. 6.15** Assessment of the collateral ligaments of the stifle joint for lateral stability. (source: Gaby Ernst, Saland, Switzerland)

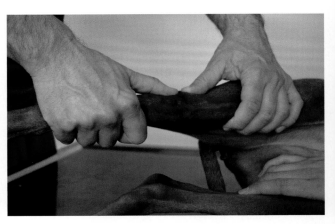

▶ **Fig. 6.16** Assessment of the collateral ligaments of the stifle joint for medial stability. (source: Gaby Ernst, Saland, Switzerland)

🗭 Findings and Differential Diagnosis

- medial hypermobility
  - medial collateral ligament rupture, detachment usually occurs at the femur; in small dogs, cranial cruciate ligament rupture (p. 201) can also result in increased medial instability
- lateral hypermobility
  - lateral collateral ligament rupture
  - fibular head fracture

Patellar Luxation Testing

Assessment of patellar luxation and reduction should be conducted across the normal range of hindlimb positions and joint angles. With one hand, the examiner grasps the leg at the tarsus. This hand is used to flex and extend the limb and to bring about internal and external rotation. The other hand is rested on the patella.

Initially, the resting position of the patella is determined (▶ Fig. 6.17). If the patella is in its normal position, the examiner attempts to luxate it medially and laterally. For anatomical reasons, medial luxation can be induced most readily when the hip and stifle joints are extended and the tibia is rotated internally (▶ Fig. 6.18). Lateral patellar luxation is most likely to be induced when the hip and stifle joints are flexed and the tibia is externally rotated (▶ Fig. 6.19).

The patella is then reduced, while subjecting the limb to various movements and manipulations.

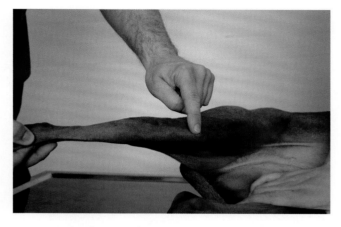

▶ **Fig. 6.17** Identification of the position of the patella. (source: Gaby Ernst, Saland, Switzerland)

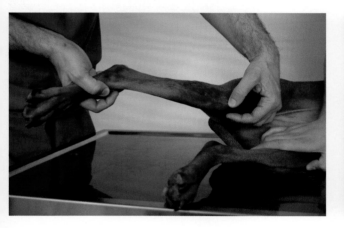

▶ **Fig. 6.18** Medial luxation of the patella: this is most easily induced when the hip and stifle joints are extended and the limb is rotated internally. (source: Gaby Ernst, Saland, Switzerland)

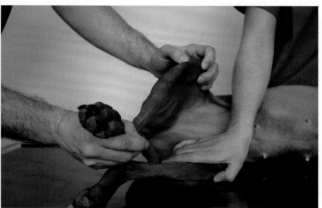

▶ **Fig. 6.19** Lateral luxation of the patella: this is most easily induced when the hip and stifle joints are flexed and the limb is rotated externally. (source: Gaby Ernst, Saland, Switzerland)

☑ Findings

In order to obtain meaningful data (▶ Table 6.4, ▶ Fig. 8.38), the following should be noted:
- Dogs should be examined in **all physiologically normal positions** (standing, recumbent, normal range of flexion, extension and rotation).
- Forces applied to the limb to induce luxation should be in the normal **physiological range**.

- The recorded finding should correspond to the **highest observed grade of abnormality**, based on the table below.
- If the patella can be pushed towards the trochlear ridges but cannot be fully luxated (a so-called riding patella), a result of „0" is recorded.
- Both medial and lateral luxation must be attempted [92].

▶ **Tab. 6.4** Findings.

Finding	Position of Patella	Induction of medial/lateral Patellar Luxation	Reduction of Patella
PL 0	in the trochlea	impossible	–
PL 1	in the trochlea	possible	spontaneous reduction
PL 2	in the trochlea	possible	patella springs back into trochlea when limb is manipulated (rotation of tibia, flexion and extension of joints)
PL 3	outside the trochlea	already luxated	patella remains luxated when the limb is manipulated, patella can only be reduced manually
PL 4	outside the trochlea	already luxated	patella cannot be returned to the trochlea by manipulation of the limb or manual reduction

Cranial Drawer Test

To perform the cranial drawer test, the index finger and thumb of one hand are used to grasp the patella and the region surrounding the lateral sesamoid bone of the gastrocnemius respectively. The other hand is used to grasp the tibial tuberosity and the head of the fibula (▶ Fig. 6.20). The cranial drawer test should be performed with the stifle joint slightly flexed (5–15°), rather than in full extension. The tibia is pushed cranially, without flexing or extending the joint. Movement of the tibia relative to the femur is assessed and any pain is noted (▶ Fig. 6.21).

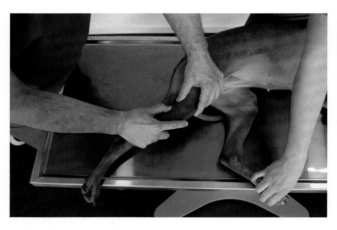

▶ **Fig. 6.20** Positioning of the hands and fingers for the cranial drawer test for diagnosis of cruciate ligament rupture. (source: Gaby Ernst, Saland, Switzerland)

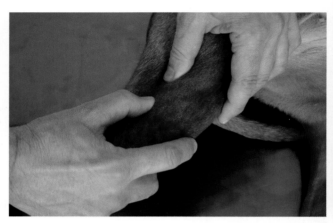

▶ **Fig. 6.21** The hand grasping the tibia pushes the tibia cranially to test for instability and pain. (source: Gaby Ernst, Saland, Switzerland)

◪ Findings and Differential Diagnosis
- instability: movement of the tibia relative to the femur
  - cranial or caudal cruciate ligament rupture (p. 201)
- instability with reduced restriction of cranial movement of the tibia
  - cranial cruciate ligament rupture (p. 201)
- instability with abrupt restriction of cranial movement of the tibia
  - caudal cruciate ligament rupture (p. 201)
- joint is stable but pain is elicited when the cranial drawer test is performed together with slight internal rotation of tibia
  - partial cranial cruciate ligament rupture (p. 201)
  - complete cranial cruciate ligament rupture (p. 201) with meniscal entrapment

Tibial Compression Test

The alternative to the cranial drawer test is the tibial compression test. The inside of one hand is pressed against the patella and the tip of the index finger is placed on the cranial border of the tibial tuberosity. The other hand grasps the metatarsal bones (▶ **Fig. 6.22**). The stifle and tarsal joints are then fully extended, whereupon the tarsal joint is flexed. Due to the recipro-cal arrangement of the cranial and caudal muscles of the crus, flexion of the tarsal joint brings the tibia into compression. If the cranial cruciate ligament is ruptured, the proximal tibia moves cranially, which is felt at the tip of the index finger (▶ **Fig. 6.23**).

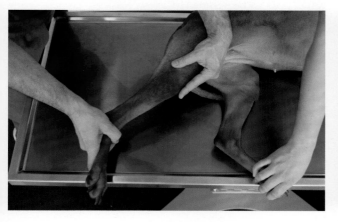

▶ **Fig. 6.22** Positioning of the hands and fingers for the tibial compression test for diagnosis of cranial cruciate ligament rupture; the tarsal and stifle joints are placed in extension, then the tarsal joint is flexed. (source: Gaby Ernst, Saland, Switzerland)

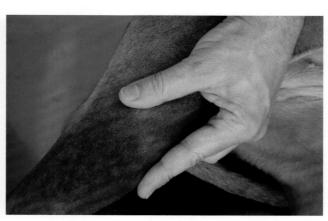

▶ **Fig. 6.23** Tibial compression test: if the cranial cruciate ligament is ruptured, the proximal part of the tibia moves cranially when the tarsal joint is flexed. (source: Gaby Ernst, Saland, Switzerland)

✎ Findings and Differential Diagnosis

- tibia moves cranially
  - cranial cruciate ligament rupture (p. 201)
- tibia does not move cranially
  - normal stifle joint
  - partial cruciate ligament rupture (p. 201)
  - caudal cruciate ligament rupture (p. 201)
  - cranial cruciate ligament rupture (p. 201) with meniscal entrapment
  - extensive fibrosis of the joint capsule

Assessment of the Menisci

Deep palpation between the tibia and femur may permit detection of a meniscus lesion (▶ Fig. 6.24). Folding of the meniscus leads to repeatable crepitation and elicitation of pain on flexion and extension of the stifle joint, occurring consistently at the same joint angle. The absence of this typical meniscal click does not confirm that the meniscus is normal.

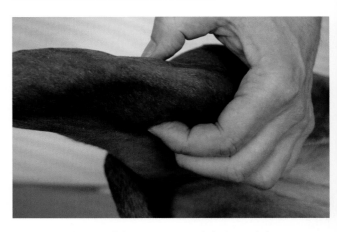

▶ **Fig. 6.24** Palpation of the menisci. Particularly the medial meniscus may be injured following cruciate ligament rupture. (source: Gaby Ernst, Saland, Switzerland)

Findings and Differential Diagnosis
- crepitation and pain
  - folded or entrapped caudal horn of the medial meniscus

Overview of Common Findings and Video Demonstration

The following table (▶ **Table 6.5**) provides an overview of common findings in this region.

▶ **Tab. 6.5** Overview of findings.

Location/Test	Finding	Interpretation	Frequency
flexion and extension	swelling	• cruciate ligament rupture	+++
		• partial cruciate ligament rupture (pain particularly on internal rotation)	+++
		• meniscal lesion following cruciate ligament rupture	++
		• joint fracture	+
		• bite wound	+
		• avulsion of extensor digitorum lateralis	+
		• osteochondritic lesion on lateral femoral condyle (usually young dogs)	+
		• insertional patellar tendinitis (Osgood-Schlatter disease, usually affects young dogs)	+
		• patellar luxation	+++
		• polyarthritis	+
	crepitation	• cruciate ligament rupture or chronic partial cruciate ligament rupture	+++
		• poorly healed joint fracture	+
		• untreated osteochondritic lesion	+
		• joint erosion in German Shepherd Dogs	+
		• patellar fracture	+
assessment of collateral ligament	medial hypermobility	• medial collateral ligament rupture, usually at the femur	+
		• in small dogs, cranial cruciate ligament rupture can also result in increased medial instability	+
	lateral hypermobility	• lateral collateral ligament rupture	+
		• fibular head fracture	+
cranial drawer test	pain when test performed together with slight internal tibial rotation	• partial cruciate ligament rupture	+++
		• complete cranial cruciate ligament rupture with meniscal entrapment	+++
	instability: tibia moves relative to femur	• cranial or caudal cruciate ligament rupture	+++
	instability with reduced restriction of cranial movement of tibia	• cranial cruciate ligament rupture	+++
	instability with abrupt restriction of cranial movement of tibia	• caudal cruciate ligament rupture	+
tibial compression test	tibia moves cranially	• cranial cruciate ligament rupture	+++
	tibia does not move cranially	• normal stifle joint	
		• partial cruciate ligament rupture	+++
		• caudal cruciate ligament rupture	+++
		• cranial cruciate ligament rupture with meniscal entrapment	+++
		• extensive joint capsule fibrosis	++
meniscus testing	crepitation and pain	• folded or entrapped caudal horn of medial meniscus	++

Refer to ▶ **Video 6.4** for a video showing examination of the stifle of a dog in recumbency.

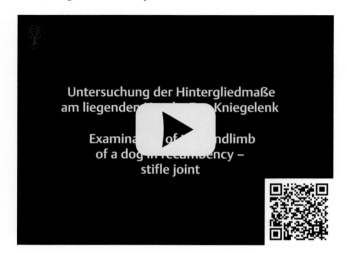

▶ **Video 6.4** Examination of the hindlimb of a dog in recumbency – stifle joint. This sequence includes location and assessment of the stifle joint, including the collateral ligaments, menisci and the patella, induction of patellar luxation, the cranial drawer test and the tibial compression test. (source: Tele D, Diessenhofen, Switzerland)

6.2.5 Femur

The femur is palpated from distal to proximal. The bone is readily palpable distally and medially. At the proximal end of the femur, the greater trochanter can be palpated on the lateral side (▶ Fig. 6.25).

The quadriceps femoris and the ischiocrural muscles are tested for induration and pain (▶ Fig. 6.26).

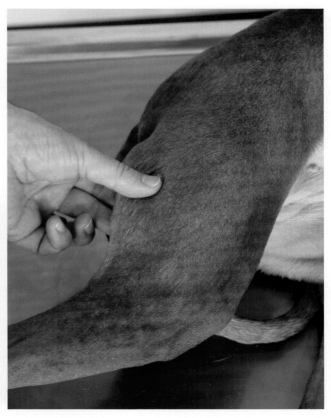

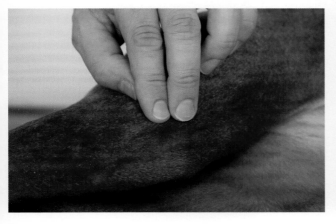

▶ **Fig. 6.25** Only the distal portion of the femur is readily palpable. (source: Gaby Ernst, Saland, Switzerland)

▶ **Fig. 6.26** Fibrosis of the ischiocrural muscles results in induration and pain. It is particularly common in German Shepherd Dogs. (source: Gaby Ernst, Saland, Switzerland)

> **⚡ Findings and Differential Diagnosis**
> - pain and crepitation
>   - fracture
>   - neoplasia (p. 194)
> - pain
>   - panosteitis (p. 188)
>   - hypertrophic osteodystrophy (p. 189)
> - muscle induration
>   - contracture following trauma
>   - fibrosis of ischiocrural muscles
>   - compartment syndrome

Overview of Common Findings and Video Demonstration

The following table (▶ Table 6.6) provides an overview of common findings in this region.

▶ **Tab. 6.6** Overview of findings.

Location	Finding	Interpretation	Frequency
femur	pain	• panosteitis	+
		• hypertrophic osteodystrophy	+
	pain and crepitation	• fracture	+ + +
		• neoplasia	+ +
	muscle induration	• contracture following trauma	+
		• fibrosis of ischiocrural muscles	+
		• compartment syndrome	+

Refer to ▶ **Video 6.5** for a video showing examination of the femur of a dog in recumbency.

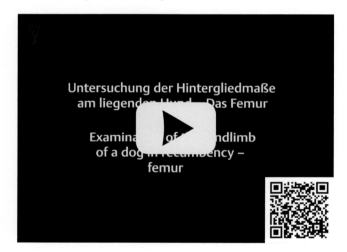

▶ **Video 6.5** Examination of the hindlimb of a dog in recumbency – femur. This sequence includes palpation of the thigh muscles – semimembranosus and semitendinosus („hamstring muscles"), biceps femoris and quadriceps – and the femur. (source: Tele D, Diessenhofen, Switzerland)

6.2.6 Hip Joint

Flexion and Extension of the Hip Joint

With one hand placed over the hip joint and the other grasping the distal femur, the hip joint is moved in all directions (▶ Fig. 6.28, ▶ Fig. 6.29). It should be possible to extend and flex the hip joint to such an extent that the femur is almost parallel to the vertebral column. The pectineus is palpated while the joint is being manipulated (▶ Fig. 6.27).

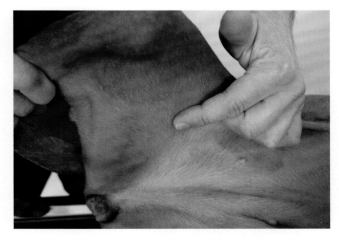

▶ **Fig. 6.27** Palpation of the pectineus. Contracture secondary to coxofemoral osteoarthritis or hip dysplasia leads to restriction of the range of motion of the hip joint and pain on direct digital palpation. (source: Gaby Ernst, Saland, Switzerland)

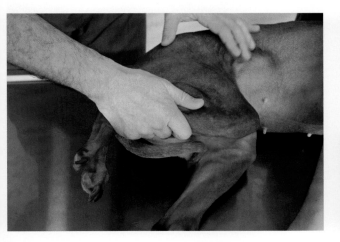

▶ **Fig. 6.28** Flexion of the hip joint. The examiner's thumb is positioned over the greater trochanter to assess the reaction of the hip joint during manipulation. (source: Gaby Ernst, Saland, Switzerland)

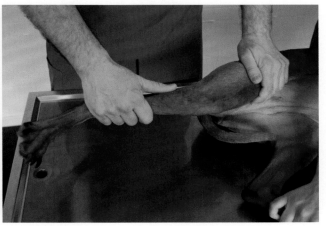

▶ **Fig. 6.29** In healthy dogs, the femur should be approximately parallel to the backline when the hip is fully extended. (source: Gaby Ernst, Saland, Switzerland)

🗒 Findings and Differential Diagnosis

- hypomobility, pain
  - hip dysplasia (p. 212)
  - Legg-Perthes disease (p. 210)
  - luxation (p. 218)
  - neoplasia (p. 194)
  - iliopsoas strain
  - cauda equina compression syndrome
  - intervertebral disc disease in lumbar vertebral column
- crepitation
  - coxofemoral osteoarthritis (p. 212)
  - joint fracture
  - femoral neck fracture
  - neoplasia (p. 194)
  - luxation (p. 218)
- pain in pectineus
  - hip dysplasia (p. 212)
  - coxofemoral osteoarthritis (p. 212)

Rotation of the Femur

With the femoral shaft at 90° to the longitudinal axis of the pelvis, the femur is rotated internally through 45° and externally through 90° (▶ Fig. 6.30, ▶ Fig. 6.31). It should be possible to abduct the femur to an angle of approximately 90° to the tabletop.

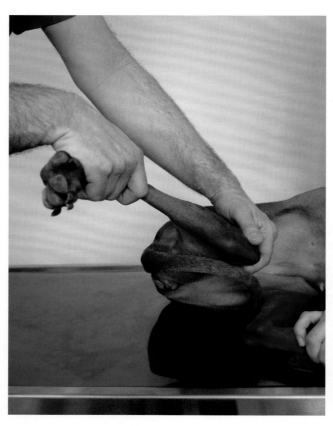

▶ **Fig. 6.30** Internal rotation of the femur for assessment of hip joint mobility. The femur should reach an angle of 45° to the tabletop. (source: Gaby Ernst, Saland, Switzerland)

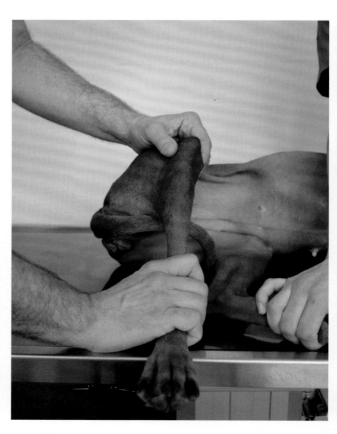

▶ **Fig. 6.31** External rotation of the femur for examination of hip joint mobility. The femur should reach an angle of 90° to the tabletop. (source: Gaby Ernst, Saland, Switzerland)

⚡ Findings and Differential Diagnosis

- reduced rotation
  - coxofemoral osteoarthritis (p. 212)
  - Legg-Perthes disease (p. 210)
  - neoplasia (p. 194)
- excessive rotation
  - hip joint luxation (p. 218)
  - femoral head fracture

Testing for Luxation

The examiner places his thumb in the small depression between the greater trochanter and the ischial tuberosity. The femur is then rotated externally. If the hip is not luxated, the two bony prominences move closer together, trapping the examiner's thumb between them. If the hip is luxated craniodorsally, the head of the femur is able to move cranially and no pressure is exerted on the examiner's thumb (▶ Fig. 6.32).

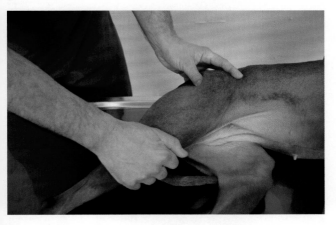

▶ **Fig. 6.32** Positioning of the examiner's hands for testing for craniodorsal hip joint luxation. (source: Gaby Ernst, Saland, Switzerland)

✿ Findings and Differential Diagnosis
- gap between the greater trochanter and ischial tuberosity stays the same or increases
  - craniodorsal luxation (p. 218)
  - femoral head fracture
- gap between the greater trochanter and ischial tuberosity decreases, placing pressure on the examiner's thumb
  - no luxation

Ortolani Test

The Ortolani test is used to assess the depth and shape of the acetabulum, and the congruence of the femoral head. The femur is first positioned at 90° to the longitudinal axis of the pelvis. The examiner places the thumb of one hand on the greater trochanter to detect movement associated with luxation. The other hand is used to grasp the femur at the stifle joint and direct the movement of the leg.

The femur is maximally adducted, then force is applied by the hand on the stifle in an attempt to luxate the femoral head dorsally. Without reducing the force on the long axis of the femur, the femur is slowly abducted until, if the joint has been subluxated by the dorsally directed force, the femoral head springs back into the acetabulum (▶ Fig. 6.33, ▶ Fig. 6.34, ▶ Video 6.6). This movement is detected by the hand placed on the trochanter.

As the Ortolani test places considerable strain on the dorsal acetabular rim, it is contraindicated in dogs under 5 months of age, in which the joint margins are fragile.

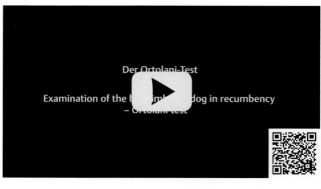

▶ **Video 6.6** Ortolani-Test. This sequence demonstrates the principle of the Ortolani test using a model skeleton.

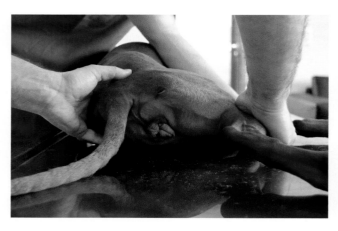

▶ **Fig. 6.33** Ortolani test. The femur is adducted and then pushed dorsally. If the joint is unstable, this manipulation results in dorsal subluxation of the hip joint. (source: Gaby Ernst, Saland, Switzerland)

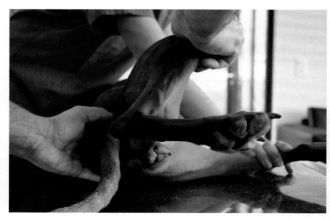

▶ **Fig. 6.34** Ortolani-Test. The femur is abducted under axial pressure until the femoral head springs back into the acetabulum. (source: Gaby Ernst, Saland, Switzerland)

⚡ Findings and Differential Diagnosis

- no detectable reduction of the femoral head, no pain, normal range of movement
  - normal hip joint
- no detectable reduction of the femoral head, pain, hypomobility
  - low grade hip dysplasia (p. 212)
  - coxofemoral osteoarthritis (p. 212)
- detectable reduction of the femoral head
  - hip dysplasia (p. 212)

Bardens Test

The Bardens test is used as an alternative to the Ortolani test in dogs under 5 months of age. Initial positioning of the dog is the same as for the Ortolani test, with the femur at 90° to the longitudinal axis of the pelvis. The examiner then places both hands around the muscles in the proximal third of the thigh (► Fig. 6.35) and lifts the thigh vertically in an attempt to pull the femoral head upwards out of the hip joint (► Fig. 6.36).

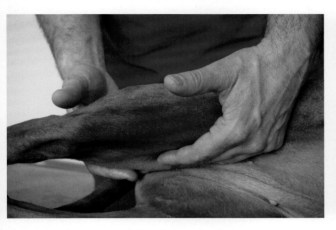

► **Fig. 6.35** Bardens test. The examiner's hands are placed around the muscles in the proximal third of the thigh. (source: Gaby Ernst, Saland, Switzerland)

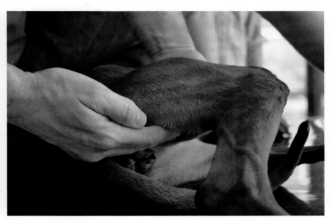

► **Fig. 6.36** Bardens test. The examiner lifts the thigh in an attempt to pull the femoral head out of the acetabulum. (source: Gaby Ernst, Saland, Switzerland)

Findings and Differential Diagnosis
- no movement indicative of luxation
  - normal hip joint
  - low grade hip dysplasia (p. 212)
- movement indicative of luxation
  - hip dysplasia (p. 212)

Overview of Common Findings and Video Demonstration

The following table (▶ **Table 6.7**) provides an overview of common findings in this region.

▶ **Tab. 6.7** Overview of findings.

Location/Test	Finding	Interpretation	Disease frequency
hip joint	pain in pectineus	• hip dysplasia	+++
		• coxofemoral osteoarthritis	+++
	pain and/or heat	• hip dysplasia	+++
		• Legg-Perthes disease	+
		• luxation	++
		• neoplasia	+
		• iliopsoas strain	+
		• cauda equina compression syndrome	+++
		• intervertebral disc disease in lumbar vertebral column	+
	hypomobility	• hip joint dysplasia	+++
		• Legg-Perthes disease	+
		• luxation	++
		• neoplasia	+
		• iliopsoas strain	+
		• cauda equina-compression syndrome	+++
		• intervertebral disc disease in lumbar vertebral column	+
	crepitation	• coxofemoral osteoarthritis	+++
		• joint fracture	+
		• femoral neck fracture	++
		• neoplasia	+
		• luxation	++
testing for luxation	gap between greater trochanter and ischial tuberosity remains the same or increases	• craniodorsal luxation	++
		• femoral head fracture	+
	gap between greater trochanter and ischial tuberosity decreases, placing pressure on examiner's thumb	• no luxation	
Ortolani test	no detectable reduction of femoral head, no pain, normal range of movement	• normal hip joint	
	no detectable reduction of femoral head, pain, hypomobility	• low grade hip dysplasia	+++
		• coxofemoral osteoarthritis	+++
	detectable reduction of femoral head, pain and hypomobility	• hip dysplasia	+++
Bardens test	no movement indicative of luxation	• normal hip joint	
		• low grade hip dysplasia	+++
	movement indicative of luxation	• hip dysplasia	+++

Refer to ▶ **Video 6.7** for a video showing examination of the hip joint of a dog in recumbency.

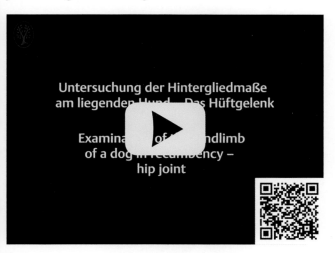

▶ **Video 6.7** Examination of the hindlimb of a dog in recumbency – hip joint. This sequence includes assessment of hip joint stability (including luxation testing), palpation of the pectineus, the Ortolani test for hip dysplasia (positive Ortolani sign) and the Bardens test. (source: Tele D, Diessenhofen, Switzerland)

6.3
Forelimb

6.3.1 Digits, Metacarpus and Carpus

Overall Evaluation

The skin of the paw and the interdigital region is inspected and the digital pads are palpated (▶ Fig. 6.37). The digits and metacarpals are then grasped and latero-medially compressed to check for a pain response. The paws, joints and metacarpals are examined for abnormal surface contours (▶ Fig. 6.38).

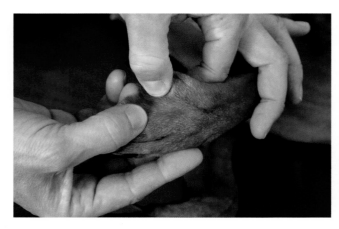

▶ **Fig. 6.37** Examination of the skin and interdigital region of the front foot. (source: Gaby Ernst, Saland, Switzerland)

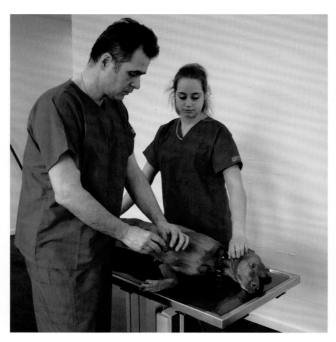

▶ **Fig. 6.38** Assessment of the metacarpals for pain, heat and abnormal surface contours. (source: Gaby Ernst, Saland, Switzerland)

⚙ Findings and Differential Diagnosis
- reddening of the interdigital skin
  - allergy
- abnormal surface contours
  - neoplasia (p. 194)
- pain, heat
  - neoplasia (p. 194)
  - fracture
  - luxation
  - foreign body

Examination of the Digital Joints

The joints are examined for evidence of heat and surface irregularities. Each individual joint is flexed, extended, adducted and abducted (▶ Fig. 6.39). While one hand is used to examine joint mobility, the other tests for heat, swelling, crepitation, axial deviation, hypomobility and hypermobility. Any pain responses should be noted. The sesamoid bones of the flexor tendons are examined by hyperextending the metacarpophalangeal joints (▶ Fig. 6.40).

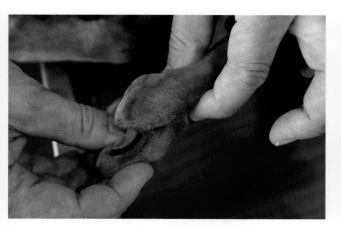

▶ **Fig. 6.39** Examination of the digital joints using the same technique as in the hindlimb. (source: Gaby Ernst, Saland, Switzerland)

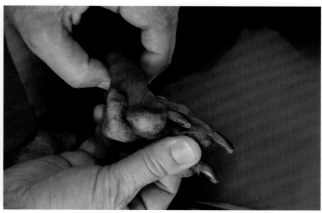

▶ **Fig. 6.40** As in the hindlimb, each of the sesamoid bones in the flexor tendons of the forelimb should be examined. The metacarpophalangeal joints are hyperextended to check for a pain response. (source: Gaby Ernst, Saland, Switzerland)

Findings and Differential Diagnosis

- crepitation
  - joint fracture
- heat
  - polyarthritis (p. 191)
  - allergy
- axial deviation
  - collateral ligament rupture
  - fracture
- hypomobility
  - sesamoid bone fragmentation (p. 220)
  - chronic joint disorder

- hypermobility
  - flexor or extensor tendon rupture
  - joint capsule tear
  - nerve lesion
- pain
  - joint fracture
  - polyarthritis (p. 191)
  - sesamoid disease (p. 220)
  - joint capsule/ligament trauma

Carpus

The intercarpal bones are normally immobile. The bones are palpated and the short ligaments are assessed by extending, flexing, abducting and adducting the carpal joint (▶ Fig. 6.41).

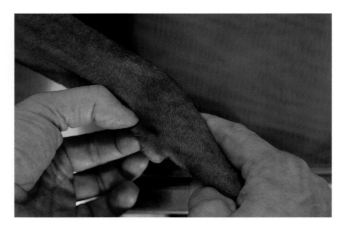

▶ **Fig. 6.41** Examination of the carpal bones. (source: Gaby Ernst, Saland, Switzerland)

> ### 🔲 Findings and Differential Diagnosis
>
> - hypermobility
>   - luxation
>   - fracture
> - painful, unstable accessory carpal bone
>   - accessory carpal bone fracture

Overview of Common Findings and Video Demonstration

The following table (▶ Table 6.8) provides an overview of common findings in this region.

▶ **Tab. 6.8** Overview of findings.

Location/Test	Finding	Interpretation	Frequency
overall evaluation	reddening of interdigital skin	• allergy	+
	abnormal surface contours	• neoplasia	+
	pain, heat	• neoplasia	+
		• fracture	+ +
		• luxation	+
		• foreign body	+ +
examination of digital joints	heat	• polyarthritis	+ +
		• allergy	+
	pain	• joint fracture	+ +
		• polyarthritis	+ +
		• sesamoid disease	+
		• joint capsule/ligament trauma	+ +
	painful and unstable accessory carpal bone	• accessory carpal bone fracture	+
	hypomobility	• sesamoid bone fragmentation	+
		• chronic joint disorder	+
	hypermobility	• flexor or extensor tendon rupture	+
		• joint capsule tear	+ +
		• nerve lesion	+
	crepitation	• joint fracture	+ +
	axial deviation	• collateral ligament rupture	+ +
		• fracture	+ +
carpus	hypermobility	• luxation	+
		• fracture	+ +

Refer to ▶ **Video 6.8** for a video showing examination of the region from the digits to the carpus of a dog in recumbency.

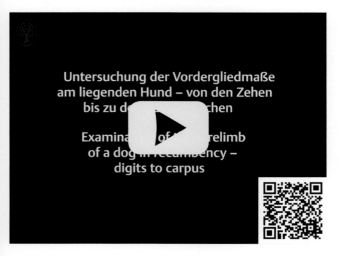

▶ **Video 6.8** Examination of the forelimb of a dog in recumbency – digits to carpus. This sequence includes palpation and assessment of the digits and digital joints (including sesamoid bones) and palpation of the metacarpal bones. (source: Tele D, Diessenhofen, Switzerland)

6.3.2 Carpal Joint

Antebrachiocarpal Joint

The antebrachiocarpal joint consists primarily of short lateral ligaments that are assessed with the joint in extension. The normal range of abduction and adduction is 8–12°.

The joint is then maximally flexed and extended.

A small oblique ligament connects the styloid process of the radius with the palmar aspect of the intermedioradial carpal bone. It is assessed using a drawer-like movement, similar to that used in the stifle joint. Working from the lateral aspect, one hand grasps the distal antebrachium, the other the carpal bones. With the joint aligned at 180°, the hand on the carpal bones is pushed cranially (▶ Fig. 6.42, ▶ Fig. 6.43, ▶ Fig. 6.44, ▶ Fig. 6.45). In normal dogs, a drawer motion cannot be elicited.

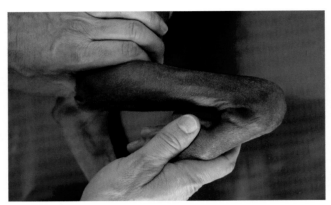

▶ **Fig. 6.42** Flexion testing of the carpus. The range of movement of the antebrachiocarpal joint is increased when the elbow joint is concurrently flexed. (source: Gaby Ernst, Saland, Switzerland)

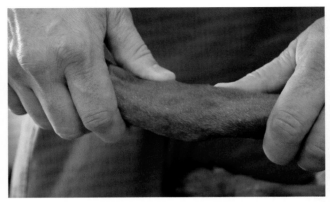

▶ **Fig. 6.44** Assessment of the structural integrity of the collateral ligaments by abduction and adduction of the carpus. (source: Gaby Ernst, Saland, Switzerland)

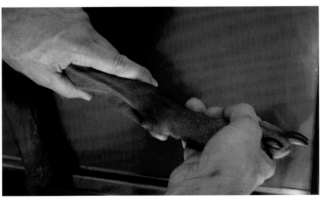

▶ **Fig. 6.43** Maximal extension of the carpus. (source: Gaby Ernst, Saland, Switzerland)

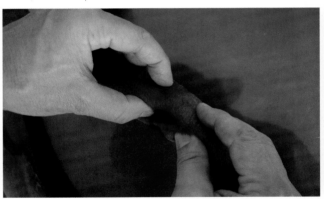

▶ **Fig. 6.45** Carpal drawer test for assessment of the oblique portion of the medial collateral ligament. (source: Gaby Ernst, Saland, Switzerland)

🗲 Findings and Differential Diagnosis

- hypermobility
  - collateral ligament rupture
  - fracture of the styloid process or bone(s) of the carpus, ligament injury of carpometacarpal or intercarpal joints
  - instability following hyperextension trauma (p. 221)
- hypomobility in extension/flexion
  - previous ligament trauma
  - fracture
- positive drawer test
  - rupture of the oblique portion of the medial collateral ligament

Assessment of the Abductor Pollicis Longus Tendon

The tendon of insertion of the abductor pollicis longus courses over the craniomedial side of the radius within a tendon sheath. It crosses the radiocarpal joint directly beneath the collateral ligament.

The tendon is assessed by direct palpation for heat, swelling and pain.

In a manipulation analogous to the Finkelstein test used in human medicine, the tendon can be placed under maximum tension by simultaneous maximal flexion and abduction of the carpal joint (► Fig. 6.46, ► Fig. 6.47). This may elicit a pain response in the tendon.

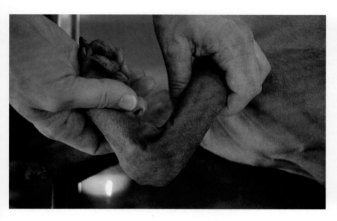

► **Fig. 6.46** Application of maximum tension to the tendon of insertion of the abductor pollicis longus by simultaneous flexion and abduction of the carpus. (source: Gaby Ernst, Saland, Switzerland)

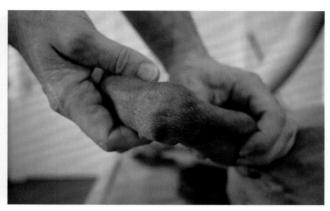

► **Fig. 6.47** Assessment of the abductor pollicis longus, cranial view. (source: Gaby Ernst, Saland, Switzerland)

⚡ Findings and Differential Diagnosis
- pain, heat and swelling in the distal medial quarter of the radius
  - tendovaginitis of the abductor pollicis longus (p.223)
  - osteosarcoma (p.194) of the distal radius
- pain elicited by specialized tendon test (modified Finkelstein test)
  - tendovaginitis of the abductor pollicis longus (p.223)

Overview of Common Findings and Video Demonstration

The following table (▶ **Table 6.9**) provides an overview of common findings in this region.

▶ **Tab. 6.9** Overview of findings.

Location/Test	Finding	Interpretation	Frequency
antebrachiocarpal joint	hypomobility in extension/flexion	• previous ligament trauma	+
		• fracture	+
	hypermobility	• collateral ligament rupture	+ +
		• fracture of styloid process or bone(s) of the carpus, ligament injury of carpometacarpal or intercarpal joints	+
		• instability following hyperextension trauma	+ +
assessment of abductor pollicis longus tendon	pain, heat and swelling in distal medial quarter of radius	• tendovaginitis of abductor pollicis longus	+ +
		• osteosarcoma of distal radius	+ +
	pain elicited by specialized tendon test (modified Finkelstein test)	• tendovaginitis of abductor pollicis longus	+ +
	positive drawer test	• rupture of oblique portion of medial collateral ligament	+

Refer to ▶ **Video 6.9** for a video showing examination of the carpal joint of a dog in recumbency.

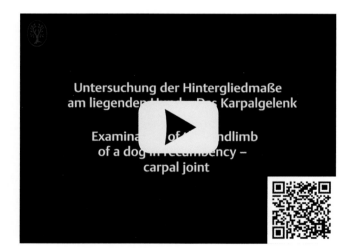

▶ **Video 6.9** Examination of the forelimb of a dog in recumbency – carpal joint. This sequence includes palpation and assessment of the carpal joint (ulnar carpal bone, intermedioradial carpal bone, accessory carpal bone) including the drawer test, and palpation and assessment of the abductor pollicis longus. (source: Tele D, Diessenhofen, Switzerland)

6.3.3 Radius and Ulna

The radius is palpable distomedially at the styloid process and proximally at the lateral aspect of the radial head. The palpable features of the ulna are the styloid process, distolaterally, and the olecranon, proximally. The radius and ulna are tested for pain on palpation and crepitation. The antebrachium is rotated to ascertain the relative mobility of both bones (▶ Fig. 6.48, ▶ Fig. 6.49, ▶ Fig. 6.50).

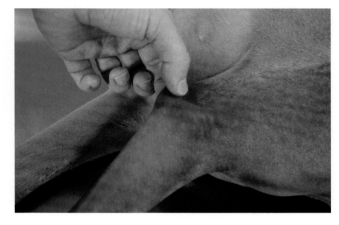

▶ **Fig. 6.48** Panosteitis frequently affects the olecranon. (source: Gaby Ernst, Saland, Switzerland)

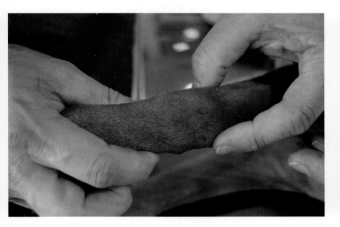

▶ **Fig. 6.49** Palpation of the medial and lateral styloid processes with the thumb and index finger. (source: Gaby Ernst, Saland, Switzerland)

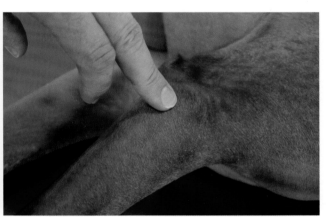

▶ **Fig. 6.50** Position of the extensor muscle group over the proximal radius. (source: Gaby Ernst, Saland, Switzerland)

🔲 Findings and Differential Diagnosis

- pain on palpation of distal third of bones
  - osteosarcoma
  - hypertrophic osteodystrophy osteodystrophyhypertrophic (p. 189)
  - retained cartilage cones (p. 190)
- pain on palpation of diaphysis
  - panosteitis (p. 188)
  - growth disorder
  - hypertrophic osteopathy (p. 189) (acropachy, paraneoplastic syndrome [lung tumor])
- pain on palpation of proximal third
  - panosteitis (p. 188)
  - elbow dysplasia (p. 224)
- valgus, exorotation and convex curvature of the radius
  - asynchronous growth of the radius and ulna following premature distal growth plate closure

Overview of Common Findings and Video Demonstration

The following table (▶ **Table 6.10**) provides an overview of common findings in this region.

▶ **Tab. 6.10** Overview of findings.

Location	Finding	Interpretation	Disease frequency
radius and ulna	pain on palpation of distal third	• osteosarcoma	+ +
		• hypertrophic osteodystrophy	+
		• retained cartilage cones	+
	pain on palpation of diaphysis	• panosteitis	+ + +
		• growth disorder	+
		• hypertrophic osteopathy	+
	pain on palpation of proximal third	• panosteitis	+ + +
		• elbow dysplasia	+ + +
	valgus, exorotation and convex curvature of radius	• asynchronous growth of radius and ulna following premature distal growth plate closure	+

Refer to ▶ **Video 6.10** for a video showing examination of the radius and ulna of a dog in recumbency.

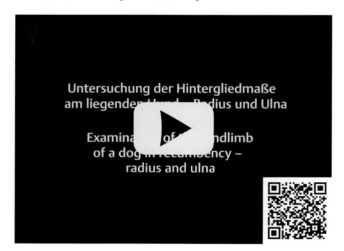

▶ **Video 6.10** Examination of the forelimb of a dog in recumbency – radius and ulna. This sequence includes palpation of the antebrachium, including the styloid processes and musculature. (source: Tele D, Diessenhofen, Switzerland)

6.3.4 Elbow Joint

Flexion and Extension

The elbow joint is fully flexed and extended (▸ Fig. 6.51, ▸ Fig. 6.52). As the joint is manipulated, the other hand is placed around the elbow to detect changes at, and within, the joint. Elicitation of pain is more intense on maximum extension than on flexion. When the joint is in maximum flexion, the anconeal process becomes palpable laterally (▸ Fig. 6.53).

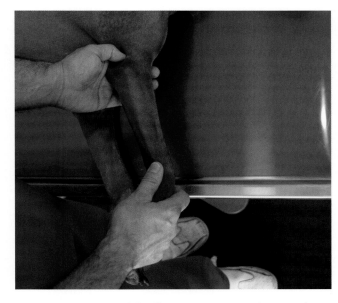

▸ **Fig. 6.51** Examination of the elbow joint in extension. (source: Gaby Ernst, Saland, Switzerland)

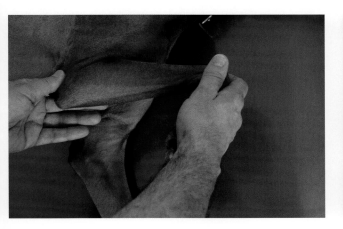

▸ **Fig. 6.52** Examination of the elbow joint in flexion. The carpus is used to manipulate the elbow joint. (source: Gaby Ernst, Saland, Switzerland)

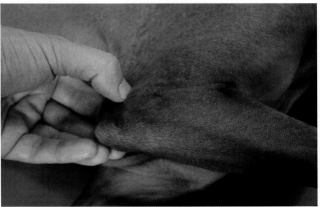

▸ **Fig. 6.53** The anconeal process can only be assessed when the elbow joint is in maximum flexion. (source: Gaby Ernst, Saland, Switzerland)

> ### ⚡ Findings and Differential Diagnosis
>
> - crepitation
>   - elbow osteoarthritis
>   - joint fracture
>   - incongruity
> - pain, heat
>   - elbow dysplasia (p. 224)
>   - elbow osteoarthritis
> - extensive effusion in the lateral compartment
>   - ununited anconeal process
>   - fracture of the lateral epicondyle (Salter Harris Type 4 fracture)

Assessment of the Collateral Ligaments

The collateral ligaments can be assessed with the elbow in extension and flexion (▶ Fig. 6.54). Maximum possible abduction and adduction of the extended joint should not exceed 10°. When the joint is flexed, the radius and ulna cross each other. In this position, external and internal rotation are limited by the medial and lateral collateral ligaments respectively. This is useful for assessing joint stability.

In most cases of collateral ligament rupture, the medial ligament is affected. Lateral luxation of the radial head occurs occasionally, manifesting as an abnormal surface contour (▶ Fig. 6.55, ▶ Fig. 6.56).

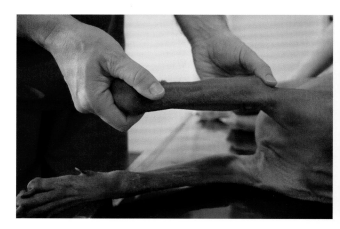

▶ **Fig. 6.54** Assessment of the collateral ligaments of the elbow via abduction and adduction of the joint. (source: Gaby Ernst, Saland, Switzerland)

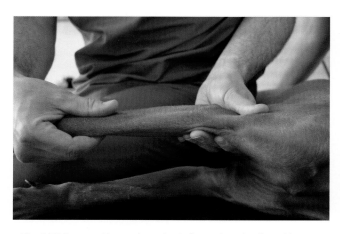

▶ **Fig. 6.55** Increased internal rotation indicates lateral collateral ligament rupture. (source: Gaby Ernst, Saland, Switzerland)

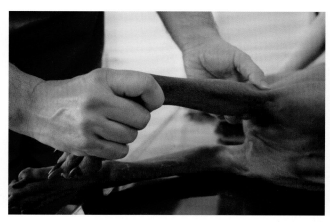

▶ **Fig. 6.56** Increased external rotation indicates medial collateral ligament rupture. (source: Gaby Ernst, Saland, Switzerland)

⚡ Findings and Differential Diagnosis

- increased external rotation of the flexed elbow joint, valgus when joint is extended
  - medial collateral ligament rupture
- increased internal rotation of the flexed elbow joint, varus when joint is extended
  - lateral collateral ligament rupture (rare)
- radial head located lateral to the humeral epicondyle, reduced elbow joint mobility, crepitation
  - lateral luxation of the elbow joint

Assessment of the Medial Compartment of the Elbow Joint

Two of the three common forms of elbow dysplasia (fragmented coronoid process, osteochondrosis of the medial humeral condyle) and their associated secondary changes („kissing" lesions on the medial humeral condyle, osteoarthritis) involve the medial joint compartment. These abnormalities are often referred to collectively as medial compartment syndrome.

The medial compartment is assessed by applying digital pressure directly to the medial coronoid process (► Fig. 6.57). Then, with the elbow in extension, the radius and ulna are rotated internally. If the medial collateral ligament is intact, this manipulation brings the medial coronoid process into direct contact with the humeral condyle. Any pain elicited by the resulting pressure on the coronoid process should be noted (► Fig. 6.58).

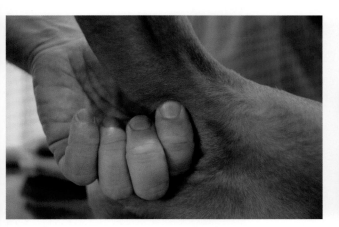

► **Fig. 6.57** Direct digital palpation of the medial coronoid process with the index finger. (source: Gaby Ernst, Saland, Switzerland)

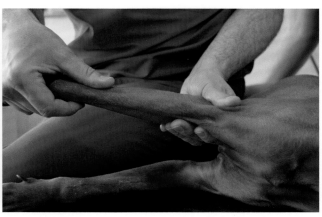

► **Fig. 6.58** Application of pressure to the medial coronoid process via internal rotation of the radius and ulna with the elbow joint in extension. (source: Gaby Ernst, Saland, Switzerland)

⚙ Findings and Differential Diagnosis

- pain on direct palpation of the medial coronoid process
  - elbow dysplasia (p. 224) (medial compartment syndrome)
  - fracture of the medial coronoid process
  - elbow osteoarthritis
- pain on internal rotation of the radius/ulna when the elbow is extended
  - fragmented medial coronoid process
  - osteochondrosis (p. 185) of the medial humeral condyle
  - elbow osteoarthritis
  - joint fracture
  - incongruity of the elbow joint

Overview of Common Findings and Video Demonstration

The following table (▶ **Table 6.11**) provides an overview of common findings in this region.

▶ **Tab. 6.11** Overview of findings.

Location/Test	Finding	Interpretation	Disease frequency
flexion and extension	pain, heat	• elbow dysplasia	+++
		• elbow osteoarthritis	+++
	crepitation	• elbow osteoarthritis	+++
		• joint fracture	+
		• incongruity	++
	extensive effusion in lateral compartment	• ununited anconeal process	++
		• fracture of lateral epicondyle (Salter Harris Type 4 fracture)	+
assessment of collateral ligaments	increased internal rotation of flexed elbow joint, valgus when elbow joint extended	• medial collateral ligament rupture	++
	increased external rotation of flexed elbow joint, varus when joint is extended	• lateral collateral ligament rupture (rare)	+
	radial head located lateral to humeral epicondyle, reduced elbow mobility, crepitation	• lateral elbow luxation	+
assessment of medial compartment of elbow joint	pain on direct palpation of medial coronoid process	• elbow dysplasia (medial compartment syndrome)	+++
		• fracture of medial coronoid process	+
		• elbow osteoarthritis	+++
	pain on internal rotation of radius/ulna	• fragmented medial coronoid process	+++
		• osteochondrosis of medial humeral condyle	+++
		• elbow osteoarthritis	+++
		• joint fracture	+
		• incongruity of elbow joint	++

Refer to ▶ **Video 6.11** for a video showing examination of the elbow joint of a dog in recumbency.

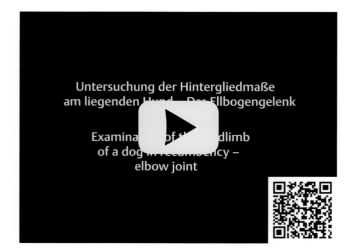

▶ **Video 6.11** Examination of the forelimb of a dog in recumbency – elbow joint. This sequence includes location of the elbow joint by palpation of the humeral epicondyle and assessment of the joint (including the collateral ligaments). (source: Tele D, Diessenhofen, Switzerland)

6.3.5 Humerus

The humerus is palpated from distal to proximal (▶ Fig. 6.59, ▶ Fig. 6.60). The radial nerve crosses the lateral aspect of the bone. Proximally, the greater tubercle and the proximal end of the humeral shaft are palpable.

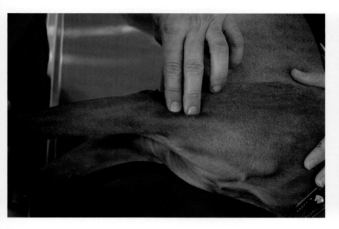

▶ **Fig. 6.59** The humerus can only be palpated directly at its distal end. (source: Gaby Ernst, Saland, Switzerland)

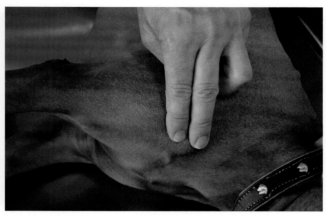

▶ **Fig. 6.60** The greater tubercle is readily palpable. (source: Gaby Ernst, Saland, Switzerland)

🔧 Findings and Differential Diagnosis

- pain on palpation
  - fracture
  - neoplasia (p. 194) of the proximal humerus
  - panosteitis (p. 188)
  - radial nerve injury
- crepitation
  - fracture

Overview of Common Findings and Video Demonstration

The following table (▶ **Table 6.12**) provides an overview of common findings in this region.

▶ **Tab. 6.12** Overview of findings.

Location	Finding	Interpretation	Frequency
humerus	pain on palpation	• fracture	+
		• neoplasia of proximal humerus	+ + +
		• panosteitis	+
		• radial nerve injury	+
	crepitation	• fracture	+

Refer to ▶ **Video 6.12** for a video showing examination of the humerus of a dog in recumbency.

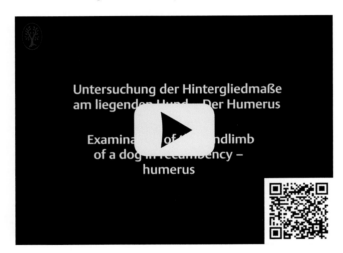

▶ **Video 6.12** Examination of the forelimb of a dog in recumbency – humerus. This sequence includes palpation of the humerus and the triceps brachii and biceps brachii, and assessment of the biceps brachii tendon for tendovaginitis. (source: Tele D, Diessenhofen, Switzerland)

6.3.6 Shoulder Region

Shoulder Joint

Examination of the shoulder joint is challenging, as it lies beneath several muscles. Cranially, the joint can be palpated medial to the biceps brachii tendon. Joint effusion is very difficult to detect. The joint should be extended and flexed and any pain noted.

The presence of an osteochondritic lesion at the caudal aspect of the humeral head can be detected by rotating the humerus internally with the shoulder slightly extended. This moves the head of the humerus laterally, allowing it to be examined indirectly beneath the overlying muscle layers (▶ Fig. 6.61, ▶ Fig. 6.62).

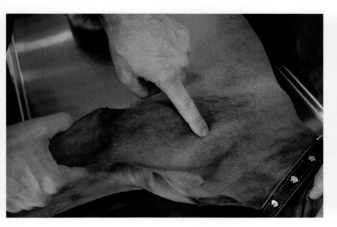

▶ **Fig. 6.61** The shoulder joint lies immediately medial to the acromion. Internal rotation of the humerus moves the head of the humerus towards the skin, allowing it to be assessed for osteochondritic lesions (index finger). (source: Gaby Ernst, Saland, Switzerland)

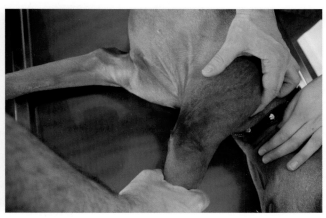

▶ **Fig. 6.62** Assessment of the shoulder joint for crepitation and stability during flexion and extension of the joint. (source: Gaby Ernst, Saland, Switzerland)

> ### ⚑ Findings and Differential Diagnosis
> - pain on palpation of the caudal humeral head
>   - osteochondritic lesion
> - swelling and pain in the cranial aspect of the joint
>   - avulsion of the biceps
>   - biceps tendinitis (p. 228)
>   - fracture of the supraglenoid tubercle
>   - shoulder joint instability or dysplasia
>   - neoplasia (p. 194) of proximal humerus
> - greater tubercle positioned distinctly distal and medial to the acromion
>   - medial shoulder luxation
> - hypomobility of the shoulder joint
>   - shoulder joint luxation
>   - joint fracture
>   - osteochondritic lesion
>   - biceps tendinitis (p. 228)
> - valgus alignment of the shoulder joint
>   - infra-/supraspinatus contracture

Assessment of the Biceps Tendon

Direct palpation of the biceps tendon is possible beneath the intertubercular ligament between the greater and lesser tubercle of the humerus. It can also be palpated more proximally, at the shoulder joint, and more distally, in the intertubercular groove.

The tendon is placed under maximum tension by flexing the shoulder joint and extending the elbow joint. The other hand is used to press on the portion of the biceps tendon located near the shoulder joint (▶ Fig. 6.63, ▶ Fig. 6.64).

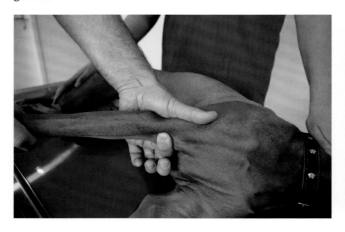

▶ **Fig. 6.63** The biceps tendon inserts on the radius. If the tendon is retracted at this location (index finger) while the shoulder is flexed, the proximal portion of the tendon is also placed under tension. (source: Gaby Ernst, Saland, Switzerland)

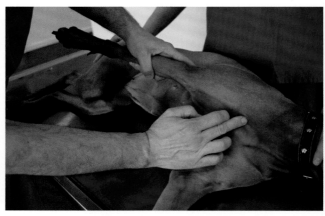

▶ **Fig. 6.64** Assessment of the biceps tendon for pain on palpation during flexion and extension of the shoulder joint. (source: Gaby Ernst, Saland, Switzerland)

⚡ Findings and Differential Diagnosis

- pain on direct pressure
  - biceps tendinitis (p. 228)
  - avulsion of the biceps tendon at the shoulder joint

Overview of Common Findings and Video Demonstration

The following table (▶ **Table 6.13**) provides an overview of common findings in this region.

▶ **Tab. 6.13** Overview of findings.

Location/Test	Finding	Interpretation	Frequency
shoulder joint	swelling and pain at cranial aspect of joint	• avulsion of biceps	+
		• biceps tendinitis	+ +
		• fracture of supraglenoid tubercle	+
		• instability or dysplasia of shoulder joint	+
		• neoplasia of proximal humerus	+ + +
	pain on palpation of caudal humeral head	• osteochondritic lesion	+ + +
	hypomobility	• luxation of shoulder joint	+
		• joint fracture	+
		• osteochondritic lesion	+ + +
		• biceps tendinitis	+ +
	greater tubercle located distinctly distal and medial to acromion	• medial shoulder luxation	+
	valgus alignment of shoulder joint	• infra-/supraspinatus contracture	+
biceps tendon test	pain on direct pressure	• biceps tendinitis	+ +
		• avulsion of biceps tendon at shoulder joint	+

Refer to ▶ **Video 6.13** for a video showing examination of the shoulder joint of a dog in recumbency.

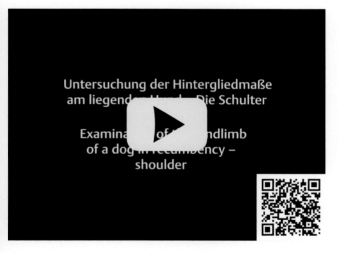

▶ **Video 6.13** Examination of the forelimb of a dog in recumbency – shoulder. This sequence includes palpation and assessment of the shoulder joint, including testing for osteochondrosis (OCD) of the humerus. (source: Tele D, Diessenhofen, Switzerland)

6.3.7 Scapular Region

Scapula

The scapula is palpated along its boundaries, and the structural stability of the scapular spine and acromion is assessed (▶ Fig. 6.65, ▶ Fig. 6.66).

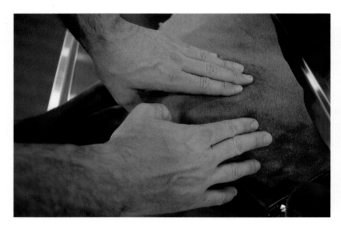

▶ **Fig. 6.65** Testing for the presence/extent of muscle atrophy caudal and cranial to the spine of the scapula. (source: Gaby Ernst, Saland, Switzerland)

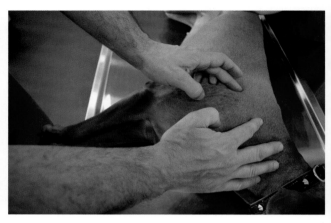

▶ **Fig. 6.66** Palpation of the scapula along its osseous boundaries. (source: Gaby Ernst, Saland, Switzerland)

🔍 Findings and Differential Diagnosis

- pain, crepitation
  - fracture
- pain, swelling
  - neoplasia (p. 194)
- axial deviation
  - healed fracture
- hard and painful muscles
  - contracture

Subscapular Region

The brachial plexus lies directly beneath the scapula. It can be reached from the cranial aspect with the tips of the fingers (►Fig. 6.67).

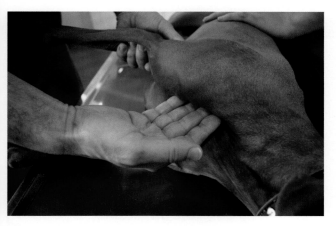

►**Fig. 6.67** Parts of the brachial plexus can be reached with the tips of the fingers. (source: Gaby Ernst, Saland, Switzerland)

Findings and Differential Diagnosis
- pain on palpation under the scapula
  - brachial plexus trauma
  - brachial plexus tumors

Overview of Common Findings and Video Demonstration

The following table (▶ Table 6.14) provides an overview of common findings in this region.

▶ **Tab. 6.14** Overview of findings.

Location	Finding	Interpretation	Frequency
scapula	pain, swelling	• neoplasia	+
	pain, crepitation	• fracture	+
	hard and painful muscles	• contracture	+
	axial deviation	• healed fracture	+
subscapular region	pain on palpation under scapula	• brachial plexus trauma	+ +
		• brachial plexus tumors	+

Refer to ▶ **Video 6.14** for a video showing examination of the scapula of a dog in recumbency.

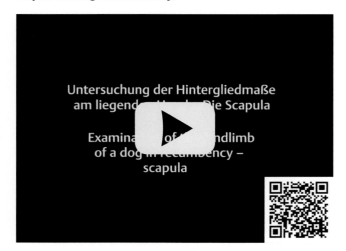

▶ **Video 6.14** Examination of the forelimb of a dog in recumbency – scapula. This sequence includes palpation of the scapula and the nerves of the brachial plexus. (source: Tele D, Diessenhofen, Switzerland)

6.4
Bibliography

[92] Koch DA, Grundmann S, Savoldelli D et al. Die Diagnostik der Patellaluxation des Kleintieres. Schw Arch Tierheilk 1998; 371–374

7 Neurological Examination

Daniel Koch, Martin S. Fischer

7.1
Introduction

When examining a lame dog, it may be necessary to distinguish between lameness and paresis. The neurological examination includes a structured sequence of tests that aims to establish a topical diagnosis. In the first instance, the lesion should be localized to the central or peripheral nervous system. A more precise localization is achieved through clinical examination. In many cases, the examination must be supplemented with diagnostic imaging – such as radiography, computed tomography and magnetic resonance tomography – and electrodiagnostic tests.

It is advisable that the neurological tests are carried out in the same order, each time an examination is performed. Dogs should be examined in a quiet environment. Anxious patients should be re-examined at another time or under different conditions to avoid misinterpretation of findings, particularly when assessing the menace response or testing for pain. In order to distinguish between a normal and an abnormal response, it is important that the dog is cooperative and unsedated. All findings should be documented in writing.

The following sample examination procedure is based on the recommendations of Jaggy [93].

7.2
Anamnesis

7.2.1 Signalment

Predispositions to certain neurological disorders are observed in various breeds of dog. These include intervertebral disc weakness in chondrodystrophic breeds (and ageing dogs), cervical spondylopathy in the Doberman Pinscher and Great Dane and degenerative myelopathy and degenerative lumbosacral disease in the German Shepherd Dog.

> **Interpretation of Signalment**
> - chondrodystrophic breeds: intervertebral disc disease: Doberman Pinscher, Great Dane: cervical spondylotic myelopathy
> - German Shepherd Dog: DLSS (p. 232), DM (p. 234)
> - toy breeds: atlantoaxial subluxation, hydrocephalus, impaired cerebrospinal fluid outflow
> - Rhodesian Ridgeback: dermoid sinus
> - American Staffordshire Terrier: thalamocerebellar degeneration
> - Bulldogs, Pug: subarachnoid diverticulum, degenerative and congenital vertebral canal stenosis

7.2.2 History

Once the owner has identified the presenting complaint, a history should be taken, focusing on the following factors:
1. course of disease (acute, chronic, progressive, recurring)
2. description of locomotion, movement on stairs, any toe dragging
3. carriage of the neck and tail, changes in body shape (particularly the backline)
4. injuries and accidents
5. behavior towards people and animals, changes in behavior, aggression, learning difficulties
6. reactions to normal stimuli, ability to negotiate familiar and unfamiliar terrain or to orientate in the dark
7. ability to take up food from the ground, ability to eat normally, any dropping of food from the jaws
8. defecation behavior
9. previous and existing disease
10. disease in litter mates
11. reaction to prescribed medications
12. vaccination status and any vaccination reactions

> **Interpretation of History**
> - peracute onset, medium-sized dog, absence of trauma
>   - fibrocartilaginous embolism/spinal cord infarction (p. 234)
> - acute onset, hindlimb paralysis, pain
>   - intervertebral disc disease
>   - other extradural compression
>   - vertebral column injury
> - low tail carriage, defecation while walking, fecal incontinence
>   - DLSS (p. 232)
>   - chronic compressive myelopathies
> - difficulty eating from the ground
>   - intervertebral disc disease
>   - wobbler syndrome
>   - atlantoaxial subluxation
> - altered mentation
>   - brain lesion

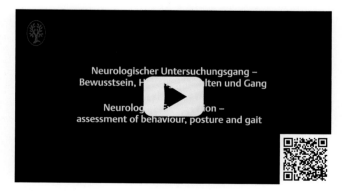

> ▶ **Video 7.1** Neurological examination in the dog: assessment of behavior, posture and gait. (source: Nicole Hollenstein, Tierfotografie)

7.3
Mentation and Behavior

The dog should be observed in a quiet environment, ideally in the open, away from distracting influences such as other dogs, people and vehicles. Mentation is considered normal if the dog reacts in an appropriate or targeted way to specific stimuli such as calls, commands, hand-clapping or pinching.

> **Interpretation of Behaviour**
> - aggression, agitation, disorientation, stereotypical movements
>   - neoplastic or degenerative encephalopathies
>   - metabolic disorders (e.g. hepatic encephalopathy)
>   - obsessive-compulsive behavioral disorder
> - apathy, stupor or coma
>   - trauma, tumor or infection of the brain
>   - metabolic disorder

7.4
Posture

Assessment of posture should also be conducted in the open, or in an alternative low-stimulus environment (▶ Fig. 7.1). It is often performed in conjunction with gait analysis; when the dog's gait is assessed, its posture is noted first. The limbs, trunk, neck and the craniocervical axis should be positioned appropriately. The animal is palpated thoroughly to detect any muscular abnormalities such as atrophy, hypertrophy or pain. The muscles of the neck, trunk and limbs are assessed via brief application of moderate pressure. It is important that the dog is relaxed throughout, to avoid misinterpretation of the response. The head is moved passively in a lateral, dorsal and ventral direction to assess the mobility of the craniocervical axis. The tail should be mobile and its carriage should be appropriate for the breed.

> **Interpretation of posture**
> - Schiff-Sherrington (spastic extension of the forelimbs, hindlimbs usually limp)
>   - deep thoracolumbar spinal cord trauma
> - opisthotonus
>   - midbrain lesion
> - myoclonia
>   - distemper
>   - encephalomyelitis (various etiologies)
> - tremor
>   - cerebellar lesion
>   - intoxication
>   - metabolic disorder e.g. hypocalcemia
> - lordosis, kyphosis, scoliosis
>   - vertebral malformation
>   - intervertebral disc disease
>   - syringomyelia
> - head tilt
>   - vestibular disorders (peripheral and central)

Refer to ▶ **Video 7.1** for a video showing assessment of posture and behavior.

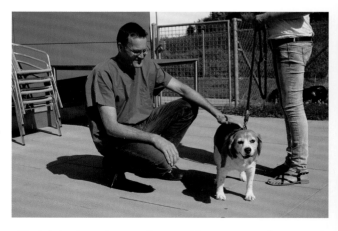

▶ **Fig. 7.1** A quiet environment is required for assessment of posture and behavior. (source: Nicole Hollenstein, Tierfotografie)

7.5
Gait Analysis

Progressive movement, or locomotion, involves repositioning of the center of gravity in a forward, backward or sideways direction. This process is regulated neurophysiologically by ascending spinocortical pathways, descending corticospinal pathways and the locomotor centers.

Dogs usually exhibit a diagonal gait. Simultaneous flexion of one hindlimb and contralateral forelimb is followed by extension of this diagonal pair of limbs. Deviation from this diagonal sequence of motion is referred to as incoordination or ataxia.

The dog is led by an assistant through the walking, trotting and galloping gaits (▶ Fig. 7.2). Each gait is assessed for changes suggestive of lameness; these may occur in one, two or all limbs. Depending on the location of the lesion, gait disturbances are described as spinal ataxia, cerebellar ataxia, vestibular ataxia or cortical ataxia. Based on the extent of the lesion, ataxia is categorized as mild, moderate or severe. In many cases, clinical signs are intensified by more challenging forms of movement, such as walking over uneven ground, stair climbing/descent and jumping over obstacles.

Jumping is particularly useful for observing the interaction between functional processes.

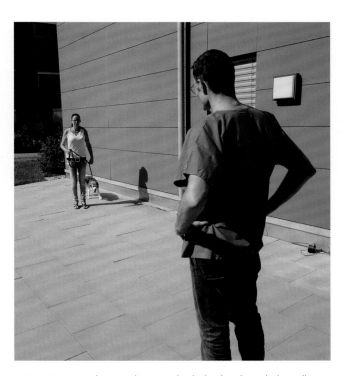

▶ **Fig. 7.2** Gait analysis. As the owner leads the dog through the walk, trot and gallop, the examiner checks for gait abnormalities, ataxias or other co-ordination disorders. (source: Nicole Hollenstein, Tierfotografie)

> 🗲 **Interpretation of Gait Analysis**
> - hypermetria, tremor:
>   - cerebellar disease
> - hemiparesis
>   - brain stem lesion
>   - cerebral lesion
> - stumbling, knuckling, toe-dragging, staggering in the hindquarters (spinal ataxia):
>   - DM (p. 234)
>   - compressive myelopathies Th3–L3
> - wide-based stance, limb spasticity, hypermetria, head tremor (cerebellar ataxia)
>   - neoplasia, inflammation of the cerebellum
>   - cerebellar degenerative and storage disorders
> - head tilt, circling, loss of balance (vestibular ataxia)
>   - inflammation of inner ear
>   - geriatric vestibular syndrome
>   - neoplasia
> - complete loss of motor function (plegia or paralysis; hemi-, para-, tetra- or mono-)
>   - severe upper or lower motor neuron lesion
> - reduced voluntary movement (paresis)
>   - medium grade upper or lower motor neuron lesion
> - compulsive movements (circling, walking along walls)
>   - focal or diffuse cerebral changes (tumors, malformations)
> - pacing gait
>   - no pathological attribution
>   - often considered normal

Refer to ▶ **Video 7.1** for a video showing evaluation of behavior, posture and gait.

7.6
Postural Reactions and Proprioceptive Testing

Postural and proprioceptive responses are assessed to detect subtle disorders of movement, to help localize the point at which a pathway has been interrupted and to identify differences between the left and right sides of the body. Except for proprioceptive positioning, the suitability of the following tests is limited to dogs up to a medium body size and to those that are sufficiently cooperative.

7.6.1 Placing Response

The placing response is assessed using the examination table in the consulting room, or a wall of similar height in an outdoor area. Visual assessment is conducted by lifting the animal and carrying it towards the surface of the table. A normal animal places its fore- and hindlimbs as it approaches the table. For the tactile version, the animal's eyes are closed or covered before it is carried towards the table. Gentle contact between the paw and the tabletop should trigger placement of the fore- and hindlimbs (▶ **Fig. 7.3**).

> ⚡ **Interpretation of Placing Response**
> - absent or markedly delayed paw placement
>   - sensory pathway lesion
>   - midbrain lesion
>   - blindness

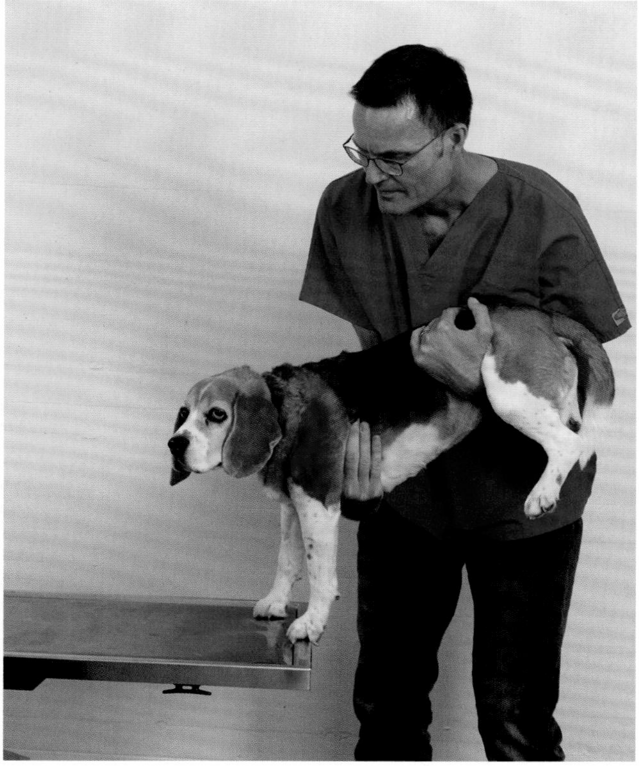

7.6.2 Extensor Postural Thrust

Extensor postural thrust is tested by lowering the dog towards the ground with its fore- and hindlimbs hanging freely until the feet lightly touch the ground. The normal response is extension and stiffening of the limbs and placement of the feet (▶ **Fig. 7.4**).

> ⚡ **Interpretation of Extensor Postural Thrust**
> - absent or delayed movement upon contact with the ground
>   - spinal cord lesion
>   - focal cerebral lesion (contralateral deficit)
>   - vestibular lesion (ipsilateral deficit)

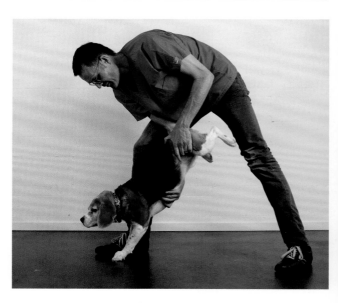

▶ **Fig. 7.4** Extensor postural thrust. The dog's limbs should be extended when they touch the ground. (source: Nicole Hollenstein, Tierfotografie)

▶ **Fig. 7.3** Placing response. The dog is carried carefully towards a flat surface; placement of the foot at touch down is assessed. (source: Nicole Hollenstein, Tierfotografie)

7.6.3 Proprioceptive Positioning

Proprioceptive positioning can be assessed on the floor or on the examination table. With the animal in a standing position, the limbs are brought into an abnormal position, e.g. simply by turning the paw onto its dorsum. Normally, the dog responds by rapidly correcting its foot position and adopting a normal stance (▶ **Fig. 7.5**). As with other tests, it is important to compare the responses on the left and right sides, and in the fore- and hindlimbs.

> **Interpretation of Proprioceptive Positioning**
> - delayed corrective response
>   - lesion in the cortex, cerebellum, brain stem, pons, medulla oblongata, spinal cord, peripheral nerves or muscles

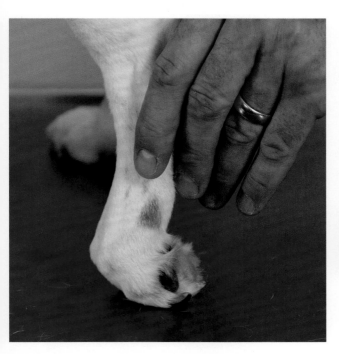

▶ **Fig. 7.5** Proprioceptive positioning. A normal dog responds by correcting its foot position immediately. (source: Nicole Hollenstein, Tierfotografie)

7.6.4 Righting Response

The righting response is tested on the ground. The examiner suspends the dog, holding the animal by the thighs (smaller dogs) or around the ribcage (larger dogs). As the dog is lowered carefully to the ground, it should first lift its head (▶ **Fig. 7.6**) and flex its neck dorsally, then extend its forelimbs.

> **Interpretation of Righting Response**
> - ventral flexion of the head
>   - vestibular disorder

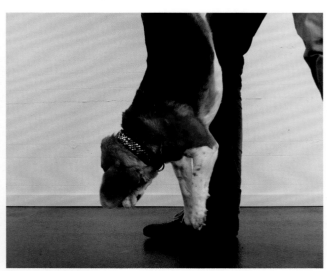

▶ **Fig. 7.6** Righting response. A healthy dog raises its head as it is lowered towards the ground. (source: Nicole Hollenstein, Tierfotografie)

7.6.5 Hemiwalking

Hemiwalking, or standing and walking on ipsilateral limbs, is tested by lifting the limbs on one side of the body (▶ Fig. 7.7). To avoid causing pain, the limbs should be grasped proximally, without abducting the leg. This test is also performed on the ground. Initially, the examiner observes how the body is supported by the grounded feet. The dog's body is then moved sideways, noting the coordination of the supporting limbs. The left and right sides are compared.

> **🗹 Interpretation of Hemiwalking**
> * uncoordinated hemiwalking
>   – cortical lesion

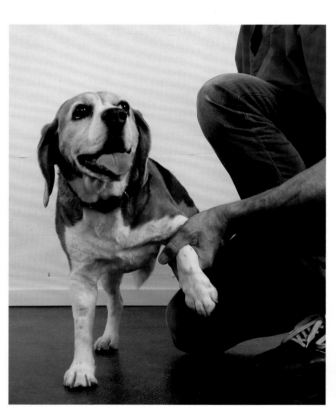

▶ **Fig. 7.7** Hemiwalking: assessment of the coordination of ipsilateral limbs. (source: Nicole Hollenstein, Tierfotografie)

7.6.6 Hopping

Hopping is assessed by lifting three limbs and moving the animal in various directions. The normal response is a hopping action with coordinated support of the animal's body weight on the ipsilateral side (▶ Fig. 7.8). Once again, the left side is compared with the right.

> **🗹 Interpretation of Hopping**
> * stumbling, weakness or collapse during hopping; steps too small or too large
>   – lesion or deficit of the cerebrum, brain stem, cerebellum or spinal cord

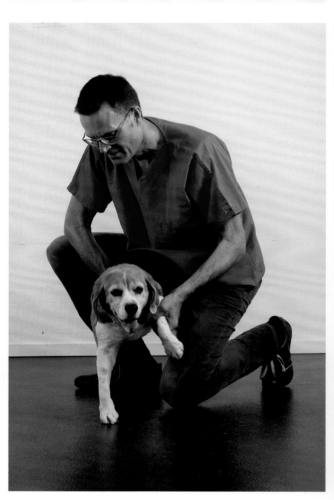

▶ **Fig. 7.8** Hopping. The dog should be able to support its weight on one leg. (source: Nicole Hollenstein, Tierfotografie)

7.6.7 Wheelbarrow Test

In the wheelbarrow test, the dog is made to stand or walk on its forelimbs. The hindlimbs are lifted carefully and the animal is gently pushed forward. The dog should be able to stand and walk on its forelimbs in a coordinated manner (▶ Fig. 7.9).

To trigger subtle deficits, the neck can be flexed slightly as the hindlimbs are raised, eliminating visual input.

> **⊘ Interpretation of Wheelbarrow Test**
> - head held low during testing
>   - cervical disorder
> - hypermetria
>   - lesion in caudal brain stem or or cerebellum
> - unsteady walking, falling, caving in, ataxia
>   - cervical disorder
>   - brachial plexus lesion

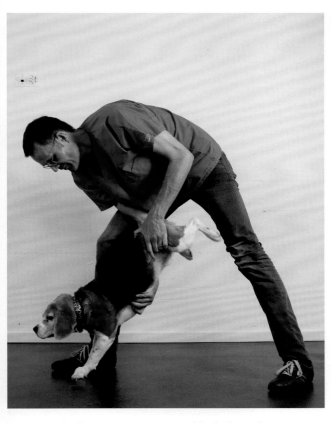

▶ **Fig. 7.9** Wheelbarrow test: assessment of forelimb coordination. (source: Nicole Hollenstein, Tierfotografie)

7.6.8 Video Demonstration

Refer to ▶ Video 7.2 for a video showing assessment of postural and proprioceptive responses.

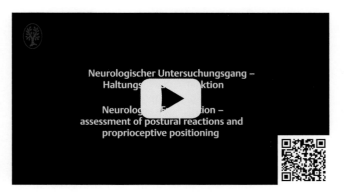

▶ **Video 7.2** Neurological examination in the dog: assessment of postural and proprioceptive responses. (source: Nicole Hollenstein, Tierfotografie)

7.7

Spinal Reflexes

Normal spinal reflex function depends primarily on the integrity of the motor and sensory nerves, the muscles and the grey matter of the corresponding spinal cord segment. Spinal reflex testing can be used to assess particular segments of the grey matter and their associated nerve roots and nerves. In the stretch (myotatic) reflexes, the muscles and their neuromuscular spindles are passively stretched, eliciting a signal that passes through a sensory nerve to the grey matter and on to a motor nerve, resulting in contraction of the relevant muscle. In surface reflexes, muscle contraction is triggered by stimulation of the skin. Pressure on the pads of the foot or the interdigital area results in reflex flexion of the limb, the so-called flexor (withdrawal) reflex.

7.7.1 Patellar Reflex

The reflex center for the patellar reflex lies between L2 and L6. The dog is placed on the examination table in lateral recumbency with its hindlimb loosely supported so that its distal end is not in contact with the tabletop. A reflex hammer is used to tap the patellar ligament gently at its midsection, between the tibial tuberosity and the patella. This triggers contraction of the quadriceps muscle and, thereby, extension of the stifle and tarsal joints (▶ **Fig. 7.10**).

7.7.2 Cranial Tibial Reflex

The reflex center for the cranial tibial reflex is located between L6 and S2. With the dog in the same position as for the patellar reflex, the tibialis cranialis is tapped with a reflex hammer, just distal to the head of the fibula (▶ **Fig. 7.11**). The normal response is flexion of the tarsal joint.

> **Interpretation of Spinal Reflexes in the Hindlimb**
> - increased response
>   - upper motor neuron lesion cranial to L4–L6
> - reduced response
>   - lower motor neuron lesion (nerve root, plexus, peripheral nerve)
>   - muscle injury

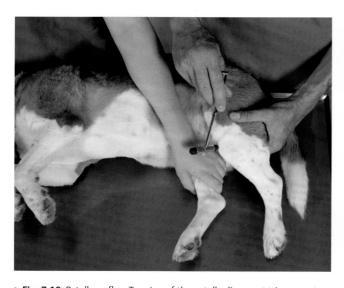

▶ **Fig. 7.10** Patellar reflex. Tapping of the patellar ligament triggers extension of the limb. (source: Nicole Hollenstein, Tierfotografie)

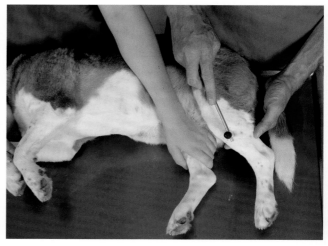

▶ **Fig. 7.11** Cranial tibial reflex. Tapping of the tibialis cranialis triggers flexion of the tarsal joint. (source: Nicole Hollenstein, Tierfotografie)

7.7.3 Flexor (Withdrawal) Reflex in the Hindlimb

The reflex center for the flexor reflex in the hindlimb is located between L4 and S3. The dog is placed in lateral recumbency. Pinching of the toes, foot pads or the interdigital skin results in sudden flexion (withdrawal) of the entire limb (▶ Fig. 7.12).

ℹ Interpretation of the Withdrawal (Flexor) Reflex
- absence of flexion/withdrawal
  - peripheral nerve lesion
- triggering of the flexor reflex elicits extension of the contralateral limb
  - upper motor neuron lesion

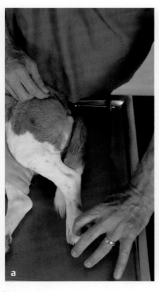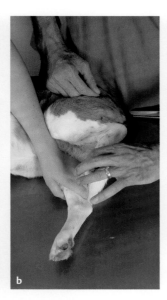

▶ **Fig. 7.12** Flexor (withdrawal) reflex in the hindlimb.
a Elicitation of the flexor reflex in the hindlimb by pinching the foot pads. (source: Nicole Hollenstein, Tierfotografie)
b Normal response: flexion of the stimulated hindlimb. (source: Nicole Hollenstein, Tierfotografie)

7.7.4 Extensor Carpi Radialis Reflex

The reflex center for the extensor carpi radialis reflex lies between C7 and Th1. The limb is supported under the elbow. Light tapping of the extensor carpi radialis below the elbow with a reflex hammer triggers slight extension of the carpus (▶ Fig. 7.13).

ℹ Interpretation of Spinal Reflexes in the Forelimb
- increased response
  - upper motor neuron lesion cranial to C5
- reduced response
  - lower motor neuron lesion (C5–T2 including nerve root, plexus, peripheral nerve)
  - muscle injury

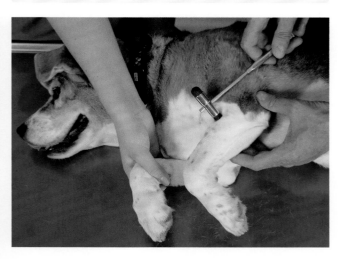

▶ **Fig. 7.13** Extensor carpi radialis reflex. Tapping of the extensor carpi radialis below the head of the radius triggers extension of the limb. (source: Nicole Hollenstein, Tierfotografie)

7.7.5 Flexor (Withdrawal) Reflex in the Forelimb

The reflex center for the flexor reflex in the forelimb is situated between C6 and Th2. The dog is placed in lateral recumbency. Pinching of the toes, foot pads or interdigital skin triggers sudden flexion (withdrawal) of the limb (► Fig. 7.14). To identify differences between the left and right sides, the spinal reflexes should be tested in all four limbs.

Interpretation of the Flexor Reflex
- absence of flexion (withdrawal)
  - peripheral nerve lesion
- triggering of the flexor reflex elicits extension of the contralateral limb
  - upper motor neuron lesion

7.7.6 Perineal Reflex

The perineal reflex center lies between S1 and S3. The dog is assessed in a standing position, with the tail slightly elevated. Touching or gentle pinching of the perineal region with forceps triggers contraction of the anal sphincter (► Fig. 7.15) and depression of the tail.

Interpretation of Perineal Reflex
- reduced anal response, open anus, incontinence
  - lesion S1–S3, pudendal nerve or pelvic nerves

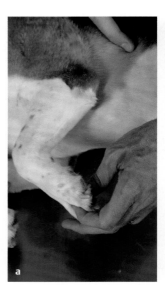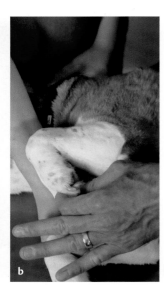

► **Fig. 7.14** Flexor reflex in the forelimb.
a Elicitation of the flexor reflex in the forelimb by pinching the foot pads. (source: Nicole Hollenstein, Tierfotografie)
b Normal response: flexion of the forelimb. (source: Nicole Hollenstein, Tierfotografie)

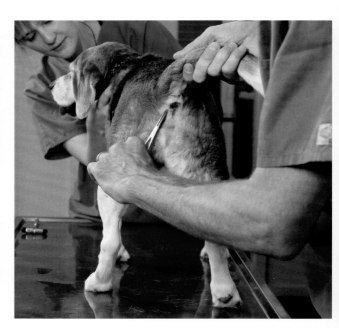

► **Fig. 7.15** Testing of the perineal reflex for assessment of the sacral spinal cord between S1 and S3. The normal response is contraction of the anal sphincter. (source: Nicole Hollenstein, Tierfotografie)

7.7.7 Panniculus Reflex

Signals produced by stimulation of nociceptors in the skin travel to the spinal cord through sensory nerve fibers. Ascending pathways transmit the stimulus through the white matter to the level of C8/Th2 where the stimulus reaches the motor reflex center. The motor neurons transmit the contractile impulse to the trunk muscles via the thoracic nerves.

The dog is examined in a standing or sitting position. Stimulation or pinching of the skin with forceps or a needle triggers contraction of the cutaneous muscles (▶ **Fig. 7.16**). Testing commences caudally at the level of L6. As in other spinal reflex tests, the left and right sides should be compared. Spinal cord lesions may cause disruption of the reflex arc caudal to the site of the lesion.

> **Interpretation of the Panniculus Reflex**
> * reduced panniculus reflex
>   – spinal cord lesion cranial to the tested region

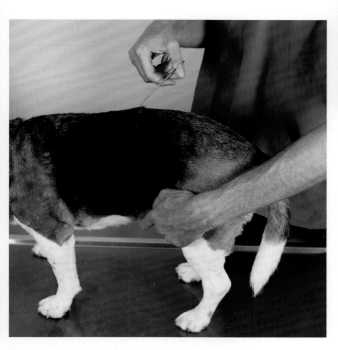

▶ **Fig. 7.16** Testing of the panniculus reflex using forceps. (source: Nicole Hollenstein, Tierfotografie)

7.7.8 Video Demonstration

Refer to ▶ **Video 7.3** for a video showing assessment of the spinal reflexes.

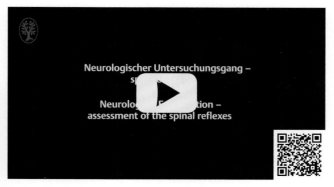

▶ **Video 7.3** Neurological examination in the dog: assessment of the spinal reflexes. (source: Nicole Hollenstein, Tierfotografie)

7.8

Cranial Nerves

When examining cranial nerve function, it is particularly important that the dog is calm. Anxious patients should be re-examined at a later stage. This is especially important for assessment of the menace response.

Cranial nerve function can be evaluated using relatively straightforward tests. Except for cranial nerves I and II, the nuclei are located in the midbrain, pons and medulla oblongata. Thus, brain stem lesions can result in single or multiple cranial nerve deficits.

Examination of the cranial nerves is best performed with the patient placed on an examination table.

7.8.1 Palpebral Reflex (V, VII)

The palpebral reflex is elicited by touching the periocular skin (▶ Fig. 7.17). Closure of the eyelids is the normal response. The components of the reflex arc are the trigeminal nerve, brain stem and facial nerve.

> **Interpretation of the Palpebral Reflex**
> - absent or reduced palpebral reflex
>   - trigeminal or facial nerve lesion
>   - lesion within the brain stem or cortex

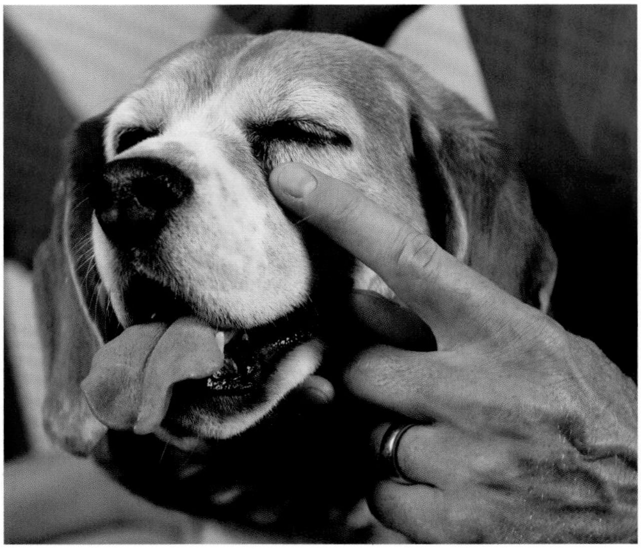

▶ **Fig. 7.17** Testing of the palpebral reflex by touching the periocular skin. (source: Nicole Hollenstein, Tierfotografie)

7.8.2 Menace Response (II, VIII)

The menace response is triggered by making a sudden gesture towards the eye with the hand (▶ Fig. 7.18). The normal response is closure of the eyelids. The neural components of the menace response are the optic nerve, cortex, cerebellum, brain stem and facial nerve.

> **Interpretation of the Menace Response**
> - lack of eyelid closure in response to a threatening gesture
>   - blindness in the tested eye
>   - facial nerve lesion

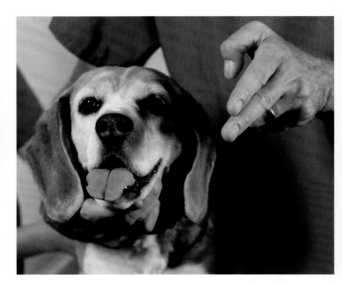

▶ **Fig. 7.18** Testing of the menace response by directing the fingers rapidly towards the eye. (source: Nicole Hollenstein, Tierfotografie)

7.8.3 Cotton Ball Test

Vision can be further assessed using the cotton ball test, in which a cotton ball is dropped within the animal's visual field. The normal response is for the animal to follow the path of the cotton ball by moving its eyes or head. This reaction depends on the integrity of the optic nerve and cerebral cortex.

> **Interpretation of the Cotton Ball Test**
> - lack of eyelid closure during menace testing and negative response to the cotton ball test
>   - blindness

7.8.4 Head Sensation (V, X)

Sensation in the cranial region is tested by lightly touching or tapping the head with the fingers (▶ Fig. 7.19). The stimulus is transmitted by the trigeminal nerve and is eventually relayed to the brain stem via the sensory cortex. The animal normally responds with a defensive movement. Near the pinna, sensory innervation is provided by the vagus nerve (▶ Fig. 7.19b).

> **Interpretation of Head Sensation**
> - absence of defensive movements
>   - trigeminal or vagus nerve lesion

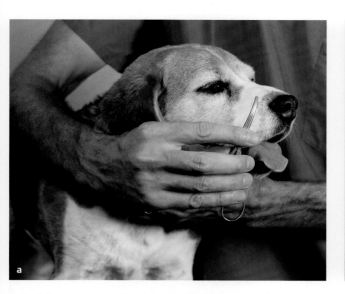
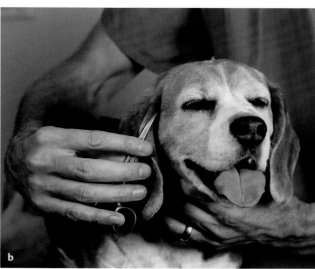

▶ **Fig. 7.19** Assessment of head sensation for evaluation of the sensory components of the trigeminal and vagus nerves.
a Evaluation of the trigeminal nerve. (source: Nicole Hollenstein, Tierfotografie)
b Evaluation of the vagus nerve. (source: Nicole Hollenstein, Tierfotografie)

7.8.5 Jaw Tone (V), Motor Function of the Tongue (XII)

Jaw tone is assessed by gently forcing the jaws apart (▶ Fig. 7.20), during which resistance should be encountered. Movement of the tongue, for which the hypoglossal nerve is responsible, should be assessed.

> **Interpretation of Jaw Tone and Motor Function of the Tongue**
> - asymmetrical tongue position, uncoordinated tongue movement during drinking
>   - nerve trauma near the tongue (tongue directed towards paralyzed side)
>   - brain stem lesion
> - paralysis of the lower jaw, atrophied temporalis
>   - deficit of motor component of the trigeminal nerve

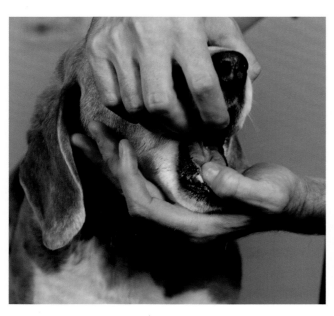

▶ **Fig. 7.20** Assessment of jaw tone and motor function of the tongue by opening the mouth. (source: Nicole Hollenstein, Tierfotografie)

7.8.6 Swallowing (Gag) Reflex (IX/X)

The swallowing reflex is elicited by palpating the pharyngeal region, with application of gentle pressure (▶ Fig. 7.21). The reflex is mediated by the glossopharyngeal and vagus nerves.

> **Interpretation of the Swallowing Reflex**
> - reduced or absent swallowing reflex
>   - myasthenia
>   - rabies
>   - tumors
>   - peripheral nerve trauma due to foreign body
>   - brain stem lesion

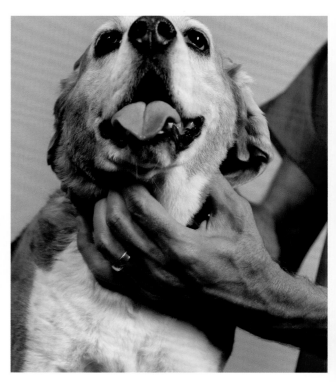

▶ **Fig. 7.21** Assessment of the swallowing reflex by gently pressing on the pharynx. (source: Nicole Hollenstein, Tierfotografie)

7.8.7 Facial Expression (VII)

The functions of the facial nerve include innervation of the mimetic muscles, or muscles of facial expression. This is evaluated by assessing overall head shape and by palpating the muscles of the head (▶ Fig. 7.22).

> **⚡ Interpretation of Facial Expression**
> - ptosis, miosis, enophthalmos, third eyelid protrusion (Horner's syndrome)
>   - damage to sympathetic innervation
>   - hypothalamic lesion
>   - nerve root trauma involving T1–T3
>   - middle ear lesion
> - asymmetry of eyelid position, nostrils or ears
>   - facial nerve lesion (particularly near ear canal)

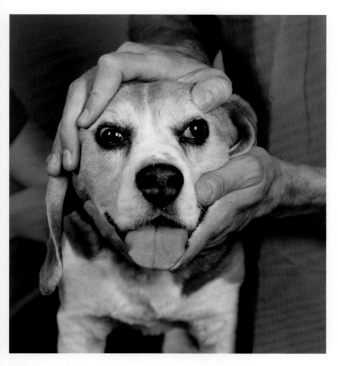

▶ **Fig. 7.22** Assessment of facial expression. (source: Nicole Hollenstein, Tierfotografie)

7.8.8 Eye Movement (III, IV, VI), Nystagmus (VIII)

Moving the head from side to side may elicit physiological nystagmus (▶ Fig. 7.23). Symmetry of eye position should also be evaluated. Abnormal bulb position is referred to as strabismus.

> **Interpretation of Eye Movement and Nystagmus**
> - ventrolateral strabismus
>   - cranial nerve III paralysis
> - medial strabismus
>   - cranial nerve VI paralysis
> - rotation of the bulb
>   - cranial nerve IV paralysis

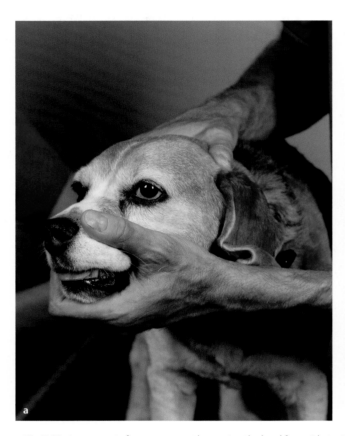
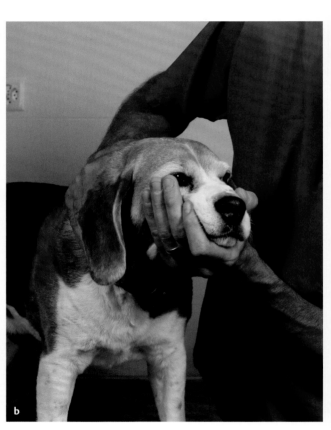

▶ **Fig. 7.23** Assessment of eye movement by moving the head from side to side. Horizontal nystagmus is a normal finding.
a Movement of the head to the right. (source: Nicole Hollenstein, Tierfotografie)
b Movement of the head to the left. (source: Nicole Hollenstein, Tierfotografie)

7.8.9 Pupillary Light Reflex (II/III)

Fibers within the oculomotor nerve are responsible for parasympathetic innervation of the iris. The nucleus receives stimulation from both sides via the optical pathways. This results in contraction of the iris sphincter. The pupil constricts on the illuminated side (direct pupillary light reflex) and on the contralateral side (indirect or consensual pupillary light reflex). The pupillary light reflex is assessed by directing light into the eye (▶ Fig. 7.24). The normal response is constriction of the pupil in the illuminated and contralateral eye. The stronger the light source, the greater is the degree of constriction.

> **Interpretation of the Pupillary Light Reflex**
> - ptosis, miosis, enophthalmos
>   - Horner's syndrome (see above)
>   - damage to sympathetic innervation
>   - hypothalamic lesion
>   - nerve root trauma involving T1–T3
>   - middle ear lesion
> - mydriasis, ventrolateral strabismus, ptosis
>   - cranial nerve III paralysis
>   - injury affecting eye, orbit, midbrain

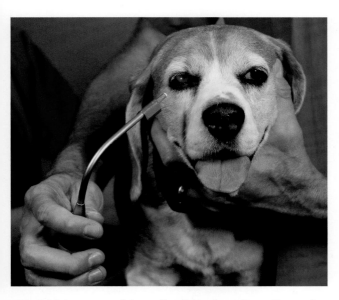

▶ **Fig. 7.24** Assessment of the pupillary light reflex: A focused beam of light is directed into the eye. The normal response is constriction of the pupil in the illuminated and contralateral eye. (source: Nicole Hollenstein, Tierfotografie)

7.8.10 Video Demonstration

Refer to ▶ Video 7.4 for a video showing examination of the cranial nerves.

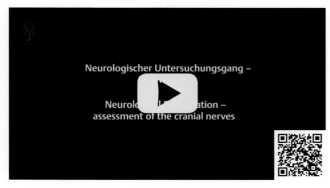

Neurologischer Untersuchungsgang –

Neurol... ...ation –
assessment of the cranial nerves

▶ **Video 7.4** Neurological examination in the dog: assessment of the cranial nerves. (source: Nicole Hollenstein, Tierfotografie)

7.9

Pain Testing

Painful stimuli (▶ **Fig. 7.25**) are transmitted along ascending pathways in the spinal cord to higher centers in the thalamus. Immediately thereafter, the cerebrum perceives the stimulus as pain, resulting in a defensive reaction by the animal and twitching in the relevant dermatome. In most cases the animal consciously turns its head to the side and attempts to bite.

Refer to ▶ **Video 7.5** for a video demonstration of pain testing.

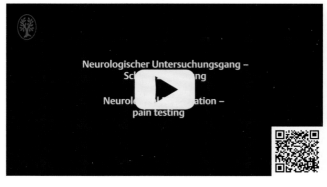

▶ **Video 7.5** Neurological examination in the dog: pain testing. (source: Nicole Hollenstein, Tierfotografie)

> **⚡ Interpretation of the Pain Testing**
> - absent response (analgesia, anesthesia)
>   – severe peripheral nerve or spinal cord lesion
> - increased or exaggerated response (hyperalgesia, hyperesthesia)
>   – nerve irritation (inflammatory or neuropathic pain)
>   – meningeal irritation (e.g. due to intervertebral disc disease)
> - self-mutilation, scratching, licking of a particular site (paresthesia)
>   – nerve damage (compressive, inflammatory, neoplastic)
>   – CNS lesion with altered perception (syringomyelia)

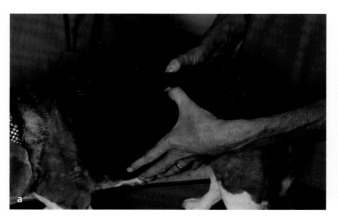
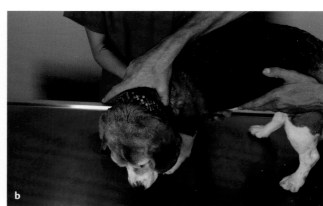
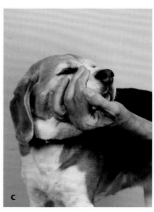
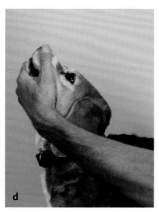
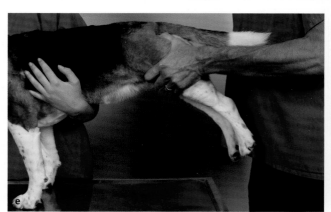

▶ **Fig. 7.25** Testing for pain by palpating the back and neck. Pain reactions manifest as conscious movement of the patient's head.
a Testing for pain in the thoracic and lumbar vertebral column. (source: Nicole Hollenstein, Tierfotografie)
b Testing for pain in the nerve roots of the cervical vertebral column. (source: Nicole Hollenstein, Tierfotografie)
c Testing for pain by flexing the neck laterally. (source: Nicole Hollenstein, Tierfotografie)
d Testing for pain by moving the neck dorsally and ventrally. (source: Nicole Hollenstein, Tierfotografie)
e Testing for pain in the lumbosacral vertebral column by hyperextending the spine. (source: Nicole Hollenstein, Tierfotografie)

7.10

Summary and Classification

7.10.1 Lesion Localization

Neurological deficits should first be localized to the peripheral or central nervous system (PNS or CNS). Within the CNS, brain lesions must be distinguished from spinal cord disorders. Finally, a distinction is made between upper and motor neuron lesions.

The first stage of localization involves the spinal reflexes (▶ Fig. 7.26). Overall reduction of spinal reflexes indicates a general PNS disorder. Otherwise the CNS is affected.

The cranial nerves permit distinction between a CNS lesion in the brain and spinal cord. Even just a single cranial nerve deficit points to a lesion in the brain. Brain lesions are further differentiated using various findings obtained during the neurological examination. With cerebral lesions, a normal gait is observed, accompanied by compulsive movements, abnormal behaviors or seizures. Brain stem lesions are usually associated with hypometria, apathy or coma, or multiple cranial nerve deficits. Signs indicative of a cerebellar lesion include hypermetria, tremor or exaggerated reactions to postural and proprioceptive tests. Lesions affecting the vestibular system result in a head tilt, vestibular ataxia, cranial nerve deficits, nystagmus or strabismus, and occasionally Horner's syndrome.

If cranial nerve function is normal, the lesion is located in the spinal cord and must be localized to a particular segment. With lesions at C1 to C5, upper motor neuron deficits (increased reflexes, spasticity) are usually evident in all four limbs; lesions near the intumescence at C6 to Th1 result in lower motor neuron deficits (reduced to absent reflexes, flaccidity) in the forelimbs and upper motor neuron signs in the hindlimbs; lesions at Th2 to L3 result in upper motor neuron signs in the hindlimbs, while the forelimbs are normal (exception: deep acute lesions producing Schiff-Sherrington syndrome); lesions involving the intumescence at L4 to S3 give rise to lower motor neuron signs in the hindlimb with normal reactions in the forelimbs.

Further, more precise localization of the cause of neurological dysfunction requires the use of additional diagnostic aids. These include diagnostic imaging, such as computed tomography or magnetic resonance tomography, laboratory tests or electrodiagnostic techniques.

Dysfunction associated with cervical, thoracic and lumbar lesions is conventionally graded according to the following system:
- Grade 1: pain only
- Grade 2: tetra-/paraparesis, ataxia, dog is ambulatory
- Grade 3: tetra-/paraparesis, loss of motor function
- Grade 4: tetra-/paraplegia, loss of superficial pain perception in the limbs
- Grade 5: tetra-/paraplegia, loss of deep pain perception in the limbs

Disorders resulting in extradural compression, such as intervertebral disc disease, progress chronologically according to the sequence described above. The prognosis deteriorates with increasing grade. Intradural lesions such as infarcts, hemorrhage or neoplasia do not necessarily progress in this sequential manner.

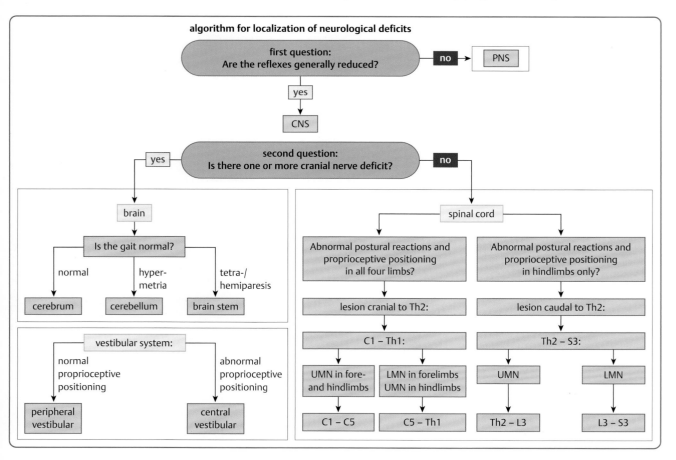

▶ **Fig. 7.26** Algorithm for localization of neurological deficits (after [93]). (source: Karin Baum)

7.10.2 Overview of Important Neurological Disorders Related to the Locomotor System

Localization: Cerebrum

The following findings are typical for a cerebral lesion
(► Table 7.1):
- mentation: normal to comatose
- behavior: aggression, anxiety, dullness
- postural and proprioceptive reactions: general reduction with diffuse lesions, contralateral deficits with focal lesions
- cranial nerves: blindness with normal pupillary light reflex
- PU/PD, abnormal pupillary responses
- cranial and cervical pain

Localization: Cerebellum

The following findings are typical for a cerebellar lesion
(► Table 7.2):
- posture: wide-based stance
- gait: ataxia, spasticity, hypermetria
- spinal reflexes: normal
- cranial nerves: reduced menace response

► **Tab. 7.1** Cerebral lesion: overview of findings.

Diagnosis	Relevant Criterion/Test	Typical Finding	Frequency
epilepsy	mentation	convulsive seizures (generalized tonic-clonic seizures, or focal with brief loss of consciousness, transient compulsive movement)	+ +
neoplasia (meningiomas, gliomas, mesenchymal tumors, ependymomas, sarcomas)	–	dependent upon location, no consistent signs (see above for general typical findings)	+ +
brain infarct	mentation	convulsive seizures	+
	gait analysis	abnormal gait, circling	
	cranial nerves	visual deficits	
hydrocephalus	general examination, facial expression	abnormal head shape	+
	mentation and behavior	learning difficulties	
	cranial nerves	ventrolateral strabismus, visual or auditory deficits	
meningoencephalitis	mentation and behavior	behavioral disorders, seizures	+
	gait analysis	gait abnormalities	
	pain testing	pain response	

► **Tab. 7.2** Cerebellar lesion: overview of findings.

Diagnosis	Relevant criterion/test	Typical finding	Frequency
neoplasia	–	dependent upon location, no consistent signs (see above for general typical findings)	+
tremor-syndrome, white dog shaker syndrome (can also affect other parts of brain)	anamnesis	white dog (West Highland White Terrier, Maltese Terrier)	+
	–	see general characteristics	
	other	exacerbated by excitement; spontaneous remission possible	
cerebellar abiotrophy	anamnesis	specific breeds	+
	posture	opisthotonus	
	gait analysis	progressive ataxia, tremor	
	cranial nerves	reduced menace response	

Localization: Vestibular System

The following findings are typical for a lesion located in the vestibular system (▶ Table 7.3):

- head tilt, tendency to fall
- peripheral vestibular system: normal proprioceptive positioning
- central vestibular system: delayed proprioceptive positioning, cranial nerve deficits other than those related to facial nerve and sympathetic innervation

Localization: Brain Stem

The following findings are typical for a brain stem lesion (▶ Table 7.4).

▶ **Tab. 7.3** Vestibular system lesion: overview of findings.

Diagnosis	Relevant Criterion/Test	Typical Finding	Frequency
otitis media/interna	anamnesis	ear pain	+ +
	posture	signs of peripheral vestibular disease, head tilt, head shaking	
	gait analysis		
	cranial nerves	facial paralysis, Horner's syndrome	
ototoxic medication e.g. systemic aminoglycosides, topical preparations	posture	signs of peripheral vestibular disease, deafness	+
	gait analysis		
idiopathic geriatric vestibular syndrome	anamnesis	dogs over 9 years	+
	posture	acute, mild to severe peripheral vestibular deficits (without Horner's syndrome and facial paralysis)	
	gait analysis		

▶ **Tab. 7.4** Brain stem lesion: overview of findings.

Diagnosis	Relevant Criterion/Test	Typical Finding	Frequency
brain stem lesion	mentation	apathetic to comatose	+
	gait	spastic paresis of all limbs, vestibular ataxia, circling to one side	+
	postural and proprioceptive reactions	deficits worse on one side with focal lesions	+
	spinal reflexes	normal to increased	+
	cranial nerves	deficits of III, IV, VI, VIII (strabismus, anisocoria, nystagmus), paralysis of lower jaw, reduced head sensation (V), unilateral facial drooping, absent menace response (VII), balance deficits (XIII), swallowing deficits (IX), altered voice, stridor (X), lingual paralysis (XII)	+

Localization: Spinal Cord (excluding Compressive Disease)

The following findings are typical for spinal cord lesions, excluding compressive disease (▶ Table 7.5):

- behavior: normal
- gait: paresis to paralysis of all limbs or hindlimbs
- reduced postural and proprioceptive reactions caudal to the lesion
- spinal reflexes: hypo- or areflexia when LMN are affected; normo- or hyperreflexia caudal to the lesion when UMN affected
- pain: rarely present

Localization: Spinal Cord (Compressive Disease)

The following findings are typical for spinal cord lesions involving compressive disease (▶ Table 7.6):

- signs/deficits occurring in the following order: pain, ataxia/proprioceptive deficits, loss of motor function, loss of superficial pain perception, loss of deep pain perception
- increased reflex responses caudal to the lesion (if UMN affected); reduced reflexes at the level of the lesion (if LMN affected); absence of panniculus reflex at the level of the lesion.

▶ **Tab. 7.5** Spinal cord lesions (excluding compressive disease): overview of findings.

Diagnosis	Relevant Criterion/Test	Typical Finding	Frequency
fibrocartilaginous embolism/ spinal cord infarct	anamnesis	young to middle-aged large breed dogs; initially painful then painless	+ +
	gait analysis	peracute onset of abnormal gait to paralysis	
	postural and proprioceptive reactions	often worse on one side	
degenerative myelopathy	anamnesis	Bernese Mountain Dog, German Shepherd Dog	+ +
	gait analysis	progressive ataxia, weakness and paresis of hindlimbs	
	spinal reflexes	reflexes normal to mildly increased in hindlimbs, crossed extensor reflex, UMN signs	
aseptic suppurative meningitis-arteritis	general examination	pyrexia, leucocytosis	+
	gait analysis	stiff gait; ataxia and paresis in chronic form	
	pain testing	cervical pain	

▶ **Tab. 7.6** Spinal cord lesion (compressive disease): overview of findings.

Diagnosis	Relevant Criterion/Test	Typical Finding	Frequency
thoracolumbar intervertebral disc disease	anamnesis	pain on palpation of disease site	+ + +
	posture	hunched back	
	gait analysis	ataxia to paralysis, depending on degree of compression	
	spinal reflexes	normal in forelimbs, increased in hindlimbs; urinary bladder difficult to express	
	pain testing	pain on flexion of neck	
cervical intervertebral disc disease (C1 to C5)	mentation and behavior	agitation, unsettled behavior	+ +
	posture	low head carriage	
	gait analysis	ataxia to paralysis, depending on degree of compression; with mild disease, deficits may only be evident in hindlimbs	
	spinal reflexes	increased in fore- and hindlimbs	
atlanto-axial subluxation	anamnesis	toy breeds, onset following mild trauma	+
	gait analysis	tetraparesis/ataxia	
	spinal reflexes	increased	
caudal cervical spondylo-myelopathy (wobbler syndrome)	gait analysis	hindlimb ataxia, spastic hypometria in forelimbs (two-engine gait), difficulty rising	+
	pain testing	restricted, sometimes painful movement of the cervical vertebrae	

Localization: Peripheral Nerves

The following findings are typical for a peripheral nerve lesion
(▶ **Table 7.7**):

- behavior: normal
- gait: paresis to paralysis
- spinal reflexes: normal to reduced or absent
- cranial nerves: several neuromuscular diseases also affect cranial nerve function
- pain: usually absent

▶ **Tab. 7.7** Peripheral nerve lesion: overview of findings.

Diagnosis	Relevant Criterion/Test	Typical Findings	Frequency
degenerative lumbosacral stenosis (cauda equina-syndrome)	anamnesis	pain on rising and jumping, pain on hyperextension (lordosis); early signs of urinary and fecal incontinence	+++
	general examination	muscle atrophy	
	posture	low tail carriage	
	gait analysis	weakness of hindlimbs, uni- or bilateral lameness	
	spinal reflexes	spinal reflexes involving ischiatic nerve, pudendal nerve and pelvic and caudal nerves reduced in advanced stages	
	pain testing	lumbosacral pain	
acute idipoathic polyradiculoneuritis	anamnesis	normal fecal and urinary continence	+
	gait analysis	acute tetraparesis	
	spinal nerves	weak to absent reflex responses	
	cranial nerves	reduced menace response and palpebral reflex	
	pain testing	normal pain perception	
neoplasia of peripheral nerves (especially nerve sheath tumors)	anamnesis	pain at tumor site	+
	posture	neurogenic muscle atrophy (usually pronounced)	
	spinal reflexes	reduced response	
brachial plexus lesion	posture	monoplegia (forelimb), abrasion of toes and dorsum of paws, dropped elbow	+
	gait analysis		
	spinal reflexes	reduced to absent reflex response	
	cranial nerves	Horner's syndrome	
	pain testing	lack of superficial and deep pain perception in affected dermatome	

7.11

Bibliography

[93] Jaggy A. Atlas und Lehrbuch der Kleintierneurologie. Hannover: Schlütersche; 2007

[94] Vandevelde M, Jaggy A, Lang J. Veterinärmedizinische Neurologie. Ein Leitfaden für Studium und Praxis. 2. neubearb. u. erw. Aufl. Berlin: Paul Parey; 2001

[95] Kornberg M. Klinisch-neurologischer Untersuchungsgang. In: Kramer M. Kompendium der allgemeinen Veterinärchirurgie. Hannover: Schlütersche; 2004

[96] Schwarz G. Neurologische Erkrankungen. In: Kohn B, Schwarz G. Praktikum der Hundeklinik. Stuttgart: Enke; 2017

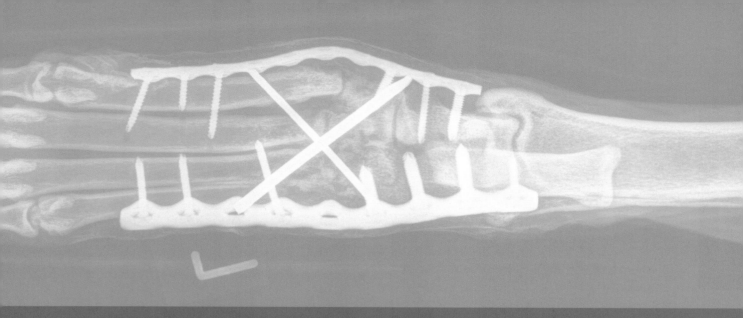

Part 3
Therapeutic Guidelines
for Common Disorders

8 Important Orthopedic Disorders

Daniel Koch, Martin S. Fischer

8.1
General Information

8.1.1 Relative Frequency

The relative frequency of joint disorders in dogs is shown in ▶ Fig. 8.1.

Approximately 70% of cases of canine lameness involve the hindlimbs and 50% are localized to the stifle joint. Dysplasias and their secondary effects (hip dysplasia and coxofemoral osteoarthritis, elbow dysplasia and elbow osteoarthritis, patellar luxation) and the complex of disorders associated with cruciate ligament rupture account for most of the orthopedic disease seen in dogs.

It may initially seem surprising that joint disorders occur so frequently in energetic, athletic and even lean dogs. A subjective comparison seems to suggest that arthropathies are considerably more common in dogs than in humans. It is important in this context to consider the influence of modern dog breeding. In striving for physical perfection and compliance with breed standards, many breed associations have unfortunately deprioritized the functional integrity of their dogs. Consequently, certain breeds are propagated with purely aesthetic objectives and the desired result is achieved in just a few generations. Natural selection is eliminated from this process; dogs can no longer seek out their preferred mate and the principle of „survival of the fittest" no longer applies.

Most joint disorders arise at the puppy stage when the dog's body weight and size are too great for the delicate juvenile articular cartilage, which quickly becomes damaged. It is often too late for corrective interventions, such as modification of food intake, medication or surgery, as the major phase of skeletal development occurs over just a few weeks. Large, overweight dogs are also overrepresented in cases of cruciate ligament rupture, which only rarely results from forceful impact on the stifle joint. Cruciate ligament rupture is thus categorized as a dysplasia or disorder of skeletal growth, rather than as an injury. The logical implication for therapy is that the problem cannot be solved by simply replacing the cruciate ligament. It is now widely recognized by surgeons that alteration of joint biomechanics or total joint replacement is required to address the animal's needs. Corrective osteotomy of the elbow, hip or stifle results in realignment of misdirected muscular forces and leads to long term therapeutic success.

8.1.2 General Therapeutic Recommendations

Analgesics/NSAIDs

Non-steroidal anti-inflammatory drugs act on the effector organ. Their duration of effect is usually 12–24 hours. If long term use is required, dogs should be monitored for kidney and liver damage. Non-steroidal anti-inflammatory drugs can be administered orally or parenterally.
- carprofen (4 mg/kg, SID or 2 mg/kg, BID)
- meloxicam (0.2 mg/kg, SID)
- robenacoxib (1 mg/kg, SID)
- mavacoxib (2 mg/kg, monthly tablet)

Opioids and opiates act on the brain. They are usually injected or administered transdermally.
- butorphanol (0.1–0.4 mg/kg, IV, IM, SC, duration of action 1–3 hours)
- buprenorphine (0.009–0.027 mg/kg; IV, IM, SC, duration of effect 2–6 hours)
- morphine HCl and other opioids (adapted from human medicine; 0.3–1 mg/kg, SC, duration of effect 2–4 hours)
- fentanyl patch (reclassified from human medicine; various concentrations, applied to the skin; effective levels reached after 12 hours, duration of effect 2–3 days)
- tramadol (1–4 mg/kg, SID to QID, PO)

Care must be taken when using corticosteroids (prednisolone or dexamethasone) as analgesics, as these have significant gastrointestinal and endocrinological side effects.

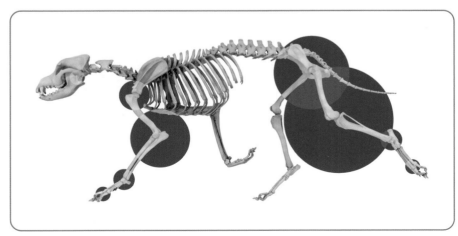

▶ **Fig. 8.1** Joint disorders in dogs. The diameter of the circle represents the relative frequency with which a particular joint is affected. (source: Daniel Koch, Jonas Lauströer, Amir Andikfar)

Therapies for Cartilage Repair and Protection

Oral chondroprotective preparations consist of 2 main groups. Chondroitin- and glucosamine-based products are derived from shark cartilage or bovine tracheas. Due to the large molecular weight of these substances, only around 10% of the oral dose is absorbed and passes to the joint. Within the joint, the active ingredients are taken up by the hyaline cartilage where they bind water and purportedly contribute to cartilage regeneration. While the effectiveness of these substances is disputed, it is generally agreed that they must be administered for at least 2 months and that only high-purity preparations will result in therapeutic levels. The second main group contains green-lipped mussel extracts. Various formulations are available under the trade name Gonex®. This group acts primarily to relieve pain and has little chondroprotective effect.

Injectable cartilage components bypass the digestive process and thus reach higher effective levels in the joints. These products include hyaluronic acid preparations and pentosan polysulfate.

Exercise Restriction

For dogs with joint, bone or muscle disorders, the recommended form of exercise prior to planned surgery, after a surgical procedure or as part of a conservative management regimen consists of short, relatively frequent walks. This allows the muscles to be used while avoiding excess strain on the joints due to consequences of fatigue. Under no circumstances should movement be curtailed excessively, as well-developed muscle mass has a stabilizing effect on proximally located joints such as the hip and shoulder.

Weight Reduction

Since around 60% of the dog's body weight is borne by the forelimbs, weight reduction is especially beneficial in cases of forelimb disorders. Depending on the disorder and the associated pathology, the effect of weight loss on the damaged cartilage cannot be overestimated. Owners should be encouraged to place overweight dogs on a weight reduction program [115].

Physiotherapy

Physiotherapy is of tremendous value in management of joint disease. The aims of physiotherapy as part of conservative therapy or post-surgical management include, but are not limited to, rapid return to normal locomotion, maintenance and accretion of muscle, an increase in the range of movement of injured or arthritic joints, removal of wound secretions and accumulated lymph and correction of abnormal loading due to chronic joint disease [99].

Collaboration between the veterinarian and the physiotherapist ideally commences before a planned surgical intervention, whereby the aims of therapy are decided jointly. Post-operative physiotherapeutic management should begin as soon as possible (e.g. 5 days post-operatively for femoral head resection, slightly later for surgical management of cruciate ligament rupture). The recovery period is shortened considerably by professional physiotherapy and associated therapeutic modalities. This approach is generally very well accepted by the animal and the owner.

8.2
Generalized Skeletal Disease

8.2.1 Osteochondrosis

Etiology and pathogenesis Osteochondrosis (OC; ▶ Fig. 8.2) is a developmental disorder of young dogs manifesting particularly in the elbow, shoulder, stifle and tarsal joints. Less commonly affected areas are the lumbosacral joint, the hip joint and the joints of the digits (forelimb and hindlimb). Proposed causal factors include rapid growth, qualitative malnutrition, excess calcium supply, genetic factors, overweight and excessive strain on the joints. There is currently no consensus on the definitive etiology.

Up to the age of about 4 months, absorption of calcium from the gut of puppies occurs in an unregulated manner. After a subsequent growth phase, calcium absorption is partially regulated by a vitamin D-dependent mechanism. Maturation of these processes governing resorption is delayed in large and giant breeds [127]. Thus, an excess supply of dietary calcium results in overly high blood calcium levels [118]. Excessive blood calcium is normalized by the action of calcitonin. A calcitonin-induced increase in chondroblast activity promotes cartilage and bone formation. Within joints, this leads to undernourishment of the excessively thick cartilage layer. Since articular cartilage only receives nutrition by diffusion from the synovial fluid , the deeper zones may become necrotic. In the presence of a heavy biomechanical load, which quickly develops in rapidly growing dogs, there is no opportunity for the delicate cartilage to recover. Other metabolic hypotheses refer to a genetically determined ossification defect that results in an excessively thick layer of cartilage with inadequate biomechanical stability.

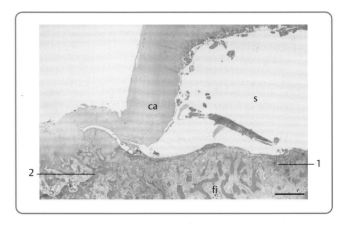

▶ **Fig. 8.2** Histological appearance of osteochondrosis: due to various metabolic factors, the chondrocytes hypertrophy, rather than undergoing normal degeneration and calcification (2). No signal is provided to osteoclasts for mineralization to commence; these cells remain inactive. This results in continuous thickening of the cartilage layer (ca). Cleavage of the thickened cartilage layer results in a subchondral fissure (s). There is also focal necrosis (1) and medullary fibrosis (fi). Bar = 620 μm. (source: Baumgärtner W. Pathohistologie für die Tiermedizin. Enke 2007)

Transarticular strain during the phase of rapid growth between 3 and 5 months is also a plausible contributing factor in the development of osteochondrosis. Under normal circumstances, the forces experienced by a joint are lower at the centre than at the periphery. Through increased loading during rapid growth, the central regions are subjected to abnormally high strain and the subchondral vascular supply is impaired. This explains the typical occurrence of OC lesions at locations such as the centre of the humeral head (shoulder joint, 74% of cases), the medial humeral condyle (elbow joint, 13%), lateral femoral condyle (stifle joint, 4%) and the ridges of the trochlea of the talus (9%). Interestingly, these joint components are located precisely at the proximal and distal end of the middle segment of the limb (humerus, tibia), where the high forces experienced by the respective joints are potentially explained by the matched motion mechanism (see Limb Kinematics (p. 18)).

The pathophysiological outcome is a weak cartilage layer that separates from the subchondral bone and may become a free-floating cartilage fragment. The fragment may establish its own blood supply via the synovial membrane and start to grow. In most cases, however, separation of the cartilage is incomplete and the uncalcified cartilage remains at its original location. Osteochondrosis is subdivided into four grades. Grade IV defects are painful and usually require surgical management. Lower grade OC lesions may heal spontaneously or remain subclinical.

Clinical signs General: Clinical signs first appear at 4–7 months of age. The history may reveal evidence of an unbalanced diet. Rapidly growing large breed dogs are most commonly affected and males are overrepresented. Osteochondritic lesions are often bilateral, but rarely occur in different joints.

Tarsal joint (p. 114): Tarsal OC usually results in obvious clinical signs. These include temporary lameness after rest , steep hindlimb conformation and marked effusion in the medial and lateral joint compartments. The OC lesion is found on the ridge of the trochlea of the talus (medial ridge in 75% of cases, lateral ridge in 25%). The majority of OC lesions are located on the proximal portion of the trochlear ridge; thus, direct digital palpation should be performed with the joint in maximum flexion to check for a pain response. Tarsal OC is rare.

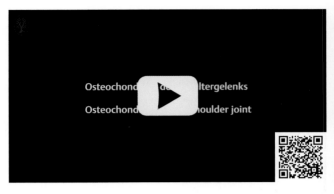

► **Video 8.1** Gait of a dog with osteochondrosis of the shoulder joint.

Stifle joint (p. 127): Joint effusion is palpable. The lateral femoral condyle is painful on palpation. Stifle joint OC is rare.

Elbow joint (p. 147): Clinical signs are indistinguishable from medial coronoid disease.

Shoulder joint (p. 153): Lameness is mild and the dog usually bears weight consistently on the affected limb. Direct palpation of the central and caudal portions of the humeral head, which is possible when the limb is rotated internally, may elicit a pain response.

Refer to ► Video 8.1 for a video showing the gait of a dog with osteochondrosis.

Diagnostic imaging and further testing

Tarsal joint Lesions cannot always be identified definitively in mediolateral and craniocaudal radiographs due to superimposition of different bones. Oblique views may be required. Radiographic findings may include a radiolucent subchondral defect on a trochlear ridge (► Fig. 8.3) and possibly a calcified joint mouse. Osteophytes may be observed on the medial and lateral joint margins, as degenerative joint changes are a common consequence of OC in the tarsal joint. If radiography is inconclusive, CT imaging may be indicated.

Stifle joint A flattened, well-delineated defect is observed in the subchondral bone on the distal surface of the lateral and,

► **Fig. 8.3** Radiograph of a tarsal joint with an osteochondritic lesion on the medial trochlear ridge of the talus.

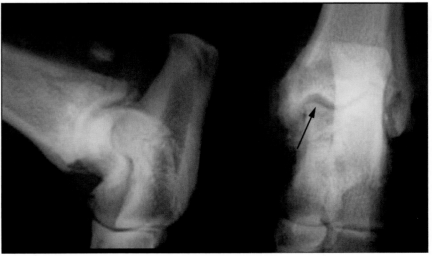

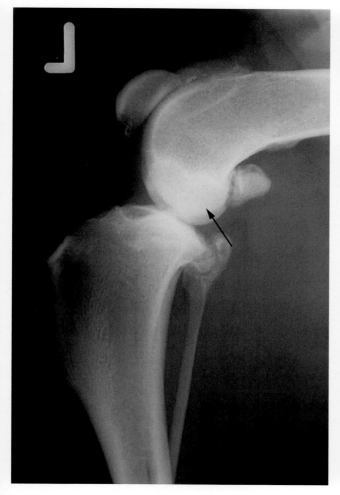

► **Fig. 8.4** Radiograph of a stifle joint with an osteochondritic lesion on the lateral femoral condyle.

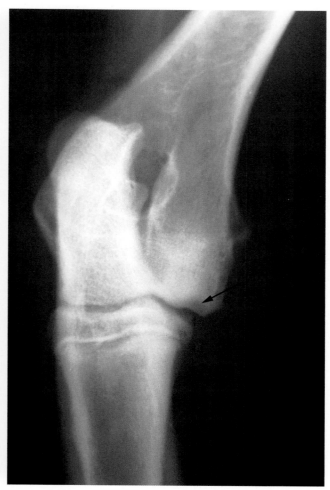

► **Fig. 8.5** Radiograph of an elbow joint showing an osteochondritic lesion on the medial humeral condyle.

rarely, the medial femoral condyle (►**Fig. 8.4**). Occasionally an oblique lateral view or an arthrogram is required.

Elbow joint Osteochondritic lesions are most readily identified in the craniocaudal view, appearing as a smooth, radiolucent bone defect on the articular surface of the medial humeral condyle (►**Fig. 8.5**). They may occur concurrently with medial coronoid process disease.

Shoulder joint The OC defect appears as a flattened cartilage defect of variable size on the caudocentral aspect of the humeral head, visible in the mediolateral view (►**Fig. 8.6**). In some cases, a slightly oblique projection is required. A free piece of cartilage may be found within the joint space.

Treatment Osteochondrosis does not always require surgical management. Conservative therapy is indicated if lameness is intermittent or radiographic changes are barely detectable. Non-surgical management is also recommended in adult dogs, in which pronounced degenerative changes are likely to render surgery unsuccessful. Appropriate measures for conservative management include long-term analgesic therapy, chondroprotective preparations, weight reduction, frequent walks of short

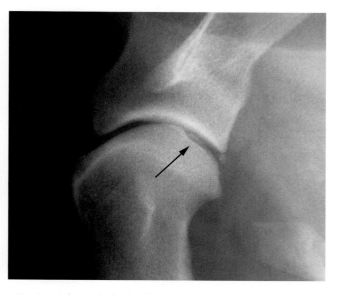

► **Fig. 8.6** Radiograph of a shoulder joint with an osteochondritic lesion on the head of the humerus.

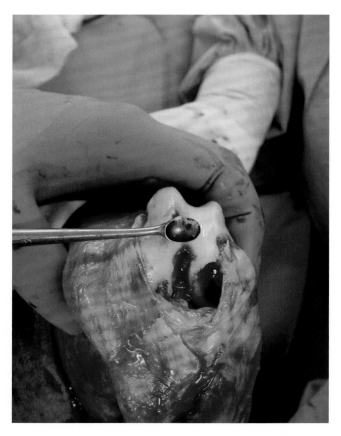

▶ **Fig. 8.7** Deep curetting of an osteochondritic lesion in the stifle joint. Fibrocartilage grows into the freshly created defect.

duration and physiotherapy. If the etiology is nutritional, the ration should be adjusted and corrected as required.

Specialist practice: Clearly visible OC lesions in young, acutely lame dogs should be managed surgically. The joint is accessed by arthrotomy or arthroscopy. The OC lesion is curetted, the defect bed is debrided and any free fragments are removed. The exposed subchondral bone can then grow into the defect, filling it with fibrocartilage within a few weeks (▶ Fig. 8.7). The younger the dog, the better is the prognosis. Shoulder OC has the best prognosis, tarsal OC the poorest. Pantarsal arthrodesis may be indicated if OC has resulted in advanced osteoarthritis.

8.2.2 Panosteitis

Etiology and pathogenesis Panosteitis occurs almost exclusively in juvenile large breed dogs. The term panosteitis is misleading, but has persisted over the years. It is sometimes also referred to as enostosis. The etiology of panosteitis is unknown. It was initially suspected to be an eosinophilic osteomyelitis, though no viruses or bacteria could be isolated from the bone. Other authors proposed an autoimmune, allergic, metabolic, parasitic or hormonal basis, without providing substantiating evidence. What is certain, however, is that panosteitis begins with the death of intramedullary fat cells near the nutrient foramen of long, tubular bones. The pathological mechanism appears to be triggered by disruption of blood supply or increased endosteal pressure. This phase is very painful. A repair process is subsequently initiated by fibro- and osteoblasts. This is useful for diagnosis as it results in an observable increase in bone density. At this stage, clinical signs may no longer be apparent, potentially complicating diagnosis by radiography. After 6–12 weeks, re-establishment of a normal medullary cavity by osteoclast activity marks the end of the disease process within the respective long bone. Other bones may subsequently be affected; generally, the same bone is not affected more than once. Panosteitis usually does not recur after the dog reaches maturity. Occasionally, disease is seen in mature dogs up to the age of 3 years.

Clinical findings Presented dogs are usually large, aged between 5 and 18 months and male. In females, an episode of panosteitis may occur during estrus. The onset of lameness is spontaneous and the dog remains lame for a few days to 3–6 weeks. Lameness does not improve as the dog warms up. Some dogs are anorexic. Bone pain can be so severe that dogs do not weight-bear on the affected limb (grade 3 or 4 lameness). The latter is rare in diseases such as elbow dysplasia. The history may reveal that lameness shifts from limb to limb. On clinical examination, a strong pain response is elicited by firm digital pressure on the long bones. The ulna is most frequently affected (42%), followed by the radius, humerus, femur and tibia [117]. As panosteitis often occurs in the proximal radius and ulna, the elbow joint (p. 147) must also be examined. Radiography should be used to rule out elbow dysplasia.

Diagnostic imaging and further testing A diagnosis of panosteitis can rarely be confirmed using radiography, as the repair process within the bone only appears around 6 weeks after the acute phase of disease. Thus, radiography is used in the first instance to eliminate elbow dysplasia as an important differential diagnosis, before providing evidence of panosteitis at a later stage. Radiographic findings include initial bone lysis, which is replaced by a hazy increase in bone density (▶ Fig. 8.8), with loss of the normal trabecular pattern, near the nutrient foramen. The endosteum returns to normal after several weeks. Occasionally, smooth or scale-like periosteal new bone is observed.

Treatment Panosteitis is self-limiting and there are no known long-term detrimental consequences. Supportive therapy comprises analgesia and reduction of food intake, as overfeeding is considered a possible causal factor, and there is often a marked discrepancy between estimated and actual body weight. Panosteitis can occur in multiple episodes affecting all four limbs.

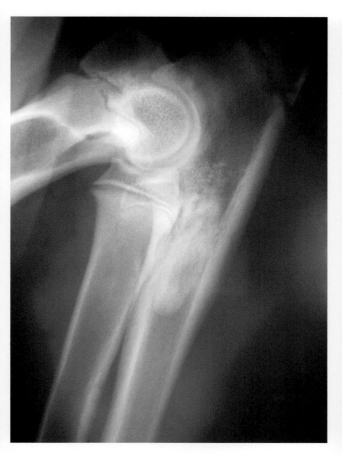

▶ **Fig. 8.8** Clearly discernible panosteitis lesion in the ulna of a 7 month old German Shepherd Dog.

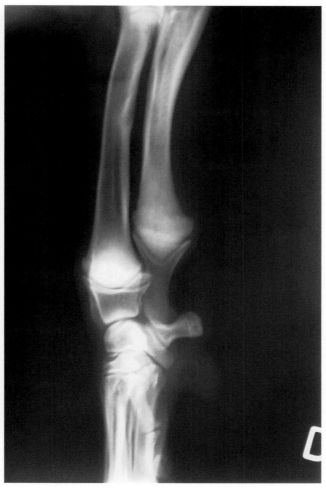

▶ **Fig. 8.9** Hypertrophic osteodystrophy: the metaphyses of the distal radius and ulna are thickened and irregular.

8.2.3 Hypertrophic Osteodystrophy

Etiology and pathogenesis Hypertrophic osteodystrophy is also referred to as idiopathic osteodystrophy, Moeller-Barlow disease or metaphyseal osteopathy. Its etiology remains unknown. Hypotheses based on dietary factors, such as vitamin C deficiency, excessive supply of vitamin D or minerals, and excess caloric intake have all been disproved. It is interesting to note that several other authors have identified RNA originating from distemper virus and *E. coli* in isolated bones, lending weight to the presumption of an infectious pathogenesis [97]. Hypertrophic osteodystrophy consistently occurs in the metaphyseal bone of puppies aged 3–5 months. The trabeculae are resorbed, the bone undergoes partial necrosis and inflammatory cells migrate to the affected area. The histological appearance resembles that of osteomyelitis. Occasionally, subperiosteal hemorrhages are also observed.

As metaphyseal disease can reduce the amount of new bone produced for longitudinal growth, it is likely to have long-term consequences. Particularly with involvement of the distal ulna (p. 103), premature growth plate closure can lead to asynchronous growth of the radius and ulna because virtually all ulnar growth occurs at the distal physis. The ulna effectively acts as a brace, while the radius can continue to grow.

Clinical findings Typically, hypertrophic osteodystrophy affects the metaphyses of both distal forelimbs. Affected young dogs become lame in just a few days. There is marked, painful swelling at the ends of the bones, accompanied by soft tissue edema (▶ Fig. 8.9). Many dogs have a history of respiratory or gastrointestinal tract infection. Most are pyrexic, anorexic, weak and dehydrated. Fatalities may occur.

Subclinical or mild forms of hypertrophic osteodystrophy can result in malalignment of the forelimb with associated lameness. The aforementioned growth disturbance manifests as bowing of the radius (p. 145), valgus, external rotation of the limb and occasionally subluxation of the elbow due to the short ulna. It is accompanied by progressive osteoarthritis of the carpus (p. 138) and elbow joint (p. 147) (▶ Fig. 8.10).

Diagnostic imaging and further testing Hypertrophic osteodystrophy most commonly affects the distal radius or the distal ulna. Radiolucent zones (or lines) and sclerotic areas are evident in the metaphyses. Sometimes a typical radiolucent line resembling the epiphyseal plate is seen in the metaphysis, immediately adjacent and parallel to the growth plate. In addition, paraperiosteal bone proliferation may be observed in the metaphyseal region. This can be smooth or irregular, and may be

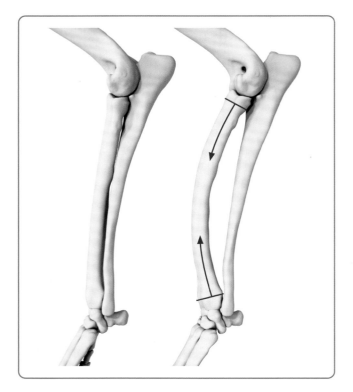

▶ **Fig. 8.10** Long-term disruption of the distal growth plate can cause bowing of the antebrachium (asynchronous growth of the radius and ulna). (source: Daniel Koch, Jonas Lauströer, Amir Andikfar)

distributed over the whole diaphysis. Ossification may be delayed in the metaphyseal region.

In the later stages of disease, premature growth plate closure may be identified by the absence of a radiolucent zone in the physis. There is bowing of the limbs, as described above. Lateral and craniocaudal radiographs of both limbs are required for definitive diagnosis and planning of corrective surgery.

Treatment Mild cases are managed with pain relief and exercise restriction.

Specialist practice: Severe cases require more potent analgesics, intravenous fluids and hospitalization. Hand feeding and even tube feeding may be required. Osteotomy can be performed for treatment of malalignment. The course of disease is highly variable.

8.2.4 Retained Cartilage Cones

Etiology and pathogenesis Retained cartilage cones are a consequence of retarded bone formation at the growth plate. They are very often located at the distal ulna (p. 103). The cause is unclear; the disease may constitute a special form or osteochondrosis. Similar changes are observed in the metaphyseal regions of other bones, where they are referred to as retained cartilage islands.

Clinical findings Cartilage cones appear during the rapid phase of growth at 3–4 months of age in large breeds. Initially, mild lameness is observed. Retained cartilage cones in the ulna

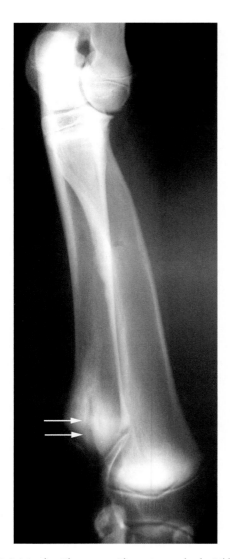

▶ **Fig. 8.11** Retained cartilage cones. The cones are clearly visible in the metaphysis of the distal ulna.

(p. 103) subsequently lead to excessive bowing of the radius, as longitudinal growth of the ulna is slowed. The animals are otherwise healthy.

Diagnostic imaging and further testing In radiographs of the ulna, cones measuring several centimeters in length are clearly visible in the distal metaphysis (▶ Fig. 8.11). They are usually found bilaterally.

Treatment Treatment is influenced considerably by the degree of limb deformity. Mild angular deformities do not require treatment, other than pain management.

Specialist practice: In the early stages of disease, an ulnar osteotomy can be performed if there is concern that severe limb deformity is likely. From the age of about 8 months, severe malalignment requires corrective osteotomy of the radius and ulna. A cautious prognosis is recommended, as elbow incongruity may result from shortening of the ulna.

8.2.5 Polyarthritis

Etiology and pathogenesis Arthritic diseases are classified as non-inflammatory or inflammatory (▶ Table 8.1). The latter category is subdivided into infectious and non-infectious forms. In dogs, by far the most common form of polyarthritis is idiopathic immune mediated polyarthritis.

Immune mediated arthritis can be idiopathic or may occur as a consequence of systemic neoplastic, infectious (staphylococci, mycoplasmas, corynebacteria, viruses, bacterial endocarditides, discospondylitides) or parasitic disease, or other serious disease (immune mediated intestinal disease, myeloproliferative disease). The pathophysiological processes are triggered, following hypersensitivity reactions, by the formation of antigen-antibody complexes and inflammatory products that are deposited in various locations, including in and around the joints. The rare erosive form of polyarthritis is further characterized by the production of chondrodestructive collagenases and proteases.

Clinical findings Polyarthritis can result in a number of clinical signs. The most common reasons for presentation are reluctance to move and a slightly stiff gait. The grade of lameness is highly variable. Pyrexia is present in most cases. Polyarthritis should thus be included as a differential diagnosis for fever of unknown origin. Typically, any swelling, heat and pain first appears in the distal joints (digital joints, carpal joint, tarsal joint). Thus, gait disturbances are often more obvious on uneven ground. Clinical signs resulting from the primary disease process may become less clinically apparent than those associated with polyarthritis.

Diagnostic imaging and further testing Diagnosis of polyarthritis is complex and expensive. The initial database comprises radiography of the most severely affected joints to eliminate a primary degenerative or traumatic etiology. In most forms of polyarthritis, diffuse joint capsule dilation is observed in the digital and metatarso- and metacarpophalangeal joints, as well as other distal joints. More proximally located joints are rarely affected. Arthritic lesions are only observed in the chronic stages of disease. If treatment is not initiated based on a presumptive diagnosis, comprehensive evaluation should include hematology, arthrocentesis of multiple joints (▶ Fig. 8.12) with joint fluid analysis, serology for possible primary disease agents (e.g. Ehrlichia, Toxoplasma, Borrelia) and investigation of other possible primary diseases. In most cases, cytology reveals a suppurative synovitis without the presence of bacteria (▶ Fig. 8.13), and antibody tests for infectious agents and tests for other diseases are negative. On this basis, a diagnosis of immune mediated polyarthritis can be made.

In the erosive forms of polyarthritis, articular changes are much clearer and there is evidence of cartilage and bone lysis. Joint capsule biopsy is recommended, in addition to arthrocentesis, to detect periarticular reactions and strengthen the diagnosis.

Treatment Treatment of polyarthritis has two components: identification and appropriate treatment of the primary disease, where possible, and management of arthritis. Erosive polyarthritides require treatment with corticosteroids (e.g. prednisolone 2 mg/kg body weight) and cytotoxic drugs (e.g. cyclophosphamide or azathioprine). Immune mediated polyarthritides can be managed with corticosteroids alone. The dose should be tapered gradually. Response to treatment is evaluated clinically and, where necessary, with repeated joint fluid analysis. The dog should be monitored for side effects of corticosteroids, and any necessary adjustments made. Alternative therapies can be considered as an alternative to corticosteroids.

The prognosis for erosive polyarthritis is usually guarded, as there is long-term damage to the joints. Immune mediated polyarthritides can be controlled with low-dose steroid therapy; in some cases therapy can be discontinued.

▶ **Tab. 8.1** Classification of arthritis [112].

Non-inflammatory	Inflammatory	
	Infectious	**Non-infectious**
• degenerative	• bacteria	• crystal-induced
• congenital	• mycoplasmas	• immune mediated
• traumatic	• protozoa	• erosive – rheumatoid arthritis – polyarthritis in Greyhounds
• neoplastic • hemophilic	–	• non-erosive – idiopathic polyarthritis – systemic lupus erythematosus – vaccination reaction – polyarthritis following meningitis

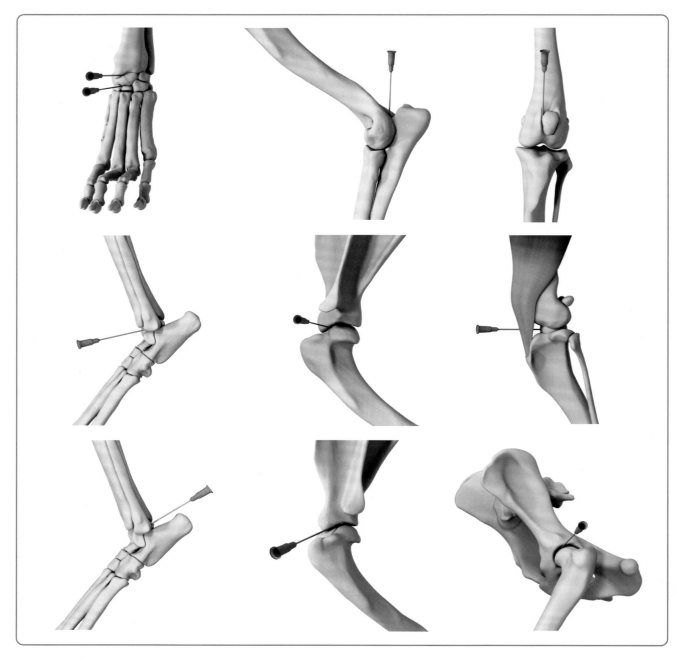

▶ **Fig. 8.12** Arthrocentesis sites in the dog. (source: Daniel Koch, Jonas Lauströer, Amir Andikfar)

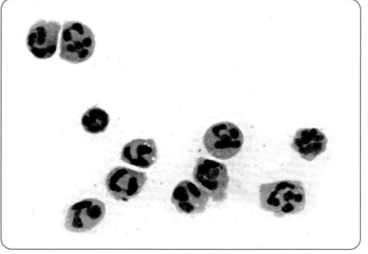

▶ **Fig. 8.13** Synovial fluid from an inflamed joint: the neutrophil count is elevated; neutrophils have segmented nuclei and eosinophilic cytoplasm (no sign of degenerative changes). Modified Wright's stain, × 100. (source: Institut für Veterinärpathologie der Vetsuisse-Fakultät Universität Zürich, Switzerland)

8.2.6 Osteomyelitis

Etiology and pathogenesis Most bone infections are of bacterial origin. Fungal osteomyelitis still occurs occasionally in the US. Sources of infection include open fractures, bone sequestra, bite wounds, spread from other sites or iatrogenic wound infection resulting from breakdown of aseptic technique or extended or repeated surgical intervention. Bone is intrinsically relatively resistant to infection. However, its defenses can be weakened (e.g. by traumatic or iatrogenic soft tissue damage with disruption of blood supply, placement of implants, systemic disease or certain deficiencies) to such an extent that bacterial colonization takes place. Many infections are caused by a single dominant organism. Around 70% are aerobes, often staphylococci. Other implicated bacteria include streptococci, *E. coli*, Pasteurella spp., Klebsiella spp., Serratia spp. and *Proteus*. Bite wounds, perforation of the gastro-intestinal tract or removal of dental calculus with concomitant surgical intervention [120] can result in microbial dissemination and colonization of bone with anaerobic bacteria (*Bacteroides*, *Fusobacterium*, Clostridia spp., *Actinomyces* and others). It should also be noted that hematogenous spread of bacteria from the umbilicus is often seen in neonates and puppies. This can have drastic consequences, as colonization of joints and highly vascularized zones of bone growth can rapidly lead to irreversible joint and bone damage.

Metatarsal fistulas have been reported in the German Shepherd Dog. These are not of osseous origin. While the etiology is unknown, the disease is steroid-responsive. Metatarsal fistulas should not be confused with classical osteomyelitis.

Clinical findings Hematogenous bacterial dissemination is almost always accompanied by fever and signs of sepsis. Affected young dogs are anorexic and lameness is evident if bones are infected. Pain and swelling is detectable on palpation.

Osteomyelitis of exogenous origin has a non-specific course. Fever is not always present. The affected body region is painful and warm. Muscular atrophy is evident and the dog is mildly lame. Where there is a history of surgery, the degree of lameness caused by developing osteomyelitis is indistinguishable from that observed during normal or slightly delayed healing. Fistulas may be observed if disease becomes chronic. These resolve with antibiotic treatment and recur after antimicrobial therapy has ceased.

Diagnostic imaging and further testing Acute osteomyelitis can be identified radiographically by the presence of a proliferative periosteal reaction (usually along the bone shaft), lysis of cortical bone and diffuse swelling in the surrounding soft tissue (▶ Fig. 8.14). In chronic osteomyelitis, the central nidus is surrounded by a sclerotic margin, representing the border with healthy bone. A sequestrum may be present. A variable degree of new bone formation in the bony periphery and soft tissue swelling are observed (▶ Fig. 8.15). Sectional imaging techniques such as computed tomography have higher sensitivity for detection of sequestra than plain radiography. Isolation of bacteria from a fistula is not diagnostic. For definitive diagnosis, bacteria must be cultured from the bone. The animal should

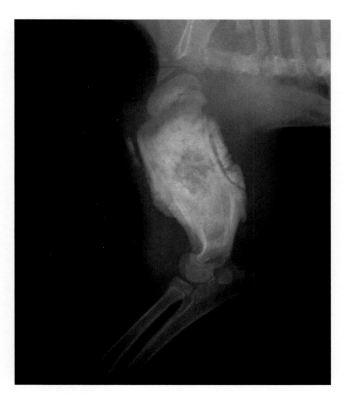

▶ **Fig. 8.14** Osteomyelitis in the humeral shaft of a 3 month-old French Bulldog. There is irregular thickening of the bone and periosteum. (source: Tony Flury, Tierklinik Lindenhof, Switzerland)

have received no antibiotics for at least 48 hours prior to sampling. Blood culture is indicated if hematogenous dissemination is suspected.

Treatment Conservative management with antibiotics is only indicated in a small number of cases, in which the lesion is very localized and the general well-being of the dog is not compromised (e.g. clindamycin 11 mg/kg SID, minimum 3 weeks duration).

Specialist practice: Many classical cases of localized osteomyelitis require targeted antibiotic therapy of at least 3 weeks duration and almost all necessitate local surgical debridement. Necrotic bone fragments are removed. Care must be taken to preserve the local blood supply. An autologous bone marrow transplant is used to fill the defect. For lesions near the trunk, omentum can be transferred into the defect. Implants near a fracture or sequestrum should be removed if they are contributing to the persistence of osteomyelitis. In this situation, it is preferable to stabilize the bone with an external fixateur or an implant with low bone-to-implant contact (e.g. locking plates). In rare cases, the infected area must be left open and flushed daily with sterile physiological fluids. The wound is closed several days later or allowed to heal by second intention. Recently developed biodegradable gentamicin-impregnated sponges can be placed in the wound. Fistula tracts should be removed. Amputation may be indicated in some cases.

Joint sepsis necessitates the removal of all implants, copious flushing or continuous irrigation (e.g. infusion with Ringer's lactate solution, 20 ml/h, egress via 1–2 drains) and prolonged

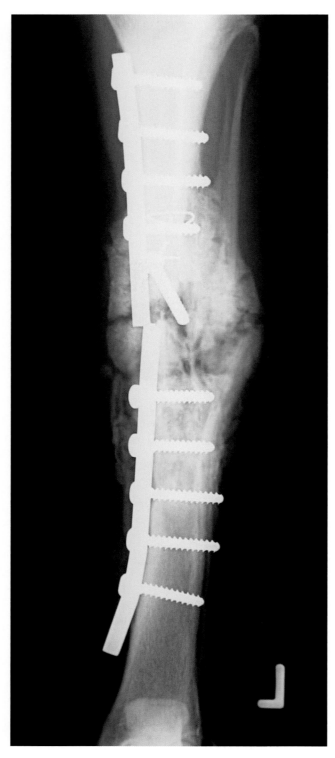

▶ **Fig. 8.15** Osteomyelitis with sequestra in a White Shepherd following iatrogenic vascular damage during fracture reduction.

antibiotic therapy, possibly supported by the use of antibiotic sponges. Subsequent placement of hip prostheses is generally contraindicated, as bacteria cannot be completely removed from the bone, and would rapidly colonize the delicate implant-bone interface, resulting in renewed instability.

Hematogenous infections are treated with intravenous antibiotics (e.g. high doses of cephalosporins, minimum 3 weeks duration) and drainage of localized abscesses. Affected puppies also require intravenous fluids and nutritional support. Delayed diagnosis is associated with a poor prognosis.

8.2.7 Bone Tumors

Etiology and pathogenesis Osteosarcoma is by far the most common tumor of the skeleton, accounting for around 80% of cases (▶ Fig. 8.16). In contrast to humans, it usually occurs in older patients. The incidence is higher in large dogs than small dogs. Predisposed locations are the distal radius, proximal humerus, distal femur and proximal tibia (away from the elbow and towards the knee). The overrepresentation of large dogs has not been definitively explained. It is assumed that tumor development is triggered by rapid bone growth or microfractures caused by high body weight and athletic activity. It has been observed that, in 5% of cases, osteosarcoma occurred in regions where another tumor was treated with radiotherapy within the previous 2–5 years [104]. In individual case reports documenting osteosarcoma in the presence of osteosynthetic plates, occurrence of the tumor at the location of the plate is probably coincidental and not a consequence of chronic, local inflammation. It should also be noted that osteosarcoma can be the primary cause of spontaneous fractures, particularly in the femur (pathological fractures). There is usually no history of substantial trauma, the fracture line is often short and lytic areas are present in the bone around the fracture site.

Other important skeletal tumors include chondrosarcoma, fibrosarcoma and hemangiosarcoma, as well as metastases from other sarcomas.

Clinical findings A typical osteosarcoma patient is a large dog aged 7–8 years. There is a history of progressive lameness that does not improve on warm-up. If microfractures occur in the affected region, acute lameness or fracture in the absence of substantial force may occur. Lameness is unresponsive to analgesics. There is usually extensive muscle atrophy in the affected limb. Tumors of the distal radius or the tibia often present as a visible and palpable swelling . Proximally located tumors may not be detected without radiography. Dogs with advanced osteosarcoma of the proximal humerus avoid touching down on the affected limb and hold the carpus and elbow in flexion. The clinical appearance resembles that of radial nerve paralysis. Tumors of the distal femur can be mistaken clinically for cruciate ligament rupture, since the gait is similar and cruciate ligament rupture can occur as a consequence of neoplasia. The regional lymph node is usually enlarged. At the time of diagnosis, around 99% of dogs have pulmonary micrometastases, thus may be observed to cough.

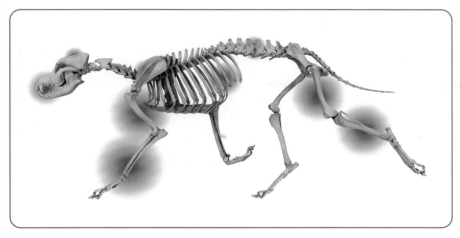

▶ **Fig. 8.16** Distribution of osteosarcoma in the dog [109]. (source: Daniel Koch, Jonas Lauströer, Amir Andikfar)

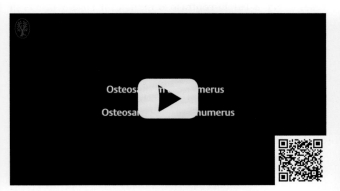

▶ **Video 8.2** Gait of a dog with osteosarcoma of the humerus.

Refer to ▶ Video 8.2 for a video showing the gait of a dog with osteosarcoma.

Diagnostic imaging and further testing Osteosarcoma is identified radiographically by the following findings: poor demarcation between normal and affected bone tissue, lysis of cortical bone, strong periosteal reaction and periosteal detachment (▶ Fig. 8.17). Osteosarcoma is usually limited to one bone and does not extend across joint boundaries. Confirmatory testing includes multiple punch biopsies of the bone, lymph node fine-needle aspiration and pulmonary radiography for detection of early metastases. If the findings are inconclusive, radiography should be repeated after 4 weeks.

Treatment As metastasis has usually already occurred at initial diagnosis, treatment is regarded as palliative. Amputation of the affected limb is associated with average survival times of about 4 months (12 months in 10% of patients).

Specialist practice: Amputation or limb-sparing tumor resection (▶ Fig. 8.18) with adjuvant chemotherapy increases survival times to 7–12 months, or one year in 33–64% of patients. Radiotherapy can be used to improve survival times or can be employed as a stand-alone form of palliative treatment [104].

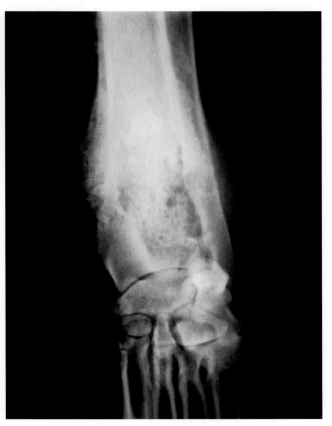

▶ **Fig. 8.17** Osteosarcoma of the distal radius in an 8 year old Leonberger.

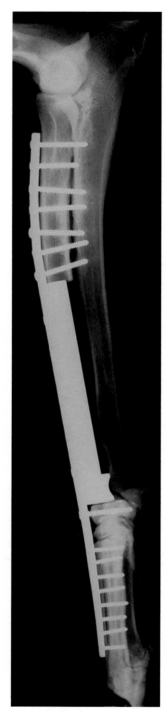

▶ **Fig. 8.18** Treatment of osteosarcoma of the distal radius with limb-sparing surgery. (source: Klinik für Kleintierchirurgie der Vetsuisse-Fakultät Universität Zürich, Switzerland)

8.2.8 Joint Tumors

Etiology and pathogenesis Joint tumors are rare but malignant. The most common is synovial cell sarcoma, which arises from undifferentiated mesenchymal cells in periarticular tissues. Most tumors consist of 2 cell lines, making histopathological diagnosis more difficult. The tumor attaches to the outside of the joint capsule but can also grow into the joint. A typical

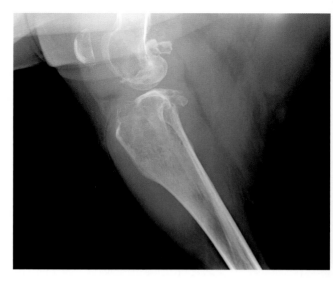

▶ **Fig. 8.19** Synovial cell sarcoma of the stifle joint. (source: Klinische Radiologie, Vetsuisse-Fakultät Universität Bern, Switzerland)

finding in advanced synovial cell sarcoma is osseous destruction in both articulating bones.

Clinical findings Diagnosis can rarely be established based on orthopedic examination alone. As tumors are frequently located at the stifle joint (p. 121), partial or complete cruciate ligament rupture is often suspected initially. Lameness is progressive, appearing mild at first, sometimes with improvement on warm up. The popliteal lymph node is slightly enlarged. The stifle joint is diffusely swollen and pain is detected on extension and on testing for cranial drawer (p. 124). There is no evidence of crepitation. Tumors of other joints, such as the tarsal joint (p. 114), elbow (p. 147) or shoulder joint (p. 153), are associated with similar, non-specific findings.

Diagnostic imaging and further testing Radiography reveals swelling of the stifle joint (▶ **Fig. 8.19**). In contrast to cruciate ligament rupture, swelling may appear irregular and may be observed in the outer periphery of the joint. With advanced disease, there is visible destruction of bones on both sides of the joint, a typical sign of synovial sarcoma. In contrast, osteosarcoma affects a single bone. The tumor tissue type is confirmed using biopsy, which may reveal other forms of joint sarcoma.

Treatment Locally resected tumors recur within 1–24 months. Amputation of the affected limb increases survival time by an average of 17 months.

Specialist practice: Adjuvant chemotherapy should be used for synovial cell sarcomas that are classified histologically as aggressive. A quarter of affected dogs have regional and pulmonary metastases which are associated with reduced survival times.

8.2.9 Hypertrophic Osteopathy

Etiology and pathogenesis Hypertrophic osteopathy is always preceded by the development of a large mass, usually a tumor or abscess, in the thorax or abdomen. It is thought that neurovascular reflexes associated with the primary disease process result in peripheral shunts, leading to local hypoxia of the bone with subsequent reactive bone formation . These periosteal reactions, resembling a string of pearls, only occur on long bones, but not in the vicinity of joints. Remission may occur following treatment of the primary disease. Hypertrophic osteopathy is also referred to as hypertrophic osteoarthropathy.

Clinical findings Hypertrophic osteopathy is very rare. Due to the involvement of a usually neoplastic primary mass, the patient is often older. Large breeds are overrepresented. Areas of swelling usually first appear in the distal forelimbs. They are palpable, painful and accompanied by edema. Mild lameness is observed in the later stages of disease.

Diagnostic imaging and further testing Radiography of the long bones reveals characteristic regular periosteal reactions (▶ **Fig. 8.20**), first appearing in varying degrees along the metacarpals and metatarsals and then along the tubular long bones. Primary disease in the thorax or abdomen must also be identified to establish a definitive diagnosis.

Treatment Treatment and prognosis are heavily dependent on the nature of the primary disease. Secondary changes in the long bones, and associated lameness, eventually regress. In most cases, however, the primary disease process is a pulmonary tumor, thus the prognosis is poor.

8.2.10 Nutritional Diseases

The effects of inappropriate nutrient supply are more pronounced in growing dogs than in adults. They are usually not the sole etiological factor, acting instead together with genetic predisposition to exacerbate other pathological processes. For further information, refer to Role of Nutrition (p. 39).

8.3 Hindlimb Diseases

8.3.1 Sesamoid Disease

Refer to information provided under Sesamoid Disease in the Forelimb (p. 220).

8.3.2 Osteochondrosis of the Tarsus

Refer to general information provided under Osteochondrosis (p. 185).

8.3.3 Tarsal Instability

Trauma

Etiology and diagnosis Many cases of tarsal instability (▶ **Fig. 8.21**) are caused by trauma. Instability is readily diagnosed via palpation and stress radiographs (stressed lateral

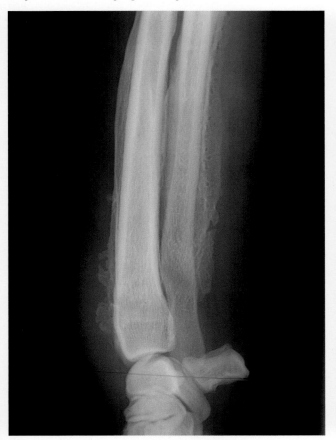

▶ **Fig. 8.20** Periosteal reaction on the radius and ulna, characteristic of hypertrophic osteopathy. The dog had multiple lung metastases of unknown origin.

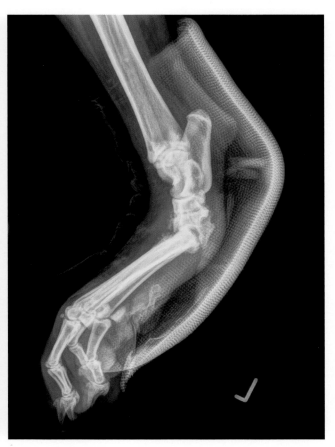

▶ **Fig. 8.21** Tarsometatarsal instability in a Borzoi. The joint has been temporarily fixed with a synthetic resin-impregnated bandage.

view, hyperextended view, hyperflexed view). The small bones consist largely of cortical bone tissue, are connected by short, taut ligaments and are relatively poorly vascularized.

Treatment and prognosis In puppies under the age of 6 months, ruptured intertarsal ligaments and luxations can be treated successfully with exercise restriction and splinting. Within a period of 6–8 weeks, fibrotic regeneration results in satisfactory joint stability. Ruptured talocrural collateral ligaments can generally be reconstructed and have an excellent prognosis. Instability resulting from avulsion fractures of the malleolus are fixed with tension band wiring.

Specialist practice: Intertarsal and tarsometatarsal luxations and ligament ruptures in dogs over 10 months of age require complex reconstructions and carry an uncertain prognosis. In many cases, they are treated directly with partial arthrodesis. Traumatic calcaneal fractures are fixed with tension band wiring or plates (▶ Fig. 8.22). Panarthrodesis may be required for management of extensive trauma, fractures of the talus and pre-existing osteoarthritis.

Spontaneous Calcaneal Fractures

Etiology and diagnosis The cause of spontaneous calcaneal fractures in dogs (▶ Fig. 8.23) is unknown. Collie-type dogs and

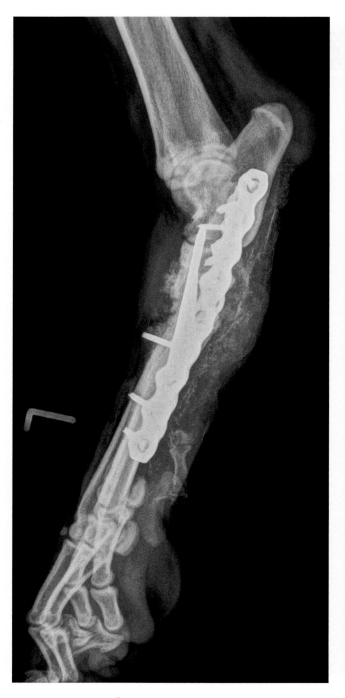
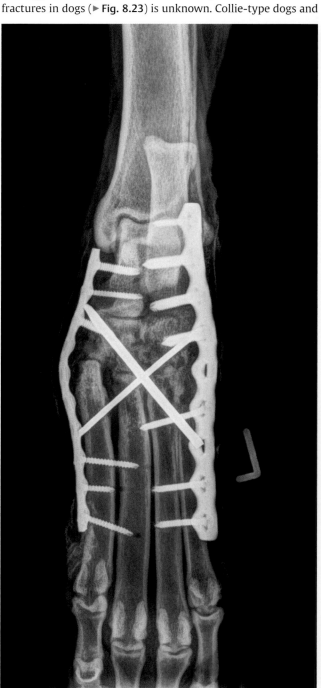

▶ **Fig. 8.22** Treatment of tarsometatarsal instability with cross pins and medial and lateral plate fixation (including use of locking screws).

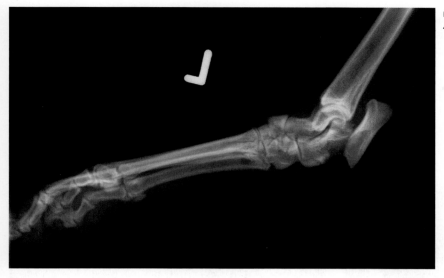

▶ **Fig. 8.23** Spontaneous calcaneal fracture in a 4 year old Border Collie.

overweight animals are predisposed. Calcaneotarsal subluxation occurs in some dogs, producing similar clinical signs. Presented dogs have no history of trauma and exhibit a partial or complete plantigrade stance in one or both hindlimbs. Not infrequently, pressure sores are present on the skin over the calcaneus, due to damage occurring on contact with the ground at touch down. The common calcaneal tendon is intact. Diagnosis can be established with radiography.

Treatment Specialist practice: Spontaneous calcaneal fractures cannot be managed successfully with conservative methods such as splints or orthoses, due to the occurrence of pressure necrosis in the skin, bone and even the common calcaneal tendon. In addition, the tensile forces exerted by the powerful musculature interfere with healing. A return to normal locomotion can only be achieved by debridement of the bone fragments and appropriate arthrodesis, including plate fixation, external fixateurs and tension band wiring, for a minimum of 6 months (▶ **Fig. 8.24**).

Common Calcaneal Tendon Rupture

Etiology and diagnosis The common calcaneal tendon (p. 89) (formerly Achilles tendon) has three components: the tendon of the gastrocnemius, the tendon of the flexor digitorum superficialis and the combined terminal tendon of the biceps femoris, gracilis and semitendinosus. The gastrocnemius makes up the greatest proportion of the compound tendon. With the exception of the flexor digitorum superficialis, all of the muscles insert on the calcaneus. The flexor digitorum superficialis forms the so-called calcaneal cap and passes to the digits.

Calcaneal tendon rupture can result from sharp and blunt trauma, and from chronic administration of corticosteroids, which weakens the connective tissue and leads to spontaneous tears. Dogs with a ruptured common calcaneal tendon have a plantigrade stance (▶ **Fig. 8.25**). The stumps of the tendon can readily be palpated as distended areas near the calcaneus. Rupture often occurs in racing dogs.

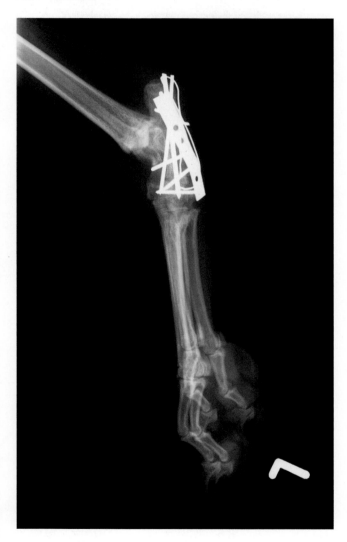

▶ **Fig. 8.24** Fixation of the calcaneus with a combination of tension band wires and a plate to compensate for the tensile forces exerted by the common calcaneal tendon.

Treatment Specialist practice: treatment for common calcaneal tendon rupture involves primary repair of the tendon stumps. For best results, these should be sutured individually (Kessler [locking loop], Bunnell or three-loop pulley suture patterns; ▶ Fig. 8.26, ▶ Fig. 8.27). The tendon can be reinforced with synthetic or biological (porcine intestinal submucosa) mesh. Additional support with an external fixateur or splint for 4–6 weeks is strongly recommended.

Calcaneal Cap Luxation

Etiology and diagnosis The calcaneal cap (p.89) is formed by the flexor digitorum superficialis. Lateral luxation occurs almost exclusively in Shelties (▶ Fig. 8.28). The cause is unknown, though the sulcus at the caudal end of the calcaneus is relatively shallow in affected dogs. The resulting gait resembles that observed with patellar luxation. In a relaxed state, the calcaneal cap can be manually luxated and reduced [125].

Treatment and prognosis There are three options for stabilization, depending on the degree of severity: fixation of the calcaneal cap to the paratendinous tissue using non-absorbable suture material; forced reduction by placement of a wire loop through the caudal end of the calcaneus and around the calcaneal cap (▶ Fig. 8.29); deepening of the calcaneal sulcus. The prognosis is good.

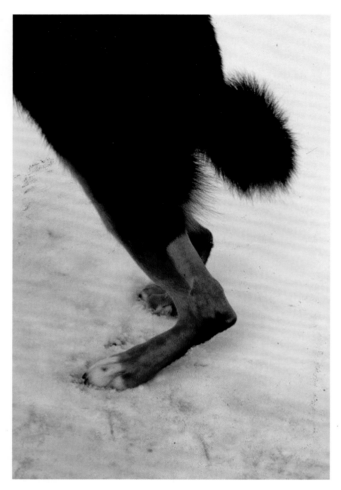

▶ **Fig. 8.25** Plantigrade stance in a dog with a ruptured common calcaneal tendon.

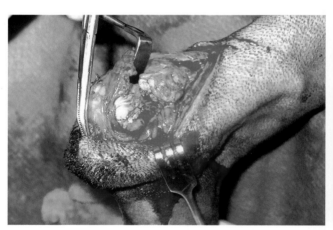

▶ **Fig. 8.26** Surgical approach for treatment of common calcaneal tendon rupture: at the site of rupture, the ends of the tendon are frayed and thickened.

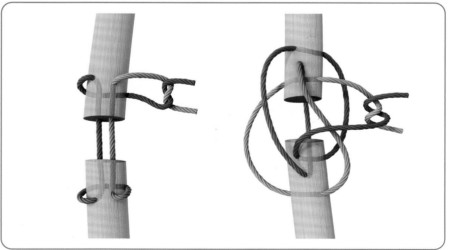

▶ **Fig. 8.27** Two suture patterns commonly used for tendon repair: locking loop (left) and three-loop pulley pattern (right). (source: Daniel Koch, Jonas Lauströer, Amir Andikfar)

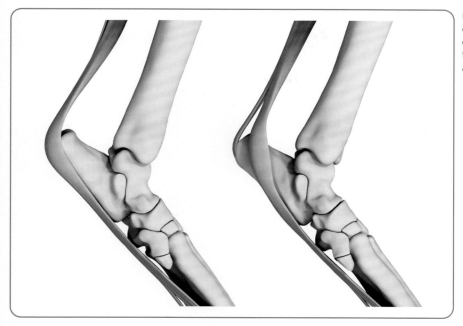

▶ **Fig. 8.28** Calcaneal cap luxation primarily occurs in a lateral direction. The cap is a component of the flexor digitorum superficialis. (source: Daniel Koch, Jonas Lauströer, Amir Andikfar)

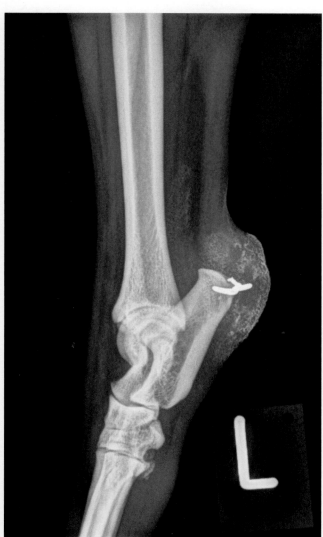

▶ **Fig. 8.29** Reduction of the calcaneal cap and alignment of the tendon by means of a wire loop passing through the calcaneus.

8.3.4 Cruciate Ligament Rupture

Etiology and pathogenesis In humans, anterior cruciate ligament rupture is usually the result of external influences (e.g. football or skiing injuries). Strong forces acting on the lower leg or uncontrolled rotation result in sudden tearing of the thick, anterior cruciate ligament (p. 91). It was long thought that the same occurs in animals, brought about by repeated jumping or exuberant play on an uneven surface.

Critical scrutiny of the pathogenesis of cranial cruciate ligament rupture in dogs has yielded information pointing to an etiology other than physical activity: excised cruciate ligament remnants exhibit evidence of degeneration over time; tearing is usually partial, progressing to complete rupture; there is no history of forceful impact on the stifle joint; canine stifle joint biomechanics are different to those of the human knee; the heavier the dog, the more frequent the occurrence of cranial cruciate ligament rupture; breeds such as the Rottweiler, Newfoundland Dog and Staffordshire Bull Terrier are overrepresented; if one stifle joint has been affected, it is not uncommon for cruciate ligament rupture to occur in the other stifle as well; radiographically, arthritic changes are already evident at the time of an „acute" rupture [105], [131].

In the US and Europe, the biomechanical basis of cranial cruciate ligament rupture is the subject of debate, resulting in different approaches to treatment. A logical and clinically meaningful derivation is based on recognizing the quadriceps as the main force transmitter of the stifle joint (▶ Fig. 8.30). Vector analysis indicates that a portion of the muscle exerts tension in a vertical direction, relative to the tibial plateau (F_{JC}), while a cranially directed portion exerts a continuous shear force (cranial tibial thrust, CTT) on the cranial cruciate ligament. This force rises with increases in the following parameters: body size and degree of overweight (e.g. Rottweiler, Newfoundland Dog, Labrador), steepness of the hindlimbs (e.g. Boxer, many fighting dogs), activity of the dog, narrowness of the proximal tibia and steepness of the tibial plateau [108], [122]. As a result,

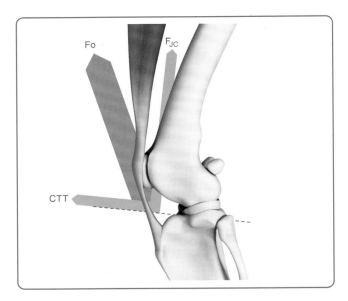

▶ **Fig. 8.30** Summary and simplified schematic illustration of the principal forces in the stifle joint. The primary force transmitter, the quadriceps femoris, pulls slightly cranially and proximally; the resulting shear force is neutralized by the cranial cruciate ligament. F_Q = force exerted by quadriceps, CTT = cranial tibial thrust, F_{JC} = joint compressive force. (source: Daniel Koch, Jonas Lauströer, Amir Andikfar)

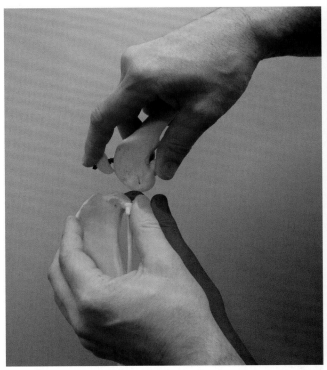

▶ **Fig. 8.31** Schematic illustration of the cranial drawer test for diagnosis of cranial cruciate ligament rupture.

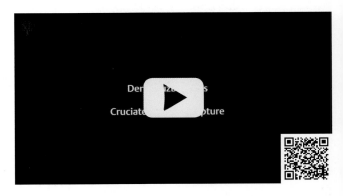

▶ **Video 8.3** Cruciate ligament rupture – abnormal gait and positive cranial drawer test.

the cranial cruciate ligament first becomes partially torn and subsequently ruptures completely.

Meniscal damage usually involves the caudal horn of the medial meniscus, since the mobility of the medial meniscus is limited by its attachment to the medial collateral ligament. In addition, considerable rotational movement occurs during the touch down phase. This may be responsible for causing preliminary damage to the cranial cruciate ligament, as well as traumatic injury of the meniscus in an unstable stifle joint.

Clinical findings Dogs with a ruptured cruciate ligament typically exhibit temporary lameness after rest, without a definitive history of trauma. The hindlimb is carried in flexion; sometimes only the tip of the foot makes contact with the ground. It is not uncommon for lameness to be episodic with varying degrees of severity. This is indicative of the frequency of partial cruciate ligament injury (p. 121). Wastage of the limb muscles is evident, and there is palpable joint effusion. With entrapment of the medial meniscus (p. 126), lameness becomes more obvious and may be non-weight bearing.

Cranial cruciate ligament rupture results in a positive cranial drawer sign. This is most readily detected with the dog in recumbency and the limb slightly flexed. If rupture is partial, the stifle joint is stable, but pain is elicited by the cranial drawer test (p. 124) and by internal rotation of the tibia (▶ Fig. 8.31). The cranial drawer test may also be negative in the presence of severe osteoarthritis or complete cranial folding of the caudal horn of the medial meniscus. The alternative method, the so-called tibial compression test (p. 125) is performed by flexing the tarsal joint while holding the stifle joint in extension. If the cranial cruciate ligament is ruptured, the reciprocal apparatus maintained by the tension in the common calcaneal tendon forces the proximal tibia to move cranially. This test is difficult to perform in large dogs.

In dogs with medial patellar luxation (p. 123), cranial cruciate ligament rupture commonly occurs in advanced age, as the ligament is weakened by increased internal rotation of the tibia.

Caudal cruciate ligament rupture is extremely rare and usually results from trauma. Distinguishing between caudal and cranial rupture is not necessarily straightforward, but is possible for an experienced examiner. As assessment is made of the way in which cranial movement of the tibia is „stopped". If the caudal cruciate ligament is ruptured, the taut cranial cruciate ligament brings movement of the tibia to an abrupt halt. If the cranial cruciate ligament is ruptured, the "stop" is softer, because cranial movement is restricted by the joint capsule.

Refer to ▶ **Video 8.3** for video showing the gait of a dog with cruciate ligament rupture.

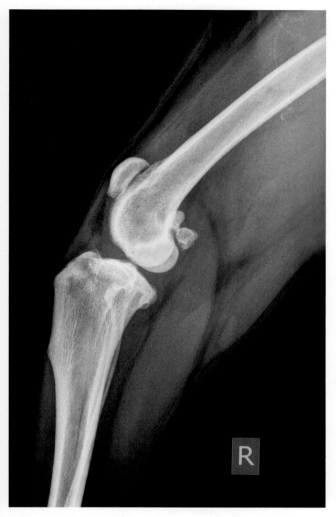

► **Fig. 8.32** Radiograph (lateral view) of a stifle joint in which the cranial cruciate ligament is completely ruptured. Findings include effusion in the cranial and caudal stifle joint compartments, early osteoarthritis and subluxation of the tibia.

Diagnostic imaging A clinical diagnosis can be established based on a positive cranial drawer test. Radiography is used to confirm the diagnosis in the case of partial rupture and to exclude other diseases such as neoplasia. Radiographic findings associated with cranial cruciate ligament rupture include joint effusion in the cranial and caudal compartments of the stifle joint (► Fig. 8.32). The increased volume of synovial fluid results in compression of the infrapatellar fat pad, which loses its triangular radiographic outline. The sesamoid bone of the popliteus may be displaced caudally. If disease is chronic, osteoarthritic changes may be evident at the distal pole (apex) of the patella, along the femoral trochlea, at the cranial and caudal ends of the tibial plateau and along the medial and lateral borders of the joint capsule. Subluxation of the tibia is occasionally observed.

Treatment In small dogs (as in cats of normal body weight), capsular fibrosis and muscular support often compensate quite effectively for stifle joint instability. Surgery is thus not neces-

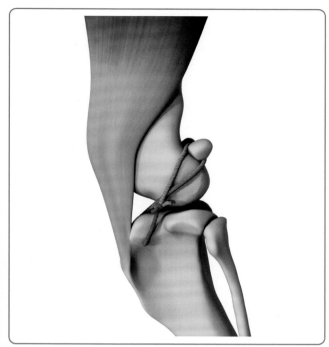

► **Fig. 8.33** Schematic illustration of suture placement for extracapsular stabilization of the stifle joint following cranial cruciate ligament rupture (de Angelis method). (source: Daniel Koch, Jonas Lauströer, Amir Andikfar)

sarily indicated. Fibrosis can also be enhanced surgically by capsular and fascial imbrication.

In dogs over 5 kg body weight, cranial cruciate ligament rupture should be managed surgically, since untreated rupture rapidly leads to severe osteoarthritis and a pronounced reduction in quality of life. Several surgical techniques are available. Factors determining the method of choice include the weight of the patient, economical considerations, available equipment and the experience of the surgeon.

As in humans, transposition of strong muscle fascia or tendon components can be performed in animals to replace the cranial cruciate ligament. It is important that replacement of the ligament is anatomically correct. The ends are sutured or screwed in place. This technique was commonly employed in the early stages of modern small animal orthopedics. The introduction of synthetic materials and improved methods for attachment to bone has allowed its continued successful use, mainly in small dogs.

The cranial cruciate ligament can also be replaced by extracapsular placement of thick synthetic sutures (extracapsular repair). The suture is positioned in a figure of eight between anchor points in the proximal tibia and behind the lateral and medial sesamoid bones (► Fig. 8.33). Up to 3 sutures are placed. Suitable suture materials include stainless steel, fishing line or non-absorbable polyester. This artificial form of ligament replacement generally produces good long term results in small dogs, even though the distance between the anchor points varies during flexion and extension, the natural torsion of the stifle joint is not accounted for and shear forces continue to exert considerable strain on the artificial ligament post-operatively.

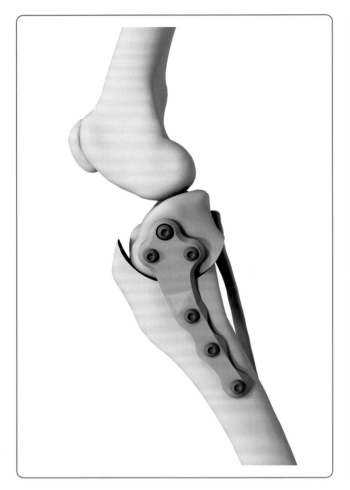

► **Fig. 8.34** Tibial plateau leveling osteotomy (TPLO): a curved osteotomy is performed at the proximal tibia and the tibial plateau is rotated and fixed. (source: Daniel Koch, Jonas Lauströer, Amir Andikfar)

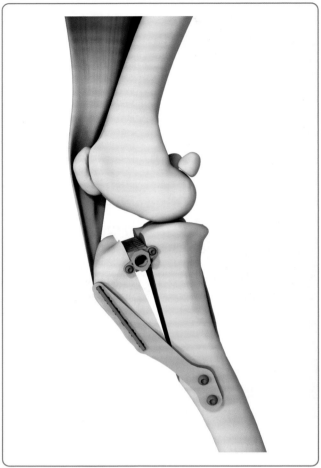

► **Fig. 8.35** Tibial tuberosity advancement (TTA): the proximal portion of the tibia is enlarged, minimizing shear forces in the stifle joint. (source: Daniel Koch, Jonas Lauströer, Amir Andikfar)

Specialist practice: Alternative methods are based on changing the biomechanics of the stifle joint, thus eliminating the need to replace the cruciate ligament. These techniques involve elevation of the tibial plateau (tibia plateau levelling osteotomy, TPLO; ► **Fig. 8.34**) [123] or cranial displacement of the attachment of the patellar ligament (tibial tuberosity advancement, TTA; ► **Fig. 8.35**, ► **Fig. 8.36**) [116]. In both methods, the force that would otherwise be counteracted by the cruciate ligament is reduced, virtually to nil. Thus, reconstruction of the cruciate ligament becomes redundant. These osteotomy-based techniques are currently the method of choice in heavy dogs and dogs with severe osteoarthritis. Post-operative care is simpler than for procedures involving cruciate ligament replacement, and within just 6 weeks there is no longer a risk that suture failure will compromise the success of the operation.

Irrespective of the method used, post-operative management should include analgesia and treatment with chondroprotective preparations (primarily chondroitin sulfate, minimum 2 months duration). Physiotherapy, strict weight control and moderate exercise are also important in the first few months after surgery. The recovery time following TTA or TPLO is around 3 months. Successful treatment may even render dogs sufficiently fit for performance activities or guard duty.

8.3.5 Patellar Luxation

Etiology and pathogenesis The causes of patellar luxation (PL) are incompletely understood. Morphometric evaluation of the limbs and pelvis has yielded no definitive information [130], except that luxation can result from obvious trauma or growth-related deformity of the hindlimbs, or altered hindlimb conformation (e.g. following femoral head resection). Empirically, the trend towards miniaturization of dog breeds has increased the occurrence of medial patellar luxation, while lateral luxation is relatively rare. Affected small breeds include the French Bulldog, Pug, Poodle, Pekingese, Jack Russell Terrier, Chihuahua, Pomeranian, Maltese Terrier, Papillon and the Bolonka. Overrepresented large breeds include the Flat Coated Retriever, Appenzeller Mountain Dog, Newfoundland and the American Cocker Spaniel. In the Kooikerhondje, heritability has been calculated at around 27% [129].

Luxation usually occurs within the first year of life. Initial luxation leads to joint effusion, pain and acute lameness. Subsequent luxations are less painful, though – depending on the severity and frequency of luxation – the retropatellar and femoral articular cartilage becomes markedly worn; within months to years, there is irreversible cartilage damage with pronounced

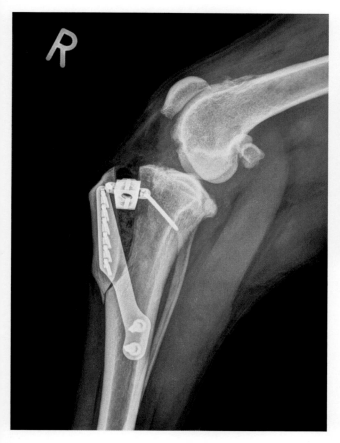

▶ **Fig. 8.36** Post-operative radiograph following TTA.

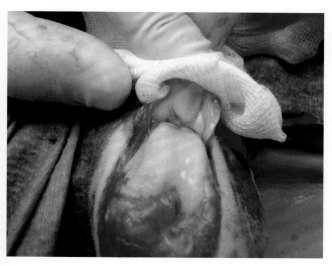

▶ **Fig. 8.37** Shallow femoral trochlea with cartilage wear on the medial trochlear ridge and beneath the patella in a Poodle with medial patellar luxation.

PL is classified into four grades (▶ **Fig. 8.38**). Grading follows the American standard: Grade 1 – patella is normally located in the trochlea and reduces spontaneously following luxation; Grade 2 – reduction can be achieved by manipulation of the limb (flexion, extension, rotation); Grade 3 – the patella is located lateral or medial to the trochlea, reduction can only be achieved by digital manipulation of the patella; Grade 4 – the patella can no longer be returned from the luxated position to its normal location.

flattening of the femoral trochlea (▶ **Fig. 8.37**). With lateral luxation, there is additional damage to the attachment of the extensor digitorum longus. When the patella is luxated, the functional unit consisting of the tibial tuberosity, patellar ligament, patella and quadriceps femoris cannot prevent the limb from buckling on touch down. Thus, the affected limb is not used and is held in a flexed position. Through shaking and rotational movements of the hindlimb, the patella can return spontaneously to its correct position, whereupon the gait becomes normal. This manifests as the intermittent lameness typical of PL. In chronic cases, a new groove is formed on the distal femur, allowing the quadriceps mechanism to maintain relatively normal limb function.

Clinical findings Intermittent lameness with periods of normal locomotion and three-legged lameness is considered pathognomonic. Important, though uncommon, differential diagnoses include calcaneal cap luxation in Shelties and neurological disorders, as suspected in Jack Russell Terriers. The grade of luxation is determined by examining the dog in standing and recumbent positions, and by manipulating the leg through the normal range of rotation, flexion and extension. With the dog in recumbency, the examiner grasps the tarsus with one hand and manipulates the limb, while using the thumb or finger of the other hand to luxate the patella (p. 123). The degree of force used for this procedure should not result in pain. The recorded

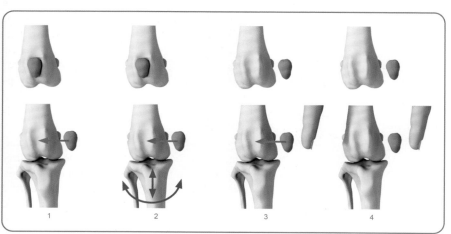

▶ **Fig. 8.38** Grading of patellar luxation. The upper row indicates the position of the patella prior to manipulation of the stifle joint (patella in the trochlea in Grades 1 and 2, patella luxated in Grades 3 and 4). The lower row illustrates the manner in which reduction is achieved (spontaneous reduction in Grade 1, manipulation of the leg in Grade 2, with the aid of digital manipulation in Grade 3, reduction not possible in Grade 4). (source: Daniel Koch, Jonas Lauströer, Amir Andikfar)

diagnosis should correspond to the highest observed degree of abnormality [110]. For example, if the patella is spontaneously luxated in the standing position, PL is classified as Grade 3, even if manipulation of the leg induces spontaneous reduction when the dog is recumbent.

Diagnostic imaging and further testing Patellar luxation is diagnosed purely on the basis of clinical findings. Since the grading of PL is heavily influenced by the skill and experience of the examiner, and is therefore quite subjective, a repeatable, standardized form of evaluation (e.g. radiographic appearance) would be most welcome. Unfortunately, radiography, CT and MRT are unable to fulfil this role.

Luxation is only rarely detected in radiographs. In congenital or acquired deformities, such as bow-leggedness (genu varum; ► Fig. 8.39) or a knock-knee stance (genu valgum), the patella may be found to lie medial or lateral to the femoral condyles in ventrodorsal views. If findings are inconclusive, oblique projections with the limb in flexion may provide information about the position of the patella and the depth of the trochlea (► Fig. 8.40). Radiography usually reveals minimal evidence of osteoarthritis and little joint effusion.

Treatment Surgery is indicated for PL in dogs that frequently exhibit a three-legged gait. The best treatments are those that re-establish the correct relative position of the patella and femur (► Video 8.4, ► Fig. 8.41, ► Fig. 8.42, ► Fig. 8.43). The preferred method is transposition (medial or lateral) of the site of insertion of the patellar ligament on the tibia and deepening of the femoral trochlea. Each of these surgical components can be performed in different ways. For the transposition procedure, osteotomy of the tibial tuberosity can be straight or slightly angled (with cranialization) and may be partial or complete. Simple and very stable fixation can be achieved using tension band wiring, though screws or a single pin are occasionally used. Sulcoplasty can be performed using wedge or block resection. It is important that the groove is deepened sufficiently to prevent spontaneous luxation of the patella. The orthopedic procedures are supplemented with soft tissue imbrication.

Refer to ► Video 8.4 for a video showing the gait of a dog with patellar luxation.

Specialist practice: An alternative approach involves placement of a patellar groove replacement prosthesis. Following osteotomy of the trochlea, a titanium prosthesis is inserted under the patella and screwed onto the femur (► Fig. 8.44). This new method is particularly suitable where cartilage erosion is severe or the trochlea is very flat. Transposition and fixation of the tibial tuberosity is not required.

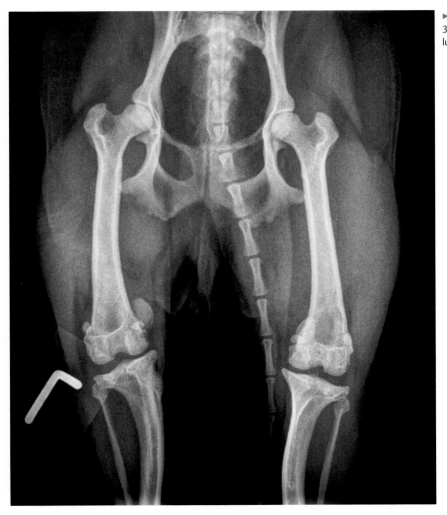

► **Fig. 8.39** Genu varum (bow-leggedness) in a 3 year old Yorkshire Terrier. Bilateral medial patellar luxation is evident.

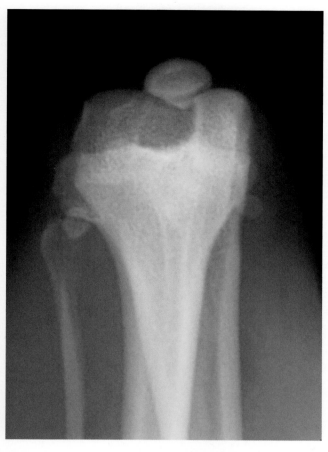

► **Fig. 8.40** Skyline view: the patella is radiographed tangentially, showing its position relative to the femur and the femoral trochlea. (source: Patrick Blättler Monnier, Frenkendorf, Switzerland)

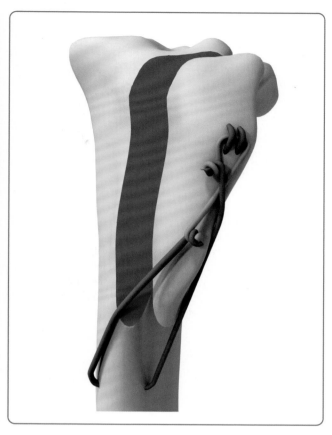

► **Fig. 8.42** Schematic illustration of transposition of the tibial tuberosity: the osteotomized tuberosity is transposed, in accordance with the severity and direction of luxation, and fixed with tension band wiring. (source: Daniel Koch, Jonas Lauströer, Amir Andikfar)

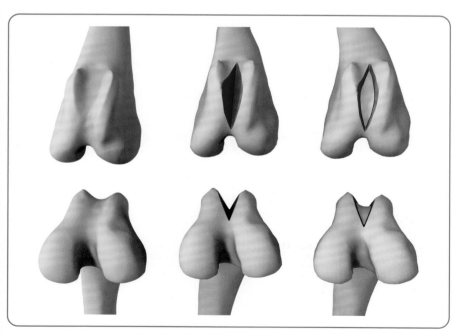

► **Fig. 8.41** Schematic illustration of wedge sulcoplasty for treatment of patellar luxation: the trochlea is deepened by performing a wedge resection, removing a thin layer of bone, and replacing the wedge. (source: Daniel Koch, Jonas Lauströer, Amir Andikfar)

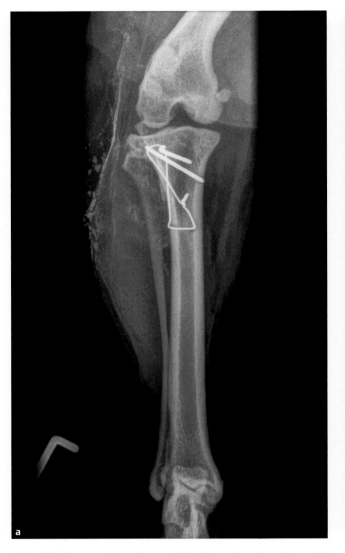
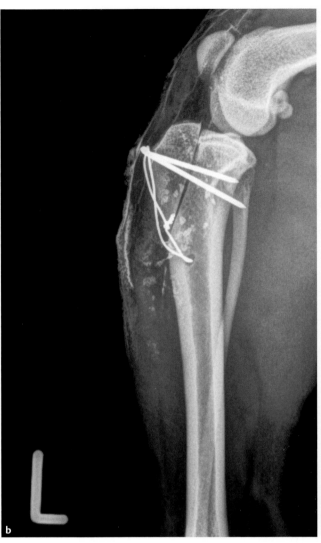

▶ **Fig. 8.43** Post-operative radiographs following wedge sulcoplasty and lateral transposition of the tibial tuberosity for treatment of medial patellar luxation.
a Craniocaudal view.
b Lateral view.

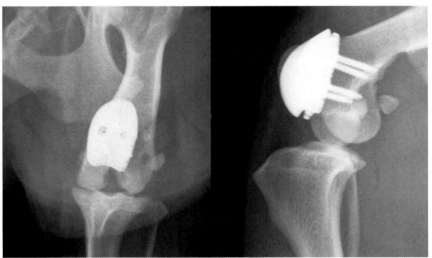

▶ **Fig. 8.44** Post-operative radiographs following placement of a patellar groove replacement prosthesis.

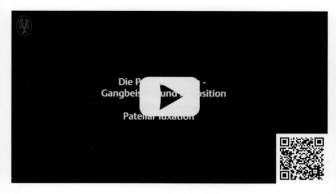

▶ **Video 8.4** Patellar luxation – abnormal gait and reduction of the patella.

8.3.6 Further Diseases of the Stifle Joint

Avulsion of the Extensor Digitorum Longus

Etiology and pathogenesis The tendon of the extensor digitorum longus (p. 91) arises from the extensor fossa of the lateral femoral condyle and disappears under the tibialis cranialis within the extensor groove of the tibia. If insufficient care is exercised during a lateral approach to the stifle joint, this tendon may be severed. It may also be damaged by a saw blade during osteotomy for treatment of cruciate ligament rupture or patellar luxation. In other cases, avulsion is caused by traumatic injury in young dogs, whereby a fragment of the femoral condyle is usually torn away along with the tendon.

Diagnosis Affected dogs are presented with hyperflexion of the digits and moderate lameness (2/4). The stifle joint (p. 121) is stable, but palpably swollen and painful. If the tendon has torn away from the site of origin, a small fragment of the lateral femoral condyle is usually detectable on radiographs (▶ Fig. 8.45).

Treatment and prognosis Left untreated, avulsion results in permanent hyperflexion of the digits, which can be managed in some cases with physiotherapy. Although the tendon is not essential for the dog's well-being and locomotion, fixation is recommended. If the tendon is attached to a large condylar fragment, the latter can be used to secure the tendon to the femur. In cases of iatrogenic injury, suturing of the tendon is indicated.

Specialist practice: In chronic cases, and where there is pronounced tendon shortening, the stump is fixed to the proximal tibia with a screw and washer. Extended external support of the stifle joint and physiotherapy are highly recommended in all cases [126].

Osteochondrosis of the Stifle Joint

Refer to general information on osteochondrosis (p. 185).

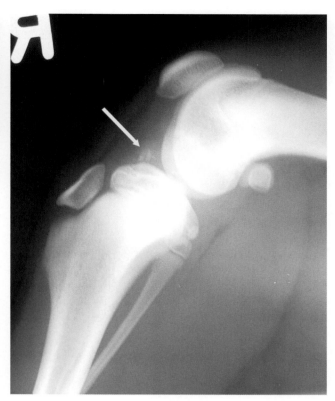

▶ **Fig. 8.45** Traumatic avulsion of the origin of the extensor digitalis lateralis from the femoral condyle. A fragment of bone that has avulsed with the tendon is clearly visible in the lateral view.

Osgood-Schlatter Disease

This relatively rare disorder is characterized by delayed fusion of the tibial tuberosity with the tibia (p. 90) or partial avulsion of the tibial tuberosity in the direction of tension exerted by the quadriceps (▶ Fig. 8.46). Also referred to as „traction osteochondritis", it is observed in children that are overweight, and in those that engage in excessive sporting activity (e.g. basketball) at a young age. In dogs, giant breeds (particularly Great Danes) are primarily affected. Patients are presented with nonspecific lameness and swelling along the patellar tendon. In dogs, the disease is better described as avulsion of the tibial tuberosity, which is readily discernible in lateral radiographic views. In all cases treated by the author, complete recovery was achieved using conservative management, including protection of the joint from excessive strain, reduction of body weight and pain relief.

8.3.7 Hamstring Fibrosis

Etiology and pathogenesis The muscles affected by hamstring fibrosis are the gracilis and the semitendinosus (p. 94). Arising from the caudal pelvis, they pass caudal to the femur to the medial aspect of the tibia (▶ Fig. 8.47). The cause of fibrosis is unknown. German Shepherd Dogs and their crosses are almost exclusively affected. Fibrosis may be promoted by the downward slope of the backline and pronounced flexion of the stifle and hip joints in these breeds. Involvement of immunological factors is also suspected. Most dogs are aged between 8 months

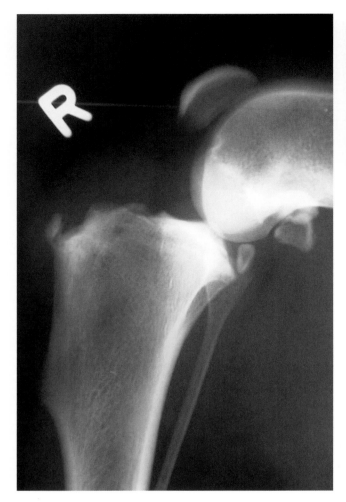

▶ **Fig. 8.46** Osgood-Schlatter disease. New bone growth is visible at the insertion of the patellar ligament at the tibia.

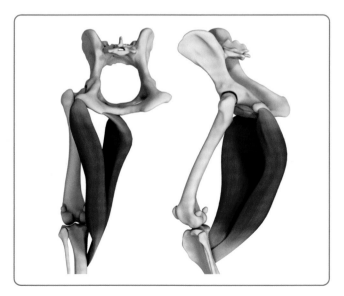

▶ **Fig. 8.47** Muscles affected by hamstring fibrosis in the German Shepherd Dog (primarily gracilis and semitendinosus): the muscles follow a diagonal, medially directed course from the pelvis to the tibia. (source: Daniel Koch, Jonas Lauströer, Amir Andikfar)

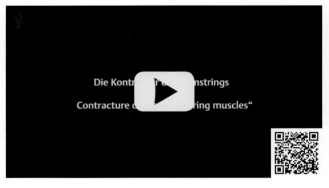

▶ **Video 8.5** Gait of a dog with fibrosis of the "hamstring muscles".

and 8 years, are very active and have a sporting history with multiple jumping- and sprinting-induced muscle injuries. These strain-like injuries result in localized inflammation, edema , hemorrhages and ultimately in fibrosis.

Clinical findings The gait of affected dogs is highly pathognomonic. Due to the disorientation of an increasing number of relatively inactive muscle fibres, the stifle joint is drawn inwards, and the tarsus outwards, during the swing phase. Stride length in the hindlimb is usually short and the musculature is generally reduced. Both hindlimbs may be affected. On palpation, the muscle groups are rough, knotted and painful. Extension of the hindlimb is restricted.

Refer to ▶ **Video 8.5** for a video showing the gait of a dog with hamstring fibrosis.

Diagnostic imaging and further testing Radiographs are not informative, unless it is necessary to exclude hip and back disorders as differential diagnoses. Ultrasound and MRT imaging, as well as biopsy, can be used to quantify the extent of fibrosis, though these measures are not required for development of a treatment plan.

Treatment Physiotherapy is the only treatment modality that has proved to be of therapeutic value. The aim is to maintain the contractility of remaining muscle tissue for as long as possible. Systemic and local cortisone and other immunosuppressive agents, as well as complete surgical removal of fibrosed muscle tissue, has been shown to provide only temporary relief. Restrictive connective tissue bands were found to recur even after total myectomy. The prognosis is thus very guarded, as healing is not possible [128].

8.3.8   Legg-Perthes Disease

Etiology and pathogenesis Legg-Perthes disease, or aseptic necrosis of the femoral head occurs in humans and in small dogs. Affected breeds include the West Highland White Terrier, Cairn Terrier, Poodle and Miniature Pinscher. The cause of Legg-Perthes disease is unknown, but is suspected to involve interruption of the blood supply at a young age. This may occur due to breed predisposition or as a result of trauma. Also relevant are differences in the vascular supply (▶ **Fig. 8.48**) of the

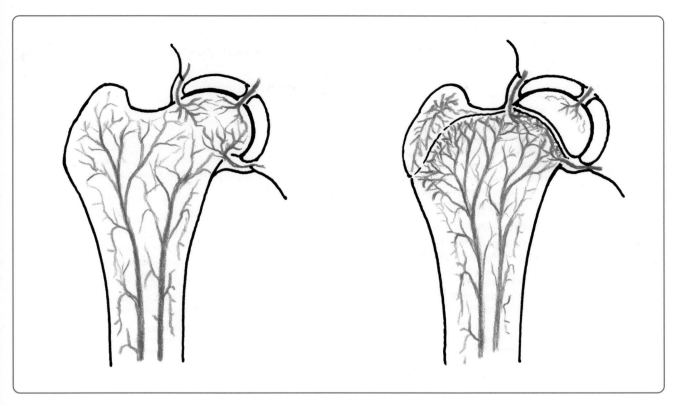

▶ **Fig. 8.48** Schematic illustration of the blood supply of the proximal femur in an adult dog (left) and in a puppy (right). (source: Matthias Haab, Departement für Pferde, Vetsuisse-Fakultät Universität Zürich, Switzerland)

proximal femur (p.94). In mature dogs, the endosteal blood supply extends to the subchondral region, while in puppies the epiphysis is largely supplied by vessels in the region near the joint. This can lead to hypovascularization-induced damage following trauma, or to arthropathy. It is interesting to note that Legg-Perthes disease is usually unilateral, lending weight to the theory that transfer of weight to the contralateral side results in improved perfusion on the more heavily weighted side. Tissue biopsy has shown that the pathophysiological changes lead to infarction of the epiphyseal and metaphyseal bone. Initially, the femoral head remains externally intact. In the interior, however, there are fibrotic changes that also extend into the growth plate of the femoral head. The articular cartilage subsequently thickens and becomes fissured and furrowed. Due to poor perfusion, the epiphysis has limited capacity for healing and undergoes visible collapse. The femoral head becomes deformed [117].

Clinical findings Signs of lameness first appear at 4–10 months of age. Dogs are usually still able to weight-bear reasonably well (lameness 2/4) and lameness does not worsen after the initial acute phase. Examination reveals muscle atrophy and pain on manipulation of the hindlimb, particularly on extension of the hip joint (p.95). Crepitus is rarely detected. Differential diagnoses include hip dysplasia, neoplasia, osteoarthritis secondary to a healed femoral head fracture and patellar luxation.

Diagnostic imaging and further testing If radiographic changes in the femoral head are mild, it may not be possible to establish a diagnosis immediately. In inconclusive cases, radiography should be repeated after 4–6 weeks. Typical findings for Legg-Perthes disease include an irregularly shaped femoral head with lytic defects, flattening of the femoral head and degenerative remodelling of the femoral head, acetabulum and femoral neck (▶ **Fig. 8.49**). Disease is often unilateral.

Treatment If a diagnosis is established early, Legg-Perthes disease can – in rare cases – be treated conservatively with anti-inflammatories, physiotherapy and possibly extracorporeal shock wave therapy for induction of neovascularization. Surgical management with femoral head resection (▶ **Fig. 8.50**) has an excellent prognosis, as the patient is usually small; thus, the newly formed connective tissue produces a very stable pseudojoint. Early introduction of physiotherapy is very important for achieving rapid muscle development and for maintaining the range of movement of the hip joint.

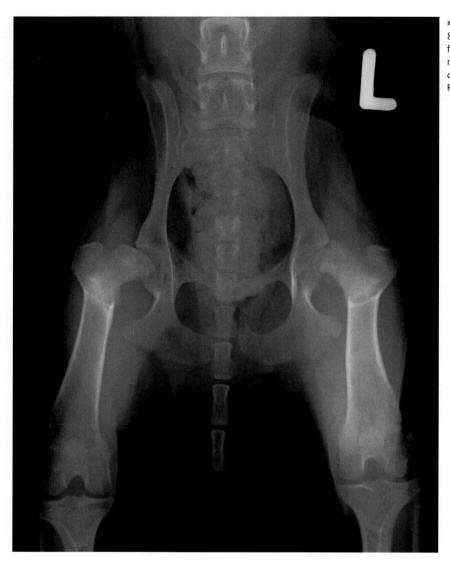

▶ **Fig. 8.49** Bilateral Legg-Perthes disease in an 8 month old West Highland White Terrier. The left femoral head is lytic and partially fractured; the right femoral head is extensively collapsed and deformed. (source: Urs Geissbühler, Klinische Radiologie, Vetsuisse-Fakultät Bern, Switzerland)

8.3.9 Hip Dysplasia and Coxofemoral Osteoarthritis

Etiology and pathogenesis The word dysplasia is derived from the Greek „dys" (bad) and „plassein" (formation, molding). Hip dysplasia(HD) is a complex disease characterized by primary laxity of the hip joint (p. 95) in young dogs. This leads to secondary degenerative changes which are referred to collectively as coxofemoral osteoarthritis.

The etiology of HD has not been determined definitively. The observation that HD is more common in progeny of dysplastic dogs indicates a genetic basis. More than 20 genes are involved. Estimates of heritability vary widely from 25–60% [101], [107], [113]. Despite intensive efforts by breeders, and more than 30 years of comprehensive progeny testing, the incidence of HD in certain breeds remains very high (over 60% in the Saint Bernard, English Setter and Gordon Setter) to high (30–50% in German Shepherd Dogs, Newfoundlands, Retrievers), while in others the disease is rare (e.g. Siberian Huskies, Collies and Belgian Shepherds) [111], [121]. These figures suggest that selec-

tion for performance promotes development of healthy hip joints.

Hip dysplasia does not necessarily result in lameness (▶ Fig. 8.51). Growth in the first months of life, feeding and husbandry play a significant role in determining whether lameness develops. Qualitatively imbalanced diets containing excess calcium lead to the development of irregularly formed joints. Dogs fed a tightly controlled ration grow more slowly than ad libitum fed litter mates, but their joints are subjected to less strain, resulting in greater hip joint stability. Moreover, they still reach their genetically determined wither height. In dogs that are genetically predisposed to HD, exposure to work- or performance-related activities at a very young age places abnormal strain on the joints, potentially leading to cartilage erosion and incipient subluxation. Most skeletal remodelling occurs in the period from 3 to 5 months of age (6 months in large breeds), during which medium sized breeds gain around 1 kg per week in body weight. It follows, therefore, that inappropriate nutrient supply and husbandry during this critical period have the greatest detrimental effect on joint development.

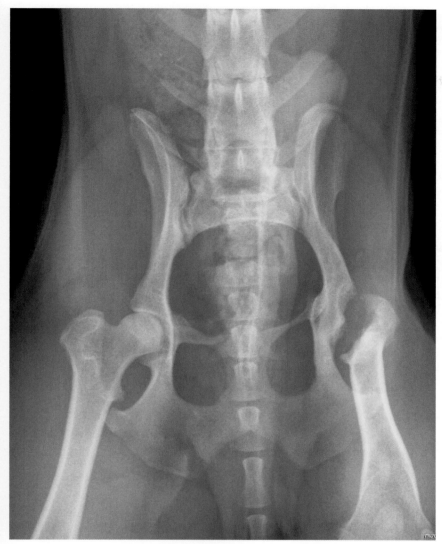

▶ **Fig. 8.50** Femoral head resection for treatment of Legg-Perthes disease in a West Highland White Terrier.

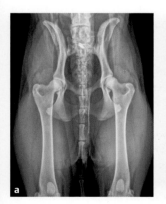
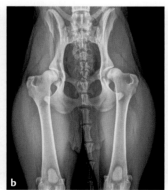
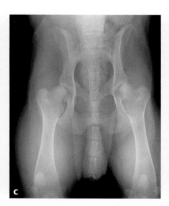
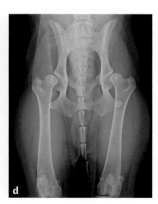

▶ **Fig. 8.51** Stages of hip dysplasia: the degree of severity increases from left to right.
a Normal hip joint.
b Mild dysplasia.
c Severe dysplasia
d Severe dysplasia with early femoral head subluxation.

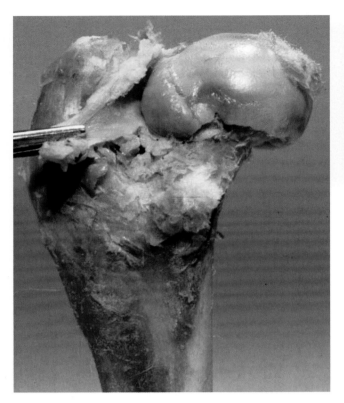

▶ **Fig. 8.52** Femoral head specimen exhibiting typical signs of coxofemoral osteoarthritis including joint capsule thickening, osteophyte development, deformation of the femoral head and cartilage wear; caudocranial view. (source: Pierre Montavon, Switzerland)

The first signs of lameness in dogs with HD are observed from 6 months of age, primarily as a result of synovitis. At this stage, there is often a marked discrepancy between body size, which has undergone a rapid increase, and muscle development, which is relatively poor. In the subsequent months, the femoral head is pushed back into the acetabulum by the increasing mass (relative to body weight) of the croup and thigh muscles. Thus, the dog's gait improves. This is also why dogs with naturally bulky hindlimb musculature, e.g. Bulldogs, Pugs and many fighting dogs, exhibit no clinical signs despite clear radiographic evidence of HD.

If joint incongruity is pronounced and muscle development is poor, HD leads to coxofemoral osteoarthritis (▶ **Fig. 8.52**). In response to joint instability, the joint capsule increases in thickness and new bone is formed around the joint. The pectineus and iliopsoas muscles hypertrophy, since their actions include stabilization of the hip joint. This may result in pain and restricted movement on abduction and extension of the hip. Progressive instability and repeated subluxation lead to degradation of cartilage on the femoral head and the cranial edge of the acetabulum. The subchondral bone is exposed and pain increases. In the acetabulum, a new, flatter articular surface develops; the original joint margins are worn away and the femoral head is thickened by the development of osteophytes. These changes constitute the typical picture of coxofemoral osteoarthritis. Generally, the degree of HD and osteoarthritis is similar in the left and right hip. In some cases, the less severely affected

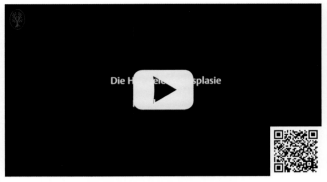

▶ **Video 8.6** Gait of a dog with hip dysplasia.

side bears more weight, and the resultant retention of muscle mass leads to improved hip joint congruity. Asymmetric disease with corresponding clinical findings may develop. Distinct asymmetry in the degree of osteoarthritis is suggestive of a disease process other than HD e.g. trauma (hip joint luxation, previous femoral head fracture), Legg-Perthes disease or infection.

Clinical findings The typical presentation is a large dog exhibiting temporary lameness after rest. The dog refuses long walks, is reluctant to jump into cars, dislikes walking on stairs and often lies with its hindlimbs flexed. Intermittent toe-dragging may be observed. During gait analysis, the stride length is found to be short and trotting may elicit strong pain, with the dog preferring to gallop.

Other clinical signs vary with age. Findings in young dogs with HD may include an unsteady gait and spontaneous luxation of the femoral head, resulting in episodes of non-weight bearing lameness (grade 4/4). Muscle development in the hindlimbs is poor. The hip joint (p.131) usually cannot be fully flexed, extended, abducted or rotated without eliciting pain. There may be a positive Ortolani (p.134)sign, which is indicative of severe HD. The Bardens test (p.135) should be used for young dogs, in which the acetabular rim is not yet fully formed.

Refer to ▶ **Video 8.6** for a video showing the gait of a dog with hip dysplasia.

In adult dogs, the clinical picture is dominated by coxofemoral osteoarthritis. Weight is transferred increasingly to the front legs, leading to greater muscle development in the forelimbs and, in some instances, secondary disorders of the shoulder, elbow and carpus. The range of movement of the hip joints is significantly restricted; full extension is rendered impossible by the thickened joint capsule, bone proliferation and permanent contraction of the iliopsoas. The pectineus prevents full abduction (▶ **Fig. 8.53**). Crepitation may be evident on manipulation of the hip joint, but subluxation is difficult to elicit.

Refer to ▶ **Video 8.7** for a video showing the gait of a dog with coxofemoral osteoarthritis.

Clinical findings are positively correlated with body size and, to a limited extent, with overweight (where present). Important differential diagnoses for HD and coxofemoral osteoarthritis include cauda equina syndrome, Legg-Perthes disease, iliopsoas strain and neoplasia of the pelvis or femoral head.

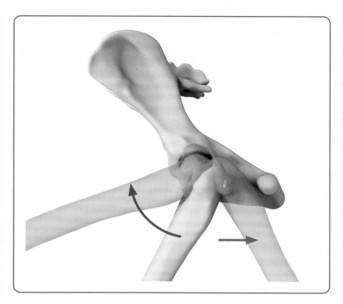

► **Fig. 8.53** Hip dysplasia and osteoarthritis result in restricted mobility of the hip joint, due to thickening of the joint capsule and contracture of the pectineus (abduction) und iliopsoas (extension). (source: Daniel Koch, Jonas Lauströer, Amir Andikfar)

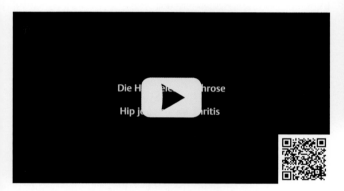

► **Video 8.7** Gait analysis in a dog with coxofemoral osteoarthritis.

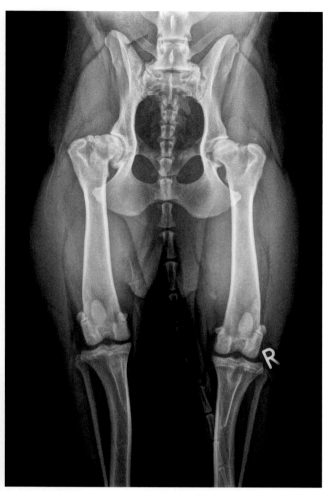

► **Fig. 8.54** Bilateral coxofemoral osteoarthritis in a 7 year old Labrador Retriever. In the left hip joint, there is marked femoral neck exostosis and pronounced flattening of the acetabulum. Joint replacement is indicated.

Diagnostic imaging and further testing Ventrodorsal hip-extended and frog leg radiographic views are widely used for classification of HD. From a clinical perspective, and for elimination of differential diagnoses, laterolateral views should also be obtained. Typical radiographic findings include (► Fig. 8.54): joint incongruity, Norberg angle less than 105°, wear of the cranial acetabular rim, subluxation of the femoral head, deformation of the femoral head and early signs of osteoarthritis. If coxofemoral osteoarthritis is present, additional findings include: osteophytes at the joint margin, flattening of the acetabulum, reduction of the radiographically visible joint space, distinct deformation of the femoral head, thickening of the femoral neck and loose fragments within the joint.

Treatment of HD If diagnosis is established early, HD can be managed successfully with conservative therapy consisting of a balanced, unsupplemented restricted diet, frequent short walks, chondroprotective preparations, analgesics and physiotherapy.

Specialist treatment of HD: early treatment of young dogs with pelvic osteotomy (triple pelvic osteotomy, TPO, or double pelvic osteotomy, DPO) plays a particularly important role in surgical management of HD (► Fig. 8.55). In this technique, the acetabulum and adjoining bone is separated from the rest of the pelvis and swiveled to increase coverage of the femoral head. Joint congruity is improved, providing the best possible protection against development of osteoarthritis. The role of this procedure is thus primarily preventative. Appropriate case selection is crucial for the success of TPO. Only dogs aged 6 to 10 months with no (or mild) osteoarthritis and a moderate degree of subluxation are good candidates for this procedure. TPO can be performed on both joints in quick succession, as morbidity is surprisingly low, even with premature screw loosening. If HD is severe, subluxation is evident or osteoarthritis is developing, hip replacement can be performed from the age of 10 months. As the prosthesis will remain in place long-term, a cementless implant should be used. In dogs under 15 kg body weight, pain can be eliminated with femoral head resection. The effectiveness of this technique is based on the development of a connective tissue bridge between the femur and the acetabulum. Good post-operative management with physiother-

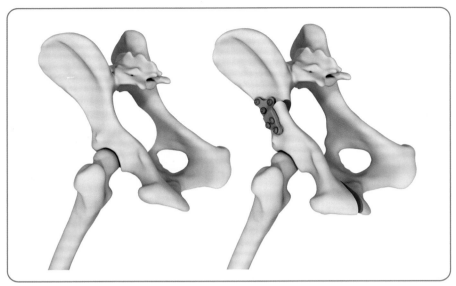

▶ **Fig. 8.55** Schematic illustration of triple pelvic osteotomy (TPO)/double pelvic osteotomy (DPO): rotation of the osteotomized pelvic segment, incorporating the acetabulum, results in increased coverage of the femoral head. (source: Daniel Koch, Jonas Lauströer, Amir Andikfar)

apy is essential for therapeutic success. Juvenile pubic symphysiodesis (JPS) should be used with caution. In this relatively simple procedure, electrocautery is used to fuse the pelvic symphysis. As a result, the pelvis only continues to grow dorsally. This procedure is very reliable when performed on dogs aged 3 to 4 months. It should be noted, though, that a definitive diagnosis of HD cannot always be established at this age. Thus, some dogs may be treated unnecessarily, and responsible breeding measures for control of HD may be circumvented if the dog is not castrated concurrently.

Treatment of coxofemoral osteoarthritis Management of body weight and physical activity is of benefit to dogs suffering from coxofemoral osteoarthritis, even in advanced age. With every kilogram that a dog does not have to carry around due to its lean condition, the owner is doing their four-legged friend a favor. Moderate, regular exercise allows for an acceptable quality of life, without placing excessive strain on the joints. Short sessions of targeted muscle training (e.g. swimming or jogging) strengthen the supportive apparatus around the hip joint and reduce the degree of lameness; the need for expensive operations may even be postponed for several years. Alternative treatment modalities for management of coxofemoral osteoarthritis may provide temporary relief in some cases.

Pain relief is achieved with oral analgesics. For good reason, non-steroidal anti-inflammatories (NSAID) are particularly popular, as they reduce joint pain and inflammation and have few side effects. Cortisone, used extensively in the past, is also very effective but results in rapid breakdown of all tissue types and leads to polyphagia, polydipsia and polyuria. Its use is therefore not recommended. An analgesic effect is also produced by glycosaminoglycans, particularly via their chondroitin sulfate content. They strengthen the articular cartilage by retaining fluid and thus delay exposure of the subchondral bone. In many severe cases of coxofemoral osteoarthritis, the above mentioned conservative measures are inadequate and surgical treatment is indicated.

In the modified pectineal myectomy technique (pectineus myectomy, iliopsoas tenotomy and neurectomy; PIN) the aim is to relieve pain by removing the pectineus, partially sectioning the tendon of the iliopsoas and neurectomizing the ventral joint capsule (▶ **Fig. 8.56**). By contracting in response to hip joint laxity, the pectineus and iliopsoas are ultimately responsible for a large proportion of the pain experienced by the patient. The PIN procedure can be performed bilaterally in one surgery. It is most successful in dogs that have mild osteoarthritis, but restricted hip joint mobility. Its duration of effect ranges from 6 months to several years.

In the rare instance that coxofemoral osteoarthritis occurs in dogs under 15 kg body weight, the femoral head can be excised. With the aid of physiotherapy, the femoral head is replaced by a connective tissue bridge that assumes the role of force transmission from the femur to the pelvis. The technique is simple and eliminates pain, usually without any residual gait abnormality. At higher body weights, it is recommended that femoral head excision only be performed on one side.

Specialist treatment of coxofemoral osteoarthritis: Replacement of the hip joint is the only permanent, satisfactory form of treatment of canine coxofemoral osteoarthritis. Increasingly, use of cementless prostheses is becoming the method of choice (▶ **Fig. 8.57**, ▶ **Fig. 8.58**). Following removal of the arthritic femoral head, the femoral shaft and acetabulum are prepared for implant placement. The artificial acetabulum (cup implant) consists of coated titanium and polyetheretherketone and is press-fit precisely into the bone. Screws are used to secure the counterpart (titanium stem) to the medial side of the femur only, thus avoiding loosening of the implant due to uneven loading of the medial and lateral femoral cortex. The connection is established by attaching the prosthetic femoral head and neck. In contrast to cemented prostheses, this method permits adjustment of the size and orientation of the components, either during surgery or several weeks thereafter. To accommodate dogs of all sizes, the cup, head-neck and stem components are available in various diameters, strengths and lengths. Within just a few days of surgery, almost all dogs exhibit improved locomotion. Lameness usually resolves within 4 to 6 weeks of surgery. While dysplasia often occurs in both hindlimbs, bilateral hip replacement is not always indicated, because dogs soon begin to bear more weight on the treated side than on the untreated contralateral side.

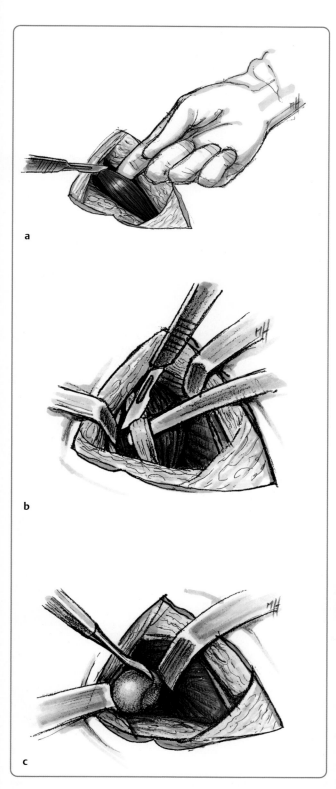

▶ **Fig. 8.56** Pectineus myectomy, iliopsoas tenotomy and joint capsule neurectomy (PIN). This procedure, performed via a ventral approach to the hip joint, reduces pain and increases the range of movement of the hip joint (left hindlimb, ventral view; top of image = cranial, right side of image = distal).
a Pectineus myectomy (source: Matthias Haab, Departement für Pferde, Vetsuisse-Fakultät Universität Zürich, Switzerland)
b Iliopsoas tenotomy (source: Matthias Haab, Departement für Pferde, Vetsuisse-Fakultät Universität Zürich, Switzerland)
c Joint capsule neurectomy (source: Matthias Haab, Departement für Pferde, Vetsuisse-Fakultät Universität Zürich, Switzerland)

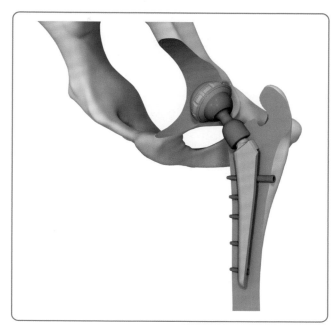

▶ **Fig. 8.57** Modular Zurich cementless total hip replacement system: the cup implant is press-fit into the acetabulum, the stem is screwed to the medial femoral cortex. (source: Daniel Koch, Jonas Lauströer, Amir Andikfar)

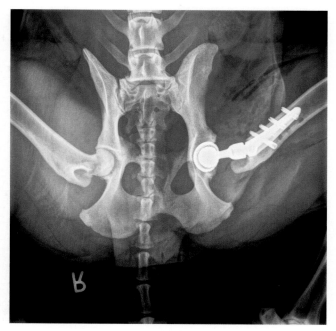

▶ **Fig. 8.58** Post-operative radiograph following total hip joint replacement using the Zurich cementless system.

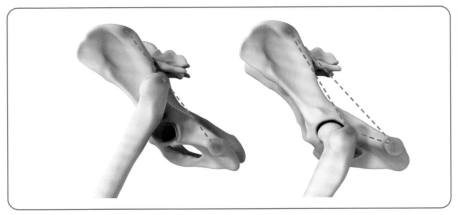

▸ **Fig. 8.59** Diagnosis of craniodorsal hip luxation with palpation: the cranially displaced greater trochanter lies on a line between the iliac crest and the ischial tuberosity. (source: Daniel Koch, Jonas Lauströer, Amir Andikfar)

8.3.10 Hip Luxation

Etiology and pathogenesis Motor vehicle collisions (hit by car) are by far the most common cause of hip luxation. Others include falls from large heights, bite wounds and spontaneous luxation due to hip dysplasia. Classification is based on the direction of luxation. Craniodorsal luxations are most common, accounting for around 80% of cases (▸ Fig. 8.59). The direction of luxation results from external rotation of the leg on impact and the strong tensile force exerted by the gluteal muscles on the greater trochanter. The joint capsule and the ligament of the head of the femur are torn. A variable degree of damage occurs at the cranial acetabular rim. In very young dogs, the traumatic force often results in avulsion of the ligament along with a small bone fragment from the femoral head, or in epiphysiolysis of the femoral head. Ventral and ventrocaudal luxations into the obturator foramen usually result from internal rotation of the leg on impact due to a fall.

Clinical findings Hip luxation results in obvious lameness, though dogs may bear weight on the affected limb after a short period of adjustment. With craniodorsal luxation, the leg appears to be shortened, externally rotated and adducted. Ventral luxation results in apparent lengthening of the leg with slight internal rotation and adduction. Palpation of the hip region reveals swelling, pain and crepitation. There is asymmetry in the triangle formed on the left and right sides by the greater trochanter, tuber sacrale and ischial tuberosity; this is used to determine the position of the femur after luxation (p. 131). In the commonly occurring craniodorsal type of luxation, the distance between the ischial tuberosity and the greater trochanter is increased. When the examiner places their thumb in the hollow between these structures and rotates the femur externally, the thumb is not compressed (see luxated (p. 133)). Varying degrees of ischiatic nerve deficit and knuckling may be observed.

Refer to ▸ Video 8.8 for a video showing the gait of a dog with a luxated hip joint.

Diagnostic imaging and further testing As in all cases of trauma, thoracic and abdominal radiographs should be taken and evaluated. Laterolateral and ventrodorsal views of the hip joints are required to confirm the diagnosis and develop a treatment plan (▸ Fig. 8.60). The radiographs should be closely

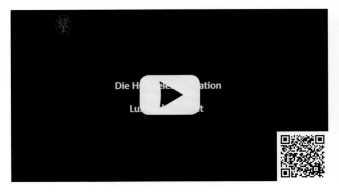

▸ **Video 8.8** Gait of a dog with a luxated hip joint.

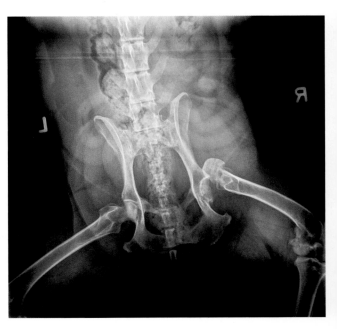

▸ **Fig. 8.60** Hip luxation in a Husky following an accident in a yard. Pre-existing coxofemoral osteoarthritis is evident.

examined for any bone fragments that remain in the acetabulum or have become forcibly detached from the acetabular rim and passed deep into the articular cavity. Radiographic findings are used to determine treatment and prognosis.

Treatment Closed (non-invasive) reduction (▶ Fig. 8.61) is indicated if the injury is recent, the acetabular rim is intact, the acetabulum is suitably deep and devoid of osteoarthritis, and there are no bone fragments in the joint. For a craniodorsal luxation, pressure is applied to the trochanter to direct the femur caudoventrally, while an assistant stabilizes the pelvis. Reduction can either be attempted with the hip extended and the femur rotated externally, or with the hip flexed and the femur rotated internally. The former spares the acetabular rim, which is very fragile in young animals, while the latter uses the acetabular rim as a lever and anchor point and may be easier to perform in strongly muscled dogs. Following successful reduction, any joint capsule remnants should be liberated from the joint space by rotating the hip joint and the hindlimb should be supported with an Ehmer sling for 10 days.

Specialist practice: Indications for open reduction include chronic luxation, unsuccessful closed reduction and the presence of bone fragments. Removal of bone fragments is performed via a craniodorsal approach, with concomitant reduction of the hip joint. The joint is stabilized with internal fixation (toggle pin – ▶ Fig. 8.62, Slocum sling – ▶ Fig. 8.63) and thorough suturing of the joint capsule. An Ehmer sling should be applied for 10 days (▶ Fig. 8.64). Fixation of Salter Harris fractures of the femoral head epiphysis can be performed using lag screws, via a ventral approach, or with long Kirschner wires, using a craniodorsal approach. In cases where there is pre-existing high grade dysplasia or severe osteoarthritis, femoral head resection (dogs 15 to 20 kg) or hip replacement (dogs over 20 kg) may be indicated. Cranio- and caudoventral luxation

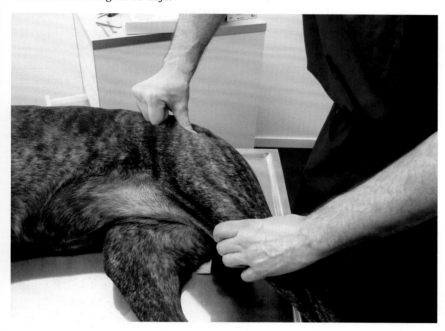

▶ **Fig. 8.61** Closed reduction of a craniodorsally luxated hip joint: the thumb of one hand guides the trochanter towards the acetabulum, while the other hand rotates the femur externally.

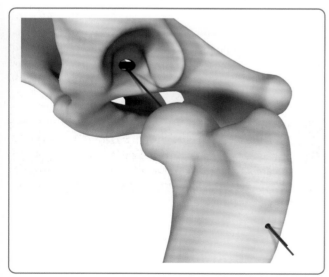

▶ **Fig. 8.62** Toggle pin technique for stabilization of the hip joint following luxation: the suture material is threaded through the femoral neck, femoral head and the acetabulum, and secured with a suture button. (source: Daniel Koch, Jonas Lauströer, Amir Andikfar)

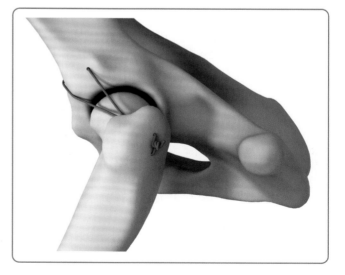

▶ **Fig. 8.63** Slocum technique for stabilization of the hip joint following luxation: the suture material is threaded through the trochanter and the bone cranial to the acetabulum. (source: Daniel Koch, Jonas Lauströer, Amir Andikfar)

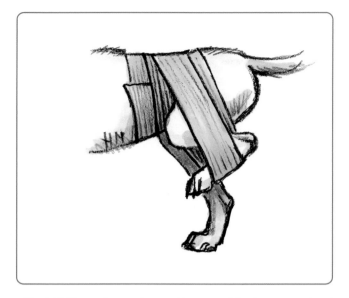

▶ **Fig. 8.64** Ehmer sling: used to provide support following open or closed reduction of craniodorsal hip luxation. (source: Matthias Haab, Departement für Pferde, Vetsuisse-Fakultät Universität Zürich, Switzerland)

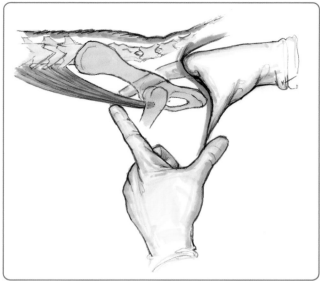

▶ **Fig. 8.66** Palpation of the iliopsoas. Palpation can be performed percutaneously or, in small to medium sized dogs, rectally. (source: Matthias Haab, Departement für Pferde, Vetsuisse-Fakultät Universität Zürich, Switzerland)

chanter. Iliopsoas strain can occur in sporting dogs in the absence of appropriate warm-up. Predisposed breeds include the Border Collie and the Belgian Shepherd [119].

Clinical findings Iliopsoas strain results in a gait similar to that seen in dogs with HD or coxofemoral osteoarthritis; these are also the most important differential diagnoses. Iliopsoas strain can be distinguished from hip joint disorders during orthopedic examination by maximally stretching the muscle (by extending the hip and rotating the femur internally) and checking for a pain response. The muscle can also be palpated directly, either rectally (cranial to the pelvis) or from the lateral aspect (▶ Fig. 8.66).

Diagnostic imaging and further testing Radiography is used to eliminate differential diagnoses. Calcification at the insertion of the iliopsoas may be observed in chronic cases. Ultrasound and MRT imaging may reveal muscle tears, hemorrhages and disruption of muscular architecture.

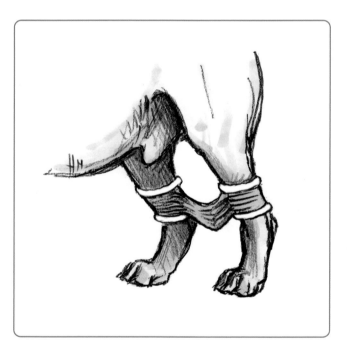

▶ **Fig. 8.65** Hobbles: used to restrict movement following pubic fractures or closed reduction of ventral hip joint luxation. (source: Matthias Haab, Departement für Pferde, Vetsuisse-Fakultät Universität Zürich, Switzerland)

should be managed with closed reduction followed by restriction of movement with hobbles (▶ Fig. 8.65).

8.3.11 Iliopsoas Strain

Etiology and pathogenesis The iliopsoas muscle (p. 97) belongs to the hip flexor group. It consists of the fleshy iliacus and the tendinous psoas major. The muscle arises from the ventral surface of the lumbar vertebrae and inserts on the lesser tro-

Treatment Treatment of iliopsoas strain requires considerable patience. Exercise restriction, anti-inflammatory drugs and targeted physiotherapy are the methods of choice. Predisposed dogs should henceforth be given adequate opportunity to warm up before training. Surgical removal of the iliopsoas is only indicated if disease is chronic and tendon calcification is evident.

8.4 Forelimb Disorders

8.4.1 Sesamoid Disease

Etiology and pathogenesis In each of the four main digits of the fore- and hindlimbs, a pair of sesamoid bones is present on

the palmar/plantar surface of each metacarpophalangeal (p.99) and metatarsophalangeal (p.85) joint. The sesamoid bones are numbered I-VIII, from medial to lateral (digits 2–5, ▶ Fig. 8.67). The tendons of the superficial and deep digital flexors pass evenly over the sesamoid bones of digits 3 and 4, while those of 2 and 5 course almost exclusively over the innermost sesamoid bones (II and VII). In heavy dogs, and during intense physical activity, bones II and VII are thus exposed to additional strain. Fractures of the palmar and plantar sesamoid bones result from trauma or fatigue, particularly in Greyhounds and other racing dogs. Degenerative changes have also been described in young large-breed dogs. This so-called sesamoid bone fragmentation has also been attributed to congenital ossification disorders, accounting for the predisposition observed in Rottweilers, Boxers and Labrador Retrievers. Sesamoid fragmentation occurs more frequently in the forelimbs (around 80% of cases), possibly due to the greater load experienced by the thoracic limbs [132].

Clinical findings Sesamoid bone fragmentation results in mild (1/4) lameness, usually occurring after heavy loading. The area around the affected sesamoid bone is thickened and hyperextension of the corresponding metacarpo-/metatarsophalangeal joint (p.138) is painful. Flexion is restricted.

Diagnostic imaging and further testing A provisional clinical diagnosis is confirmed with dorsopalmar/plantar radiographs (splayed toe view). Evaluation of the sesamoids is more difficult in mediolateral views as the bones are superimposed. Calcification of surrounding soft tissue is often observed with chronic degenerative disease. Sesamoid bone fragmentation (▶ Fig. 8.68) must be distinguished from normally occurring bipartite sesamoids.

Treatment Conservative management, comprising several weeks of exercise restriction and anti-inflammatory therapy, is recommended in mild cases where lameness occurs only after intensive strain. Otherwise, the affected sesamoid bone is surgically removed, whereupon lameness should resolve within 6 weeks. It is important to be aware that the flexor tendon subsequently passes over the joint without the protection of a sesamoid bone, which can lead to secondary changes and hyperflexion of the joint. Amputation of the toe is an alternative approach.

8.4.2 Carpal Hyperextension Injury

Etiology and pathogenesis Jumping or falling from large heights and, less frequently, motor vehicle accidents, can result in injury of the supportive structures of the carpus. Damage to palmar structures, such as the aponeuroses and the short ligaments between the carpal bones, results in a variable degree of carpal hyperextension (▶ Fig. 8.69). Not infrequently, both limbs are affected. Since the carpus normally exhibits slight valgus, more strain is experienced by medial than lateral structures and hyperextension trauma may be accompanied by rupture of the medial collateral ligament.

Clinical findings After the traumatic incident, the forelimb can hardly bear any weight. Hyperextension is obvious on touch

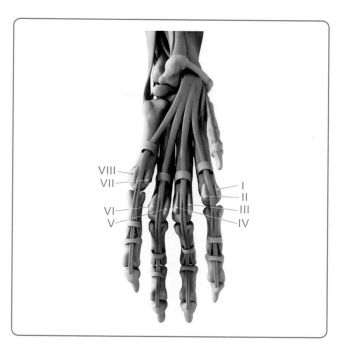

▶ **Fig. 8.67** Location of the sesamoid bones in the flexor tendons in the forelimb of the dog. The bones are numbered I-VIII from medial to lateral. Pathological changes occur most commonly in sesamoid bones II and VII. (source: Daniel Koch, Jonas Lauströer, Amir Andikfar)

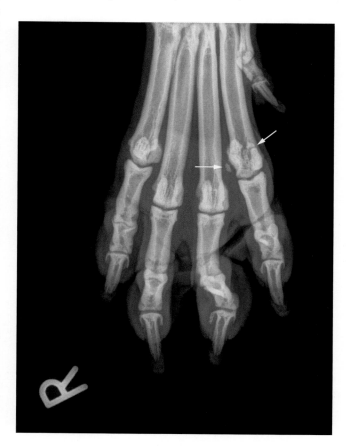

▶ **Fig. 8.68** Fragmentation of sesamoid bones I and II in a Rottweiler.

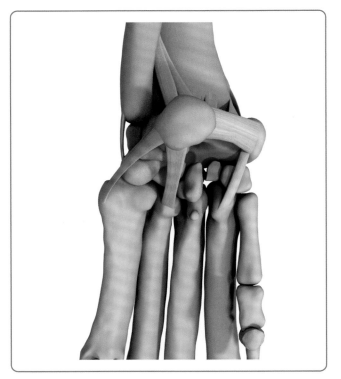

► **Fig. 8.69** Deep structures of the carpus, palmar view. Hyperextension trauma often results in rupture of the short ligaments of the intercarpal or carpometacarpal joints. (source: Daniel Koch, Jonas Lauströer, Amir Andikfar)

down. The carpus (p. 140) is markedly swollen. The suspected diagnosis is confirmed on palpation if, with the elbow extended, the carpus can be extended by more than 10–15°.

Diagnostic imaging and further testing The degree of instability and the presence of collateral ligament rupture is determined radiographically with dorsopalmar views (including stressed views, with abduction and adduction of the carpus, for assessment of the medial and lateral ligaments) and a lateral view in hyperextension (► Fig. 8.70, ► Fig. 8.71).

Treatment Conservative management with splinting is only indicated in dogs under 6 months of age, in which stabilization of the joint by fibrosis occurs relatively quickly. Suturing can be used for primary care of ruptured straight and oblique radiocarpal ligaments.

Specialist practice: treatment of intercarpal instability requires partial arthrodesis, usually necessitating fusion of the region from the intermedioradiocarpal bone to the metacarpal bones. Long-term fixation is achieved with plates, pins or an external fixateur. Panarthrodesis is indicated when there is extensive ligament rupture with involvement of the antebrachiocarpal joint, recurrence following ligament suturing, or marked carpal osteoarthritis. The technique is performed using specialized plates that are screwed to the carpus on its dorsal, medial or plantar aspect (► Fig. 8.72). In all cases, fusion is accelerated by the removal of articular cartilage and the introduction of autologous bone marrow. Post-operative support is required for 6 to 12 weeks; customized ortheses are associated with lower mor-

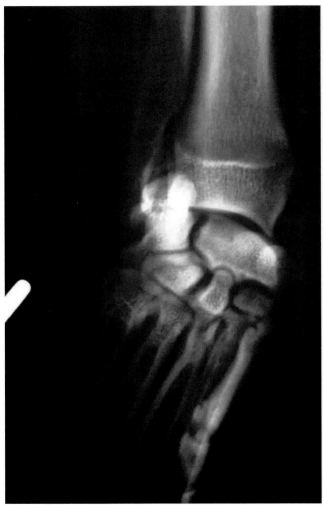

► **Fig. 8.70** Intercarpal and radiocarpal trauma with medial ligament rupture; radiography reveals increased valgus.

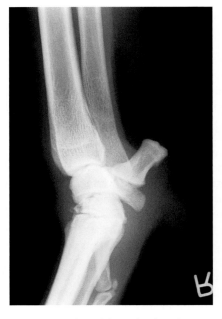

► **Fig. 8.71** Carpometacarpal instability with palmar ligament damage; hyperextension is evident.

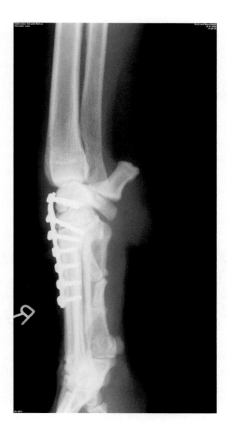

► **Fig. 8.72** Treatment of carpometacarpal instability with dorsal plate fixation.

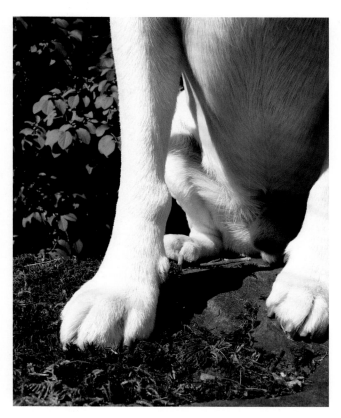

► **Fig. 8.73** Typical clinical appearance of tendovaginitis of the abductor pollicis longus: a firm, relatively painless swelling proximal and medial to the carpus in a 6 year old Labrador. (source: Klinik für Kleintierchirurgie der Vetsuisse-Fakultät Universität Zürich, Switzerland)

bidity than splint dressings and provide scope for more flexible management. Fusion of the small, poorly vascularized bones takes 4–8 months. Following partial arthrodesis, the gait should return to normal. Even with panarthrodesis, any lameness should be barely perceptible. Difficulty jumping over obstacles may be observed, since the carpus can no longer be flexed.

8.4.3 Tendovaginitis of the Abductor Pollicis Longus Muscle

Etiology and pathogenesis The abductor pollicis longus arises laterally on the proximal radius (p.101). Its ensheathed terminal tendon crosses the extensor carpi radialis on the distal radius before passing under the medial collateral ligament and inserting on the base of the first metacarpal bone (► **Fig. 5.35**). At the level of the antebrachiocarpal joint, the tendon contains a sesamoid bone that aids in stabilizing the joint. The cause of tendovaginitis of the abductor pollicis longus is incompletely understood. As in the corresponding disorder in humans (de Quervain's disease) it is thought that chronic inflammation is triggered and maintained by overuse. The tendon becomes increasingly constricted within its sheath. Chronic tendon strain may result in thickening and partial ossification of the tendon sheath.

Clinical findings Dogs with tendovaginitis of the abductor pollicis longus are usually large and over 2 years of age. Forelimb lameness is initially very mild (1/4), occurring particularly when dogs are rested briefly following intense activity. The typical finding is a rough, almost spherical swelling on the me-

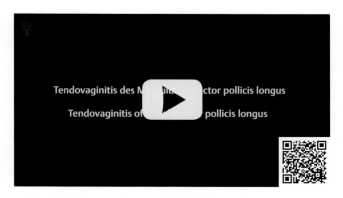

► **Video 8.9** Tendovaginitis of the abductor pollicis longus – gait analysis and clinical assessment.

dial aspect of the distal radius (► **Fig. 8.73**). Pain is not always elicited on firm palpation, but flexion and abduction of the carpus is painful (p.143) and the range of flexion is increasingly reduced. The carpus is otherwise stable. Disease may be bilateral, though the degree of swelling is not necessarily correlated with the severity of lameness and pain.

Refer to ► **Video 8.9** for a video showing gait analysis and clinical assessment.

Diagnostic imaging and further testing Radiographic changes are present in almost all cases. These include osseous

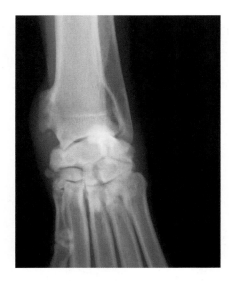

▶ **Fig. 8.74** Radiographic changes in a dog with chronic tendovaginitis of the abductor pollicis longus: bone proliferation at the medial aspect of the distal radius with no evidence of neoplasia.

proliferation on the medial and dorsal side of the distal radius (▶ **Fig. 8.74**). The medial styloid process may appear broadened. There is little or no evidence of degenerative changes in the radiocarpal joint. The most important differential diagnosis is neoplasia of the distal radius. Tendovaginitis of the abductor pollicis longus is distinguished from neoplasia by the absence of lytic zones, the uniform density of the new bone, and the restriction of osseous proliferation to the medial and distal radius. If radiography is inconclusive, CT may be indicated.

Treatment Management is divided into three stages. Mild, acute disease responds very well to exercise restriction and anti-inflammatory therapy. If lameness persists, depot corticosteroids are injected into the tendon sheath and the limb is bandaged. Injection can be repeated after 3 weeks; this should result in long-term improvement. If there is extensive osseous proliferation, or the response to corticosteroid injection is poor, surgery is required. The surgical procedure involves incision of the indurated tendon sheath, removal of as much fibrotic and osseous material as possible and release of the tendon. Tenotomy is not recommended, as the tendon acts similarly to a collateral ligament. Following surgery, a splint is applied for several weeks. The results of surgical debridement are usually good [106].

8.4.4 Elbow Dysplasia

Etiology and pathogenesis The etiopathogenesis of elbow dysplasia (ED) remains to be fully elucidated. This is complicated by the fact that the term elbow (p. 104) dysplasia incorporates various elbow disorders involving different pathogenetic mechanisms. The latter has arisen from a radiological perspective, as the pathophysiological processes involved in these disorders usually result in osteoarthritis of the elbow joint.

Today, the term ED includes 4 main disorders and a variety of uncommon elbow abnormalities. The main disorders are fragmented medial coronoid process (FMCP), ununited anconeal

process (UAP), osteochondrosis of the medial humeral condyle (OC) and elbow joint incongruity (INC). A genetic basis is implicated (heritability 0.27–0.77) [98], [107]. Nutrition and husbandry during the puppy stage can serve either as contributing or mitigating factors. Particularly significant in this regard is body weight, two thirds of which is supported by the forelimbs. Overweight up to the age of 7 months, i.e. in the phase of highest turnover, can cause subclinical disease to become clinical.

Early impressions of the pathogenesis of ED were based on research into osteochondrosis. Cartilage on predisposed articular surfaces was considered to be qualitatively inadequate and excessively thick, resulting in insufficient nourishment by the synovial fluid. This still applies in the case of osteochondrosis of the medial humeral condyle (in its location directly opposite to the medial coronoid process). Excess calcium supply in the first 4–5 months of life has been shown to have a detrimental effect on cartilage [118], while an oversupply of protein plays no part in the development of ED. Indeed, a definitive body of evidence for the cause of osteochondrosis has not yet been established. In addition to generalized problems associated with rapid growth and inadequate nutrient supply, the typical sites of OC (elbow, caudocentral humeral head, distal lateral femoral condyle, trochlear ridges of the talus) suggest that abnormally high load-bearing by these joint components during the growth phase may also play a role.

With respect to FMCP and UAP, most authors consider malformation of the trochlear notch to be the underlying cause. During the rapid phase of growth, considerably more bone and cartilage must be laid down at the trochlear notch than at the humeral condyle in order to maintain elbow joint congruity. Consequently, the trochlear notch can take on an ellipsoid shape. This exposes the distal (processus coronoideus) or proximal process (processus anconaeus) to a high degree of stress, resulting in fissuring, fragmentation or failure to fuse with the olecranon.

Force transmission in the elbow occurs predominantly on the medial side. Thus, the medial coronoid process is distinctly larger, and is subjected to greater stress, than its lateral counterpart. In view of this, the term medial coronoid disease (MCD) has increasingly been adopted in recent years, since pressure-induced abrasion of the medial coronoid process is more common than fragmentation (▶ **Fig. 8.75**) The elbow is also exposed to considerable rotational forces during the stance phase. It has not yet been determined whether these play a role in the pathogenesis of ED.

In a small number of cases, ED results from asynchronous growth of the radius and ulna („short radius syndrome"). The medial coronoid process is forced to bear most of the load and becomes fragmented. OC and FMCP can occur concurrently in the same joint. The term "kissing lesions" is used to describe scuffing of the medial humerus, resulting from a short radius. Breeds predisposed to FMCP and OC include all Retrievers, Bernese Mountain Dogs, Rottweilers and other rapidly growing breeds.

Clinical findings Diagnosis of ED can be challenging. Clinical findings may lead to a high index of suspicion, but cannot be used to eliminate panosteitis as a cause of lameness. Character-

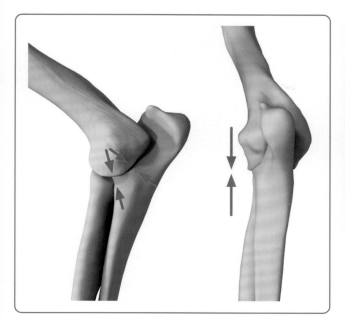

▶ **Fig. 8.75** Recent research indicates that elbow dysplasia is caused by increased pressure in the medial compartment. (source: Daniel Koch, Jonas Lauströer, Amir Andikfar)

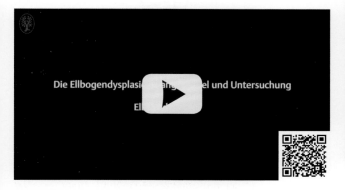

▶ **Video 8.10** Elbow dysplasia – abnormal gait and diagnosis.

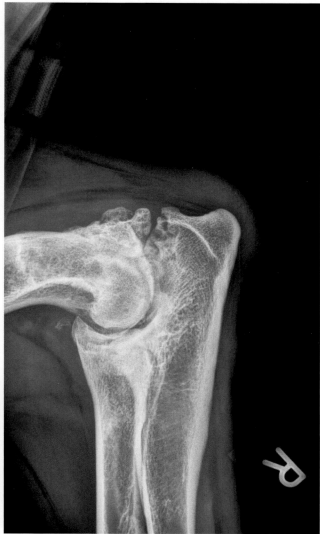

▶ **Fig. 8.76** Typical radiographic appearance of ununited anconeal process (e.g. in growing German Shepherd Dogs and Great Danes).

istic features of ED include: onset between 4 and 8 months, dogs are large and rapidly growing, the course of disease exhibits slight progression, lameness improves on warm-up, valgus disease – to reduce pressure on the medial elbow compartment (p. 149) – is frequently bilateral, pain is elicited by extension and rotation of the elbow (p. 147), palpable joint effusion is present along the medial and lateral humeral epicondyles, pain is elicited by firm palpation of the medial coronoid process and possibly the anconeal process. UAP results in the most pronounced ED-induced lameness; FMCP is the most commonly occurring form of ED.

Refer to ▶ **Video 8.10** for a video showing the gait of a dog with ED.

Diagnostic imaging and further testing Orthogonal radiographs should be taken (mediolateral, craniocaudal with slight pronation), though radiography is not always sufficiently sensitive. The most readily identifiable form of ED is UAP (▶ **Fig. 8.76**). Fusion of the anconeal process with the olecranon

normally occurs by 4 to 5 months of age. In some cases, OCD is also relatively easily discernible in craniocaudal views as subchondral lysis and sclerosis in the distal medial humeral condyle (▶ **Fig. 8.77**). Radiographic diagnosis of MCD is considerably more difficult. While the coronoid process can be visualized reasonably clearly on special projections (slightly supinated mediolateral view, oblique craniocaudal view), lesions are often undetectable or unclear. Indistinct delineation of the coronoid process (mediolateral and craniocaudal view; ▶ **Fig. 8.78**, ▶ **Fig. 8.79**) and wearing and proliferation of bone (craniocaudal view) suggest coronoid pathology, but do not confirm the diagnosis. Fissuring of the coronoid process is rarely observed and is often artifactual. Conversely, the absence of radiographic changes does not rule out ED. Arthroscopy and CT are thus the methods of choice for diagnosis of MCD, if clinical and radiological assessment is inconclusive (▶ **Fig. 8.80**). Elbow joint incongruity can only be identified if there is clear radiographic evidence of a step within the joint, since the relationship of the radius, ulna and humerus is heavily influenced

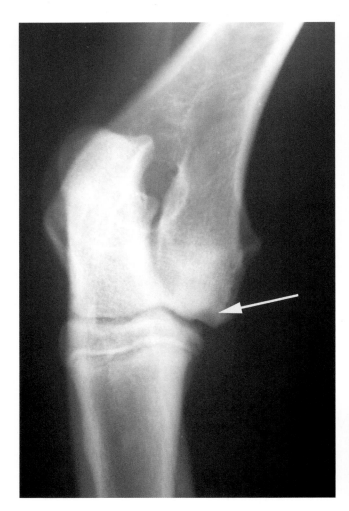

▶ **Fig. 8.77** Osteochondritic lesion on the medial humeral condyle.

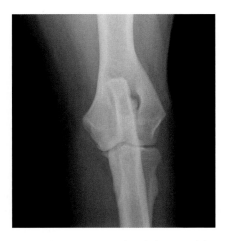

▶ **Fig. 8.78** Radiographic appearance of medial coronoid disease (cranio-caudal view). The coronoid process is poorly delineated.

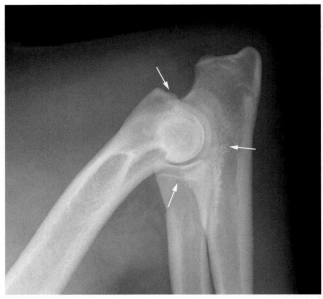

▶ **Fig. 8.79** Radiographic appearance of medial coronoid disease (lateral view): poor delineation of the coronoid process, early signs of sclerosis of the trochlear notch and osteophyte development on the anconeal process.

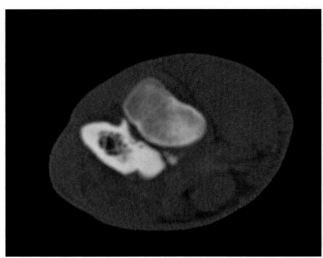

▶ **Fig. 8.80** CT image (transverse section) of the left elbow of a Labrador Retriever at the level of the medial coronoid process. Fragmentation and marked sclerosis of the coronoid process is evident. (source: Urs Geissbühler, Klinische Radiologie, Vetsuisse-Fakultät Bern, Switzerland)

by patient positioning. Even specialist radiologists can only identify incongruity with a high degree of sensitivity when the step defect exceeds around 4 mm [114].

Treatment Conservative management plays a role in the treatment of ED. In mild or inconclusive cases, or where diagnosis has been delayed and arthritic changes are present, non-surgical therapy serves to modulate disease progression, thereby delaying the onset of lameness and pain for as long as possible. Conservative methods (which are also suitable for post-operative management) include: weight reduction (beneficial be-

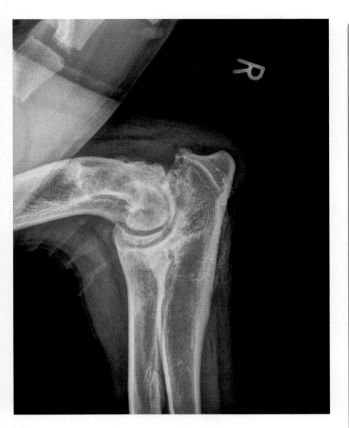

▶ **Fig. 8.81** Excision is the treatment of choice for ununited anconeal process.

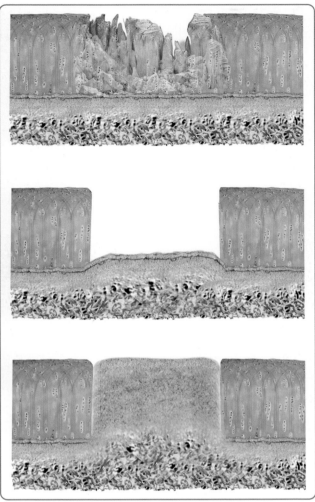

▶ **Fig. 8.82** Curettage of osteochondritic lesions. This procedure allows the underlying bone to repair. (source: Daniel Koch, Jonas Lauströer, Amir Andikfar)

cause 60% of the body weight is borne by the forelimbs), exercise modification (shorter and more frequent), physiotherapy (warm-up/exercise preparation, maintenance of muscle mass and mobility), chondroprotective preparations (to delay cartilage destruction) and anti-inflammatory therapy (to reduce joint effusion, facilitate muscle maintenance through weight-bearing and improve overall well-being). Long-term anti-inflammatory therapy can be used if the response is good and there are no side effects. The aim is to keep the dog free of pain and lameness for the longest possible time.

Specialist practice: Surgical management of ED has many levels and is specific to the form of dysplasia. Treatment of UAP usually involves excision of the ununited bone fragment (▶ Fig. 8.81). This results in loss of one of the components that stabilizes the joint in rotation. If the anconeal process is large, screw fixation together with load-altering osteotomy can be attempted. This approach carries a cautious to poor prognosis, because fixation is difficult and failure of fusion with the olecranon is not uncommon.

Medium-sized to large osteochondritic lesions are treated with curettage (▶ Fig. 8.82) and debridement of the surrounding, low-quality cartilage, leaving perpendicular cartilage walls. The subchondral bone can then grow into the defect and form replacement fibrocartilage which, under ideal conditions, is stable under pressure. Arthroscopy or arthrotomy can be used for this procedure.

The choice of treatment for MCD, the most common form of ED, is heavily influenced by contemporary research and avail-

able surgical apparatus. Classical therapy involves generous excision (using hammer and chisel) of the medial coronoid process via a medial arthrotomy (▶ Fig. 8.83). While the introduction of arthroscopy has aided the diagnosis of ED, and permits minimally invasive treatment of both elbow joints in the same anesthetic, it also entails the risk that too little of the coronoid process is removed. If MCD is accompanied by an obvious step in the elbow, ulnar ostectomy can be performed in dogs under 8–10 months of age to reduce the pressure on the medial coronoid process. In rare cases, this procedure can be carried out early enough to prevent dogs from developing clinical signs. Osteosynthesis is not required.

Recently, new surgical techniques have been developed, primarily for the purpose of reducing pressure in the medial compartment. These include partial tenotomy of the biceps brachii at the ulna (biceps ulnar release procedure, BURP) and corrective osteotomy of the humerus (sliding humerus osteotomy) or the ulna (proximal abducting ulnar osteotomy). Procedures for partial or total replacement of the elbow joint are now available in some specialistic centers [100], [102], [103], [124].

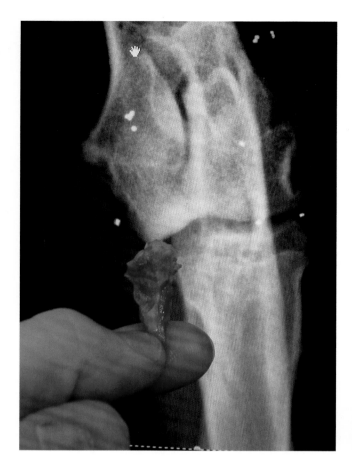

► **Fig. 8.83** The classical treatment for overloading of the medial coronoid process is subtotal coronoid ostectomy .

8.4.5   Biceps Tendinitis

Etiology and pathogenesis The biceps arises from the scapula (supraglenoid tubercle) by a long tendon that passes over the craniomedial aspect of the shoulder joint (p. 107) and subsequently courses through the intertubercular groove on the proximal humerus (p. 106). It is held within the groove by a transverse band. The synovial sheath of the tendon of origin is continuous with the joint capsule. The muscle belly extends from the medial to the cranial aspect of the humerus. Near the elbow joint, the muscle is continued by a bipartite tendon of insertion. The larger part attaches to the medial aspect of the ulna (ulnar tuberosity) and the smaller part inserts medially on the proximal radius (radial tuberosity, ► Fig. 5.42; ► Fig. 5.44, ► Fig. 5.46).

Biceps tendinitis involves the proximal portion (tendon of origin) and the synovial sheath. Causal factors include direct or indirect trauma, migrating joint mice resulting from OCD, degenerative disorders of the shoulder and pronounced transfer of weight to the forelimbs. Biceps tendinitis usually occurs in medium-sized to large dogs

Clinical findings Establishment of a definitive diagnosis is challenging. Lameness is often subtle and may be observed only when movement commences and again at the end of a long walk. On orthopedic examination, pain is elicited on firm palpation of the tendon   (p. 154)over the humerus with the

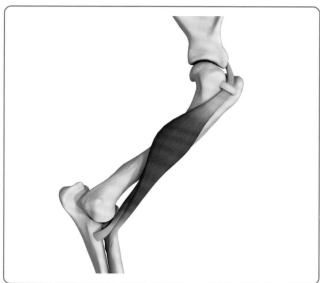

► **Fig. 8.84** Biceps tendinitis results in pain in the region of the shoulder joint or the intertubercular band. (source: Daniel Koch, Jonas Lauströer, Amir Andikfar)

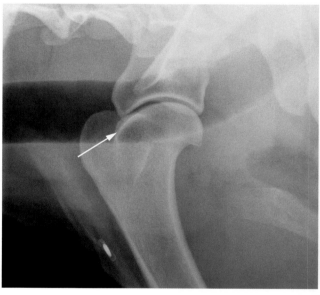

► **Fig. 8.85** Opacity in the intertubercular region may be indicative of biceps tendinitis.

shoulder flexed and the elbow in extension (► Fig. 8.84). In this position, the tendon passing over the shoulder is subjected to maximum tension and can be readily palpated with the thumb, medial to the greater tubercle.

Diagnostic imaging and further testing Mediolateral radiographs can be diagnostic, but only in clear cases. Findings include arthritic changes on the caudal margin of the humeral head, joint mice, osteolysis of the supraglenoid tubercle and opacity in the intertubercular groove (► Fig. 8.85). Contrast radiography may yield additional information, particularly with respect to the biceps tendon sheath, though sonography is the

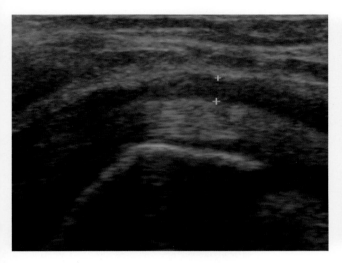

▶ **Fig. 8.86** Longitudinal section of the left biceps tendon at the level of the intertubercular groove in a 10,5 year old male neutered Labrador cross. The architecture, length and echogenicity of the fibrous components are normal. The zone between the markers indicates thickening and hypoechogenicity of the wall of the synovial sheath. (source: Urs Geissbühler, Vetimage, Switzerland)

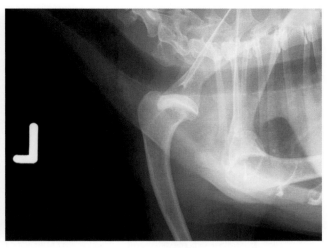

▶ **Fig. 8.87** Medial shoulder joint instability in a toy poodle following a fall on stairs.

modality of choice for evaluating the tendon. Using sonography, the tendon can be examined in its entirety, and the integrity of the tendon of origin near the shoulder joint can be assessed (▶ Fig. 8.86).

Treatment A conservative approach should be used initially for treatment of biceps tendinitis. Non-steroidal anti-inflammatory therapy and exercise restriction for 6 weeks is sufficient in many cases. Injection of cortisone into the joint or the tendon sheath may be required. For sustained reduction of pain and inflammation, the joint should be supported with a Velpeau slingfor 10 days post-injection. The well-recognized disadvantages of cortisone must be considered when using this form of treatment.

Specialist practice: If conservative management is unsuccessful, even after repeated cortisone injection, the painful proximal portion of the biceps tendon must be surgically removed from the vicinity of the joint. This can be done using one of three techniques. Some surgeons section the tendon and allow it to slide to a distal location, where it fibroses with the humerus. This procedure can be performed arthroscopically. Others prefer to fix the tendon stump to the humerus with a screw and washer. In a third technique, the tendon is severed from the scapula, released from the intertubercular groove, and passed through a tunnel in the proximal humerus to the supraspinatus, to which it is sutured. This way, the function of the biceps is at least partly preserved.

With chronic inflammation, the biceps tendon and proximal portion of the muscle belly may become entrapped by fibrous tissue, and later bone, to such an extent that the tendon is barely mobile. In this situation, surgical release of the muscle and tendon is indicated.

8.4.6 Shoulder Joint Instability

Etiology and pathogenesis Luxation of the shoulder joint (p. 107)s rare. In most cases, luxation is medial or lateral. Congenital luxations are attributable to medial ligament laxity and deformity of the glenoid cavity, while traumatic luxations are usually lateral, but can occur in any direction.

Clinical findings Patients are unable to use the affected forelimb for locomotion, unless luxation is chronic, congenital or partial (subluxation). With lateral luxation, the limb is rotated internally; with medial luxation it is rotated externally. The relative positions of the greater tubercle and acromion indicate the direction of luxation. Luxation may be accompanied by variably manifesting nerve deficits, since the brachial plexus lies medial to the scapula.

Diagnostic imaging and further testing Mediolateral and craniocaudal radiographs of the shoulder region are used to confirm the direction of luxation (▶ Fig. 8.87). The bones and shoulder joint should also be assessed for chip fractures of the glenoid region, humeral head and acromion. Wearing of the medial glenoid cavity is a common finding in cases of chronic and congenital luxation. Arthritic changes are minimal.

Treatment Acute traumatic medial luxations without chip fractures can be managed conservatively. The joint is reduced under general anesthesia and is subsequently supported for 10 days with a Velpeau sling. For acute lateral luxations, joint reduction and application of a spica splint is recommended.

Specialist practice: for treatment of chronic shoulder luxation, translocation of the biceps tendon (medial translocation for medial luxation, lateral translocation for lateral luxation) produces the best results. In its new position, the translocated tendon serves to counteract reluxation (▶ Fig. 8.88). Reinforcement of the lateral or medial shoulder ligaments with mesh or prosthetic sutures is generally only suitable for small dogs. Relatively long-term external coaptation is indicated following all forms of surgical intervention. Markedly dysplastic or arthritic joints should be arthrodesed.

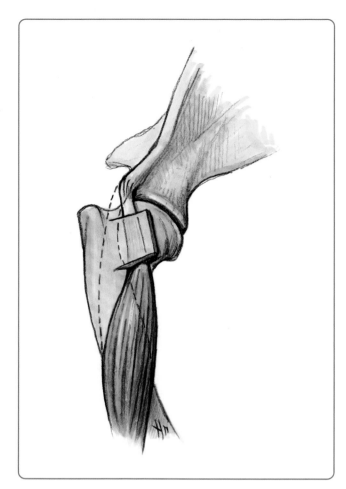

► **Fig. 8.88** Medial translocation of the biceps tendon and fixation to the proximal humerus allows the tendon to act as a collateral shoulder joint ligament. (source: Matthias Haab, Departement für Pferde, Vetsuisse-Fakultät Universität Zürich, Switzerland)

8.4.7   Osteochondrosis of the Shoulder Joint

Refer to general information on osteochondrosis (p. 185).

8.5
Bibliography

[97] Baumgartner W, Boyce RW, Alldinger S et al. Metaphyseal bone lesions in young dogs with systemic canine distemper virus infection. Vet Microbiol 1995; 44(2–4):201–209

[98] Beuing R, Mues C, Tellhein B et al. Prevalence and inheritance of canine elbow dysplasia in German Rottweiler. J Anim Breed Genet 2000; 117:375–383

[99] Bockstahler B, Millis D, Levine D, Forterre F, Tacke S. Physiotherapie auf den Punkt gebracht. Babenhausen: BE Vet; 2004

[100] Burton NJ, Ellis JR, Burton KJ et al. An ex vivo investigation of the effect of the TATE canine elbow arthroplasty system on kinematics of the elbow. J Small Anim Pract 2013; 54(5):240–247

[101] Engler J. Populationsgenetische Analysen zur Ellbogen- und Hüftgelenkdysplasie beim Labrador Retriever [Dissertation]. Hannover: Stiftung Tierärztliche Hochschule; 2009

[102] Fitzpatrick N, Yeadon R. Working algorithm for treatment decision making for developmental disease of the medial compartment of the elbow in dogs. Vet Surg 2009; 38(2):285–300

[103] Fitzpatrick N, Yeadon R, Smith T et al. Techniques of application and initial clinical experience with sliding humeral osteotomy for treatment of medial compartment disease of the canine elbow. Vet Surg 2009; 38(2):261–278

[104] Garzotto C, Berg J. Oncology: Musculoskeletal System. In: Slatter D, ed. Textbook of small animal surgery. Philadelphia: WB Saunders; 2003: 2460–2474

[105] Grierson J, Asher L, Grainger K. An investigation into risk factors for bilateral canine cruciate ligament rupture. Vet Comp Orthop Traumatol 2011; 24(3):192–196

[106] Grundmann S, Montavon PM. Stenosing tenosynovitis of the abductor pollicis longus muscle in dogs. Vet Comp Orthop Traumatol 2001; 14:95–100

[107] Hartmann P. Genetische Analysen von züchterisch bedeutsamen Merkmalen beim Berner Sennenhund [Dissertation]. Hannover: Stiftung; 2011

[108] Inauen R, Koch D, Bass M et al. Tibial tuberosity conformation as a risk factor for cranial cruciate ligament rupture in the dog. Vet Comp Orthop Traumatol 2009; 22(1):16–20

[109] Kistler KR. Canine Osteosarcoma: 1462 cases reviewed to uncover patterns of height, weight, breed, sex, age and site involvement. Phi Zeta Awards; University of Pennsylvania, School of Veterinary Medicine; 1981

[110] Koch DA, Grundmann S, Savoldelli D, L'Eplattenier H, Montavon PM. Die Diagnostik der Patellarluxation des Kleintiers. Schweizer Archiv fur Tierheilkunde. 1998;140(9):371–374.

[111] Linnmann SM. Die Hüftgelenkdysplasie des Hundes. Berlin: Veterinär-Spiegel; 2013

[112] Lübke S. Immunbedingte Polyarthritis beim Hund, eine retro- und prospektive Studie [Dissertation]. Berlin: Freie Universität Berlin; 2002.

[113] Malm S, Fikse WF, Danell B et al. Genetic variation and genetic trends in hip and elbow dysplasia in Swedish Rottweiler and Bernese Mountain Dog. J Anim Breed Genet 2008; 125(6):403–412

[114] Mason DR, Schulz KS, Samii VF et al. Sensitivity of radiographic evaluation of radio-ulnar incongruence in the dog in vitro. Vet Surg 2002; 31(2):125–132

[115] McGreevy PD, Thomson PC, Pride C et al. Prevalence of obesity in dogs examined by Australian veterinary practices and the risk factors involved. Vet Rec 2005; 156(22):695–702

[116] Montavon PM, Damur DM, Tepic S, eds. Advancement of the tibial tuberosity for the treatment of cranial cruciate deficient canine stifle. Munich: 1st World Orthopaedic Veterinary Conference; 2002

[117] Montgomery R. Miscellaneous orthopedic disease. In: Slatter D, ed. Textbook of small animal surgery. Philadelphia: WB Saunders; 2003: 2251–2260

[118] Nap RC, Hazewinkel HA. Growth and skeletal development in the dog in relation to nutrition; a review. Vet Q 1994; 16(1):50–59

[119] Nielsen C, Pluhar GE. Diagnosis and treatment of hind limb muscle strain injuries in 22 dogs. Vet Comp Orthop Traumatol 2005; 18 (4):247–253

[120] Nieves MA, Hartwig P, Kinyon JM et al. Bacterial isolates from plaque and from blood during and after routine dental procedures in dogs. Vet Surg VS 1997; 26(1):26–32

[121] Orthopedic Foundation for Animals (OFFA). Hip dysplasia statistics. Columbia; 2010

[122] Reif U, Hulse DA, Hauptman JG. Effect of tibial plateau leveling on stability of the canine cranial cruciate-deficient stifle joint: an in vitro study. Vet Surg 2002; 31(2):147–154

[123] Slocum B, Devine T. Cranial tibial thrust: a primary force in the canine stifle. J Am Vet Med Assoc 1983; 183(4):456–459

[124] Smith ZF, Wendelburg KL, Tepic S et al. In vitro biomechanical comparison of load to failure testing of a canine unconstrained medial compartment elbow arthroplasty system and normal canine thoracic limbs. Vet Comp Orthop Traumatol 2013; 26(5):356–365

[125] Solanti S, Laitinen O, Atroshi F. Hereditary and clinical characteristics of lateral luxation of the superficial digital flexor tendon in Shetland sheepdogs. Vet Ther 2002; 3(1):97–103

[126] Stöcklin P, L'Eplattenier H, Montavon PM. Avulsion of the origin of the tendon of the extensor digitalis longus muscle in a Dobermann pinscher. Schweiz Arch Tierheilkd 1999; 141(2):53–57

[127] Tryfonidou MA, van den Broek J, van den Brom WE et al. Intestinal kalzium absorption in growing dogs is influenced by kalzium intake and age but not by growth rate. J Nutr 2002; 132(11):3363–3368

[128] Vidoni B, Hassan J, Bockstahler B et al. Kontraktur des Musculus gracilis – Klinik, bildgebende Diagnostik und Therapie bei einer Deutschen Schäferhündin. Tierärztl Mschr 2008; 95:8–14

[129] Wangdee C, Leegwater PA, Heuven HC et al. Prevalence and genetics of patellar luxation in Kooiker dogs. Vet J 2014; 201(3):333–337

[130] Weber U. Morphologische Studie am Becken von Papillon-Hunden unter Berücksichtigung von Faktoren zur Ätiologie der nichttraumatischen Patellaluxation nach medial [Dissertation]. Berlin: Freie Universität; 1992

[131] Whitehair JG, Vasseur PB, Willits NH. Epidemiology of cranial cruciate ligament rupture in dogs. J Am Vet Med Assoc 1993; 203 (7):1016–1019

[132] Zabka A, Koch DA, Stocklin P et al. Ein Fall einer Sesambeinfragmentierung als Lahmheitsursache bei einer Rottweilerhündin. Schweiz Arch Tierheilkd 1999; 141(4):195–201

9 Selected Neurological Disorders

Daniel Koch, Martin S. Fischer

9.1
Distinguishing between Lameness and Paralysis

Thorough orthopedic and neurological examination usually leads to a clinical diagnosis that clearly identifies a disorder as orthopedic or neurological in nature. The key aspects of the examination in this regard are gait analysis, joint palpation and detection of any effusion and instability, palpation of the bones, postural and proprioceptive responses and assessment of spinal reflexes.

Due to the anatomical proximity of the caudal vertebral column, cauda equina and the pelvis, topical diagnosis of disorders affecting this region can be more difficult. Based purely on a pain response to palpation of the lower back, and restricted and painful extension of the hip joint, the list of differential diagnoses is long; in the worst case, this could lead to premature and incorrect interpretation and management. Differential diagnoses include lumbosacral intervertebral disc disease, compression of the cauda equina, spinal cord disease, iliopsoas strain, hip dysplasia, coxofemoral osteoarthritis, pelvic/vertebral/tail fractures, neoplasia of the skeleton or surrounding soft tissue, prostate disease and even cruciate ligament rupture. In this situation, even highly qualified and experienced practitioners need to make use of diagnostic imaging, including both conventional radiography and sectional imaging. Magnetic resonance tomography is the modality of choice for neurological disorders, since many structures of interest are located in the soft tissue; computed tomography is a second line option, as it primarily depicts osseous tissue.

A similar challenge is encountered in the forelimbs in the region of the lower cervical vertebrae and brachial plexus. In cases of unexplained forelimb lameness in older dogs, muscular or brachial plexus trauma, intervertebral disc disease and vertebral instability need to be considered alongside the classical differential diagnoses of elbow or shoulder osteoarthritis and biceps tendinitis.

The selected neurological disorders described briefly below represent possible differential diagnoses for orthopedic disorders. More detailed descriptions can be found in relevant veterinary neurology texts.

9.2
Degenerative Lumbosacral Stenosis and Cauda Equina Syndrome

Etiology and pathogenesis Degenerative lumbosacral stenosis (DLSS) is characterized by degeneration and protrusion of the lumbosacral intervertebral disc. Associated changes in the mobility of the lumbosacral joint lead to secondary degeneration

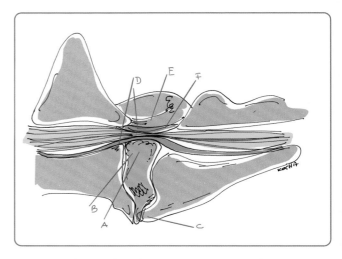

▶ **Fig. 9.1** Pathophysiology of DLSS: A Disc protrusion, B thickening of annulus fibrosus, C subluxation, D osteophytes, E joint capsule thickening, F ligament thickening.

of soft tissue structures such as the yellow ligaments (ligamentum flavum) and joint capsules of the articular process joints (facet joints). Osteophytes form at the joints between the vertebrae and at the ventral and lateral surfaces of L7 and S1. These changes result in compression (usually dynamic) of the central vertebral canal and the intervertebral foramina between L7 and S1 (▶ Fig. 9.1). Static and dynamic compression of the nerve roots of L6, L7 and the sacral nerves leads to compressive radiculopathy, which manifests clinically as cauda equina syndrome. Predisposing factors include the presence of a transitional lumbosacral vertebra, osteochondrosis of the end plate of the sacrum, discospondylitides, regional trauma and congenital primary stenosis of the vertebral canal and foramina. German Shepherd Dogs and dogs aged from 7 years are overrepresented.

Clinical findings Clinical signs of cauda equina compression syndrome usually develop over a period of months and vary in severity. Findings include difficulty rising, lameness, trembling in one or both hindlimbs, difficulty climbing stairs, toe-dragging, a downward sloping backline, and motor weakness of the tail. Feces may be deposited in multiple portions or may be dropped while walking. Dorsoflexion of the tail and lordosis of the lumbar vertebral column is painful, as extension produces dynamic reduction of the diameter of the nerve canal, resulting in increased compression. Dogs exhibit pain on firm palpation of the caudal lumbar vertebral column and often quickly sit down when pressure is applied. In advanced cases, pronounced muscle wasting, urinary and fecal incontinence and complete paralysis of the tail are observed. Total limb paralysis does not occur with DLSS.

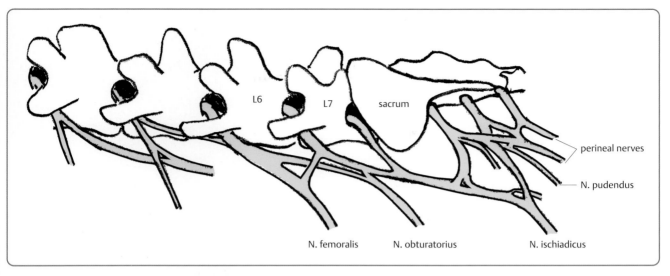

▶ **Fig. 9.2** Peripheral nerves of the lumbosacral plexus. (based on: Salomon F-V, Geyer H, Gille U. Anatomie für die Tiermedizin. 3rd ed. Stuttgart. Enke 2015)

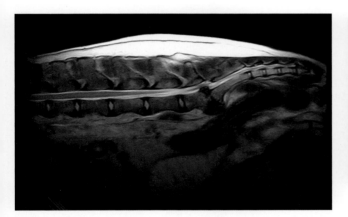

▶ **Fig. 9.3** MRT (sagittal section) image of a Labrador with DLSS (compression of the cauda equina between L7 and S1). (source: Konrad Jurina, Haar)

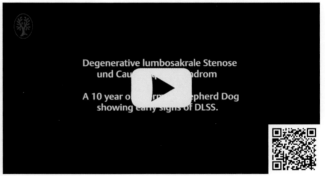

▶ **Video 9.1** 10 year old German Shepherd Dog showing early signs of DLSS.

Neurological deficits usually result from lower motor neuron compression (▶ **Fig. 9.2**). Proprioceptive positioning is often delayed. The flexion reflex and cranial tibial reflex may be reduced. Conversely, it is not uncommon for the patellar reflex to be slightly increased. Whereas this reflex arc is not directly affected, loss of the antagonistic effect of muscles innervated by the sciatic nerve on the corresponding agonists (innervated by femoral nerve; quadriceps) results in an increased reflex response (pseudohyperreflexia). Reduced anal tone and perineal reflex responses are only observed in the advanced stages of disease.

Diagnostic imaging and further testing The role of conventional radiography is to provide an overview and to permit identification of neoplasia or trauma. As an isolated finding, spondyloses do not confirm a diagnosis of DLSS; they merely indicate the presence of degenerative changes that may be clinically insignificant. The diagnostic technique of choice is magnetic resonance tomography (▶ **Fig. 9.3**) or, with some limita-

tions, computed tomography. Compression identified using sectional imaging may not correlate with clinical observations. Changes in the nerve roots of the cauda equina (see below) are a more reliable diagnostic indicator; these are often detectable with MRT. CT or MRT imaging permits precise surgical planning and targeted intervention.

Refer to ▶ **Video 9.1** for a video showing a dog with DLSS.

Treatment Medical treatment of DLSS can be attempted if there is back pain, muscle wastage and lameness without urinary and fecal incontinence. This includes weight reduction, exercise restriction, physiotherapy for muscle flexibility and improved nerve conduction, and appropriate pain relief (non-steroidal anti-inflammatories or gabapentin). Systemic corticosteroids are not recommended due to their questionable efficacy and considerable side effects. There are, however, isolated reports of successful short-term medical management of DLSS with epidural or paravertebral injection of depot corticosteroids. It should be noted that DLSS is progressive and that palliative measures do not address the underlying cause of disease.

If conservative management is unsuccessful, or clinical signs worsen, surgical decompression of the cauda equina and entrapped nerve roots is indicated. Various methods have been described. Classical dorsal laminectomy of L7 und S1 (based on localization of compression to this location by MRT), removal of hypertrophic ligaments, annulectomy/removal of protruding discs and nerve root decompression via lateral foraminotomy can be performed in isolation or in combination. Stabilization with pedicle screws, combined with bone cement or internal fixation rods, results in rapid clinical improvement, though implant failure may lead to poorer long-term results. Post-operative management includes appropriate physiotherapy and pain management. The prognosis is generally good; the reported success rate is 67–95%, depending on the severity of pre-operative findings.

9.3
Degenerative Myelopathy

Etiology and pathogenesis Degenerative myelopathy (DM) is an axonal disease characterized by necrosis in the lateral and dorsal regions of the spinal cord. It is, thus, primarily a disease of the spinal white matter. Demyelination results in axon degeneration with progressive loss of communication between the brain and the limbs. German Shepherd Dogs are overrepresented; Boxers, Hovawarts and Pembroke Welsh Corgis are also predisposed. Disease onset occurs in middle to advanced age. Degenerative myelopathy is caused by a mutation of the SOD1 gene. Dogs that are homozygous carriers of the mutation are at high risk of developing DM. The disease occurs rarely in heterozygous carriers and is observed only in a small number of very old dogs. Genetic testing is a highly effective means of controlling the disease and is currently carried out by several breed societies.

Clinical findings The course of clinical disease is slow and progressive, and includes hindlimb ataxia, weakness and paresis. Crossing of the hindlimbs under the body may be observed (▶ Fig. 9.4). There is usually no evidence of back pain. Hindlimb reflexes may be normal or increased, reflecting upper motor neuron deficits, though the patellar reflex may be absent. Urinary and fecal incontinence occurs in the later stages of disease. If disease is long-standing, forelimb function is also affected.

Diagnostic imaging and further testing Radiography and MRT imaging of the vertebral column and nervous tissue should be performed to exclude important differential diagnoses such as chronic intervertebral disc disease, neoplasia and meningomyelitis. Cerebrospinal fluid analysis is used to rule out infection. A definitive diagnosis is established by exclusion, particularly in the presence of a positive test result for the SOD1 gene mutation.

Treatment There is no effective medical therapy for DM. The diseases worsens in successive increments over a period ranging from several months to a few years. Eventually, euthanasia

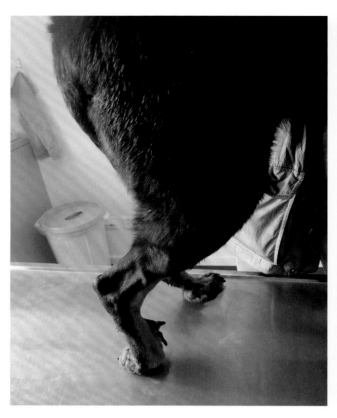

▶ **Fig. 9.4** Proprioceptive deficit in a German Shepherd Dog with DM.

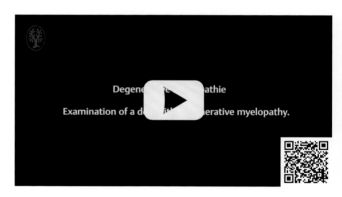

▶ **Video 9.2** Examination of a German Shepherd Dog with degenerative myelopathy.

is warranted. The ambulatory stage can be prolonged with intensive, targeted physiotherapy.

Refer to ▶ **Video 9.2** for a video showing examination of a dog with degenerative myelopathy.

9.4
Fibrocartilaginous Embolism

Etiology and pathogenesis Fibrocartilaginous material from the nucleus pulposus can pass through venous sinuses into the spinal vascular system, where it can cause ischemic or hemorrhagic infarction of the neuroparenchyma (▶ Fig. 9.5). The nerve cells undergo necrosis and the axons swell. Swelling

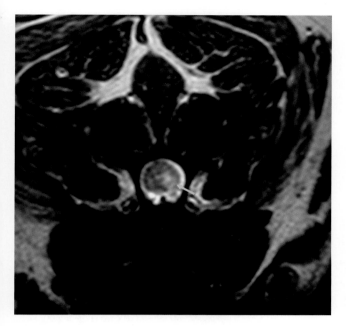

▶ **Fig. 9.5** MRT image (transverse section) of an infarct and necrosis (light structures, see arrow) in the spinal cord. (source: Schmidt MJ, Kramer M. MRT-Atlas. ZNS-Befunde bei Hund und Katze. Enke 2015)

leads to further localized damage of the surrounding spinal cord tissue. Fibrocartilaginous embolism occurs particularly in medium-sized to large young adult dogs. Most infarcts are located at the lumbosacral or cervicothoracic intumescence.

Clinical findings The onset of clinical signs is usually peracute. There is often no history of observed trauma; not infrequently, infarction occurs during playing. Clinical signs change little after the acute phase. Neural deficits reflect spinal cord damage and may be asymmetrical. The typical course of events seen with extramedullary compression (back pain, ataxia, abnormal locomotion, loss of superficial pain response, loss of deep pain response) is not observed with spinal cord infarction. Back pain is usually absent. Many patients exhibit a variable degree of paresis on presentation.

Diagnostic imaging and further testing Radiography and sectional imaging of the vertebral column is used to exclude other possible diseases such as compressive or non-compressive intervertebral disc disease, neoplasia, trauma or meningomyelitis. In MRT images, the infarct appears as a focal T2-hyperintense intramedullary lesion. Cerebrospinal fluid analysis is usually normal, though the protein content may be slightly increased. Definitive diagnosis can only be made post-mortem with histopathology.

Treatment Corticosteroids are not indicated as they have no effect on the course of disease or the prognosis. The urinary bladder should be emptied every 8 hours. Soft bedding is important for dogs with paralysis to prevent the development of pressure sores. Physiotherapy facilitates rehabilitation by preserving muscle mass and promoting perfusion. The prognosis is heavily dependent on the extent and location of the infarct. Infarcts

that do not involve the reflex centres carry a good prognosis. With lesions involving the cervical or lumbar intumescence, recovery is incomplete and more prolonged. If there is no visible improvement in neuromuscular function within 2 weeks, or a deep pain response remains absent during this period, euthanasia should be considered.

9.5
Thoracolumbar Intervertebral Disc Disease

Etiology and pathogenesis Thoracolumbar intervertebral disc disease is arguably the most common disease of the spine. Acute herniation of the metaplastic nucleus pulposus through a likewise degenerative annulus fibrosus is referred to as disc extrusion and constitutes the classic form of intervertebral disc disease seen in middle-aged dogs between the 10th thoracic and 6th lumbar vertebrae (70% of these between Th 12 and L2). The herniated nucleus causes direct, extradural compression of the spinal cord, causing the cord to swell. Chondrodystrophic breeds including the Dachshund, Pekingese, Beagle and Poodle are predisposed. In non-chondrodystrophic, larger breeds, histological changes also indicate chondroid metaplasia of the nucleus pulposus, though prolapse manifests more frequently as disc protrusion (bulging of the fibres of the annulus fibrosus) and the course of disease is more chronic/progressive.

Clinical findings Extradural spinal cord compression typically leads to a sequence of clinical signs that vary in their severity and speed of development, depending on the dynamics and extent of the disc pathology. The degree of severity is the major determinant of treatment and prognosis. The sequence is as follows: (1) back pain, (2) proprioceptive deficits and ataxia, (3) loss of motor function in the hindlimbs with limb spasticity, (4) loss of the superficial pain response (pinching of the skin of the hindlimb), (5) loss of the deep pain response (pressure on the phalanges in the hindlimbs). Compression of upper motor neurons in the thoracolumbar region causes partial to complete disinhibition of hindlimb reflexes by the brain. Thus, the patellar reflex, cranial tibial reflex and bladder sphincter tone may be increased in the presence of normal forelimb reflexes. Emptying of the often excessively full bladder is difficult. A very deep lesion between T3–L3 may cause a marked increase in forelimb muscle tone, due to the loss of an additional inhibitory centre (Schiff-Sherrington phenomenon).

Diagnostic imaging and further testing Magnetic resonance tomography is the diagnostic modality of choice (▶ Fig. 9.6). Computed tomography can be used as a second-line option. These techniques are particularly important when decompressive surgery is indicated. Conventional radiographs are of very limited value, as they do not always reveal narrowing of the intervertebral space due to prolapse of the nucleus pulposus; even if narrowing is detected, it cannot be concluded that an acute prolapse has occurred at this location. Contrast radiography (myelography) was replaced some years ago by sectional

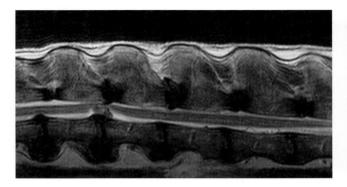

► **Fig. 9.6** MRT image of thoracolumbar disc prolapse. The nucleus pulposus usually herniates in a cranial direction. The energy of the prolapse leads to secondary swelling of the spinal cord. (source: Schmidt MJ, Kramer M. MRT-Atlas. ZNS-Befunde bei Hund und Katze. Enke 2015)

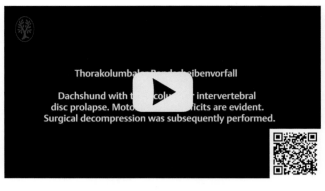

Thorakolumbaler Bandscheibenvorfall

Dachshund with thoracolumbar intervertebral disc prolapse. Motor function deficits are evident. Surgical decompression was subsequently performed.

► **Video 9.3** Dachshund with thoracolumbar intervertebral disc prolapse. Motor function deficits are evident. Surgical decompression was subsequently performed.

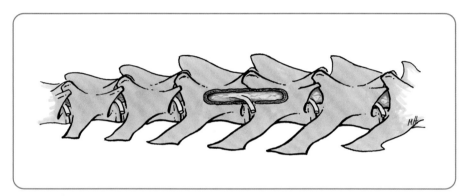

► **Fig. 9.7** Schematic illustration of pediculectomy for decompression and removal of prolapsed intervertebral disc material. (source: Matthias Haab, Departement für Pferde, Vetsuisse-Fakultät Universität Zürich, Switzerland)

imaging, as the latter is less invasive and provides more reliable results.

Treatment Dogs with back pain and proprioceptive deficits can be treated medically with analgesics, physiotherapy, and controlled and restricted exercise. The use of corticosteroids is controversial. Evidence that they reduce swelling of the compressed spinal cord is lacking. If conservative management is unsuccessful or motor function deficits appear, surgical decompression is indicated. Guided by the results of diagnostic imaging, hemilaminectomy, mini-hemilaminectomy, pediculectomy (► Fig. 9.7) or dorsal laminectomy is performed to relieve pressure on the spinal cord by opening the vertebral column and removing the prolapsed material. Lateral fenestration of the annulus fibrosus to prevent further prolapse at the same location – and, prophylactically, in the surrounding area – is recommended in the literature, as this can reduce the risk of reherniation. Following successful decompression, the patient requires intensive supportive care incorporating analgesia, physiotherapy, turning and monitoring of bladder emptying. The prognosis depends on the extent of the prolapse, the timing of decompression, surgical technique and the intensity of post-operative care. Recovery times can vary considerably between individual patients.

Refer to ► Video 9.3 for a video showing a dog with thoracolumbar intervertebral disc prolapse.

9.6
Cervical Intervertebral Disc Disease

Etiology and pathogenesis Approximately 15% of intervertebral disc prolapses occur in the cervical region, predominantly at C2–C3 and C3–C4 in small breeds. In large breeds, the lower cervical region (C5–C7) is more commonly affected. Chondrodystrophic breeds are once again overrepresented, as is the Dobermann Pinscher. In the Beagle, prolapse occurs more frequently in the cervical than the thoracolumbar region.

Clinical findings As the spinal cord has more space within the cervical vertebral column than in the more caudal regions, clinical signs only occur when the volume of prolapsed material is large. A stiff gait with low head carriage is characteristic of cervical intervertebral disc prolapse (► Fig. 9.8). Manipulation of the cervical vertebral column is very painful. Due to the exposed location of the corticospinal tracts that pass to the hindlimbs within the spinal cord, disc prolapse often leads initially to hindlimb paresis, prior to the appearance of deficits in the forelimbs.

Diagnostic imaging and further testing Sectional imaging is the preferred method for diagnosis of cervical intervertebral disc prolapse. Myelography is now used very little.

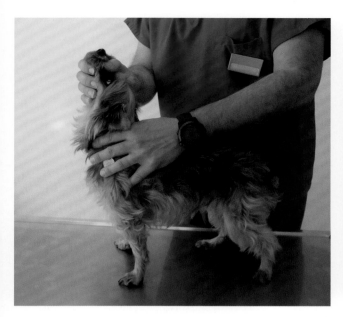

▶ **Fig. 9.8** Cervical disc prolapse: movement of the neck is painful and the head is carried low.

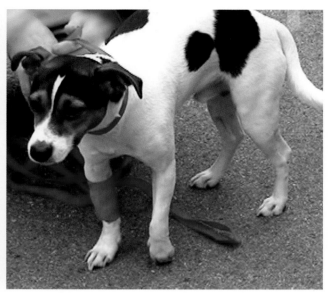

▶ **Fig. 9.9** Radial nerve paralysis: typical forelimb stance. (source: Franck Forterre, Bern)

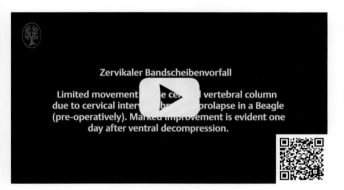

Zervikaler Bandscheibenvorfall

Limited movement ~~the ce~~ ~~l~~ vertebral column due to cervical inter~~~~ ~~b~~r~~~~ prolapse in a Beagle (pre-operatively). Ma~~rked improvement~~ is evident one day after ventral decompression.

▶ **Video 9.4** Limited movement of the cervical vertebral column due to cervical intervertebral disc prolapse in a Beagle (pre-operative assessment). Marked improvement is evident one day after ventral decompression.

Treatment Painful neck movement without neurological deficits is amenable to medical/conservative treatment, using the same approach as described for thoracolumbar prolapse. Surgical decompression (ventral or lateral) is indicated if painful neck movement persists or if paresis is present. To avoid vascular and neural damage, and to maintain a clear overview of the surgical site, the surgeon must have a detailed anatomical understanding of the approach to the vertebrae. There is less urgency associated with cervical than with thoracolumbar prolapses, because the width of the cervical vertebral canal allows the spinal cord to tolerate more swelling. For the same reason, the prognosis is usually good; very good recovery has been observed in over 90% of patients treated with ventral decompression (ventral slot technique). Post-operative treatment comprises physiotherapy, analgesia and restriction of movement.

Refer to ▶ **Video 9.4** for a video showing a dog with cervical intervertebral disc prolapse.

9.7
Brachial Plexus Injury

Cranially or laterally imposed trauma, or falls from considerable heights, can lead to stretching or avulsion of the roots of the brachial plexus or the peripheral nerves emerging from the plexus (e.g. radial nerve, ▶ Fig. 9.9). This causes monoplegia with signs of lower motor neuron damage, i.e. flaccid paralysis and reduced to absent reflex responses. The response to stimulation of the dermatome corresponding to the damaged nerve is absent or delayed. Important differential diagnoses include space-occupying hematomas of traumatic origin, predominantly unilateral cervical intervertebral disc prolapse, and nerve sheath tumors; neuritis is less common. Diagnosis is established with sectional imaging, to exclude other etiologies, and with confirmatory electromyography. Individual nerves are difficult to locate and expose. Successful repositioning, suturing and re-establishment of nerve function has only been achieved in an experimental context. Thus, the first-line treatment for dogs with brachial plexus injury is physiotherapy, with the aim of improving nerve conduction and facilitating muscular compensation. Muscle mass should be maintained as much as possible while damaged nerve fibres regrow and potentially restore innervation. Further spontaneous improvement is unlikely after 6–12 months. If proximal limb function is relatively normal, and only the carpus and digits are permanently flexed, an orthesis may be used or carpal arthrodesis attempted. Self-mutilation may warrant amputation of the limb.

9.8
Bibliography

[133] Jaggy A. Atlas und Lehrbuch der Kleintierneurologie. Hannover: Schlütersche; 2007

[134] Vandevelde M, Jaggy A, Lang J. Veterinärmedizinische Neurologie. Ein Leitfaden für Studium und Praxis. 2. neubearb. u. erw. Aufl. Berlin: Paul Parey; 2001

[135] Olby NJ, Jeffrey ND. Pathogenesis and Physiology of Central Nervous System Disease and Injury. In: Tobias KM, Johnston SA. Veterinary Surgery Small Animal. Elsevier: 2012; 374–387

[136] Schmidt MJ, Kramer M. MRT-Atlas. ZNS Befunde bei Hund und Katze. Stuttgart: Thieme; 2015

[137] Sharp NJ. Nervous System. In: Slatter D. Textbook of small animal surgery. Saunders: 2003; 1092–1286

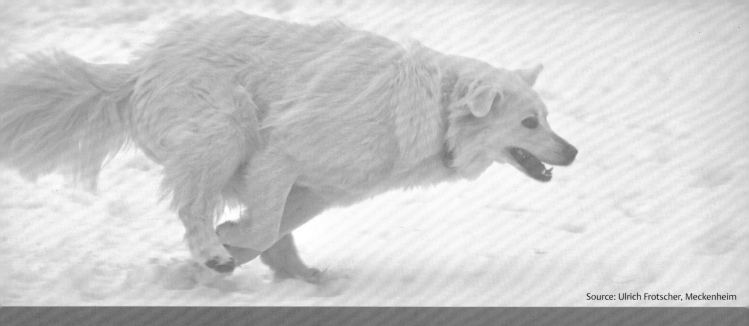

Source: Ulrich Frotscher, Meckenheim

Part 4
Appendix

10 Glossary of terms

angle of attack
Angle between the horizontal and a line drawn from the center of gravity of the body to the point of touch down.

angle of lift off
Angle between the whole limb or each individual segment and the horizontal at lift off.

angle of touch down
Angle between the entire limb or each individual segment and the horizontal at touch down.

anti-gravity muscles
Muscles that counteract gravity-induced flexion.

center of gravity
Point through which the resultant of gravitational forces experienced by the total body mass acts.

duty factor
Percentage of the total stride duration that is taken up by the stance phase; a duty factor of 50% means that the stance and swing phase are of equal duration.

dynamic stability
Model in which stable locomotion is produced by control systems (feedback loops) within the mechanics of the limb.

electromyography
Technique for measuring voltage changes in muscle as an indicator of muscle activity.

entheses
Tendon attachment zones; entheses occur in fibrous and fibrocartilaginous forms. In the former, the connective tissue attaches indirectly via the periosteum, which is joined to the bone by Sharpey's fibers or by connective tissue fibers that pass directly into the bone. Fibrous entheses are found at diaphyses and metaphyses. Fibrocartilaginous entheses occur at the epiphyses and apophyses of long bones (▶ **Fig. 1.29**). In this form of enthesis, the connective tissue transitions into initially unmineralized and then mineralized fibrocartilage, whereby the various elastic moduli (Young's moduli) of tendons and bone are equalized.

ground reaction force
Forces exerted by the ground on the body (N); measured with the aid of force plates and can be decomposed into 3 orthogonal directions in space; they are dependent on the following factors:
- distribution of body mass over the fore- and hindlimbs
- speed
- limb stiffness
- gait

idiomotion
Movement directed towards the animal's own body or towards other animals.

instantaneous center of rotation
A point where the motion of a body results from superimposition of translation and rotation; there is no identifiable fixed point around which movement takes place.

intelligent mechanics
According to the concept of intelligent mechanics, segmentation of a limb and the elastic properties of muscles allow the kinematic chain within the limb to be adjusted with very little neuronal control; i.e. cyclic locomotion can take place without a substantial contribution from the brain; even perturbations arising from uneven terrain can be compensated for with little additional energy input.

joint, force-driven
In contrast to closely interlocking pivot points, force-driven joints are formed by the transmission of forces. The movements of a force-driven joint are determined solely by prevailing forces. The pivot point of the scapula is a force-driven joint, as the connection between the scapula and the trunk is muscular.

joint, incongruent
A step is present within the joint, caused by excessive growth-related projection of the ulna above the radius (short radius).

joint, physiologically incongruent
A joint in which load is evenly distributed without localized peaks; as load increases, the areas of contact become enlarged, facilitating even distribution of stress.

kinematics
Consideration/description of the movement of a body in space without reference to the factors (forces) that cause the motion.

lift off
Moment at which the paw loses contact with the ground.

limb length, functional
Distance between the proximal pivot point of the limb and the point of touch down; i.e. varies according to the degree of bending of the joints.

matched motion
Principle of movement whereby the coupling of at least three limb segments results in amplification of the movement (distance) produced per unit of force.

myoblast mass
Embryonic muscle tissue from which muscles such as the flexors and extensors of the limbs arise.

pivot point
Fixed point around which a solid object can rotate when acted upon by a force; in the dog, the pivot point of the forelimb is in the upper third of the scapula; the pivot point of the hindlimb is in the hip joint, in the walk and trot, and also in the lumbar vertebral column in the gallop.

point of touch down
Site of contact between the paw and the ground.

propulsion, generation of
Production of forces by the body and transmission of these forces to the ground for the purpose of forward movement.

spring-mass model
Describes the horizontal and vertical movement of the centre of gravity during the stance phase of a virtual limb modelled as a linear spring.

stance phase
　Period during which a limb is in contact with the ground. The stance phase of different limbs may overlap chronologically (e.g. in the walk) or coincide (e.g. in the trot).

stance phase duration
　Time between touch down and lift off of an individual limb.

stride duration
　Time between touch down of a limb and subsequent touch down of the same limb.

stride frequency
　Number of strides per second.

stride length
　Distance traveled by the trunk between touch down of a limb and subsequent touch down of the same limb.

swing phase
　Period during which a limb is advanced (not in contact with the ground).

swing phase duration
　Time between lift off and touch down of an individual limb.

touch down
　Moment at which paw makes contact with the ground.

work, negative
　Force × distance (W), the direction of force is opposite to the direction of movement; negative work compensates for the effect of gravity.

work, positive
　Force × distance (W), force acts in the direction of movement; requires consumption of energy.

11　Video content

- Gait analysis (p. 81)
- Brief general examination (p. 83)
- Brief neurological examination (p. 83)
- Examination of the hindlimb of a dog in a standing position (p. 98)
- Examination of the forelimb of a dog in a standing position (p. 110)
- Examination of the hindlimb of a dog in recumbency – digits to tarsus (p. 115)
- Examination of the hindlimb of a dog in recumbency – tarsal joint (p. 118)
- Examination of the hindlimb of a dog in recumbency – crus (p. 120)
- Examination of the hindlimb of a dog in recumbency – stifle joint (p. 127)
- Examination of the hindlimb of a dog in recumbency – femur (p. 130)
- Ortolani-Test (p. 134)
- Examination of the hindlimb of a dog in recumbency – hip joint (p. 136)
- Examination of the forelimb of a dog in recumbency – digits to carpus (p. 141)
- Examination of the forelimb of a dog in recumbency – carpal joint (p. 144)
- Examination of the forelimb of a dog in recumbency – radius and ulna (p. 146)
- Examination of the forelimb of a dog in recumbency – elbow joint (p. 150)
- Examination of the forelimb of a dog in recumbency – humerus (p. 152)
- Examination of the forelimb of a dog in recumbency – shoulder (p. 155)
- Examination of the forelimb of a dog in recumbency – scapula (p. 158)
- assessment of posture and behavior (p. 160)
- Assessment of behaviour, posture and gait (p. 161)
- Postural and proprioceptive responses (p. 165)
- Assessment of spinal reflexes (p. 169)
- Assessment of cranial nerves (p. 175)
- Pain testing (p. 176)
- Gait of a dog with osteochondrosis of the shoulder joint (p. 186)
- Gait of a dog with osteosarcoma of the humerus (p. 195)
- Cruciate ligament rupture – abnormal gait and positive cranial drawer test (p. 202)
- Patellar luxation – abnormal gait and reduction of the patella (p. 206)
- Gait of a dog with fibrosis of the „hamstring muscles" (p. 210)
- Gait of a dog with hip dysplasia (p. 214)
- Gait analysis in a dog with coxofemoral osteoarthritis (p. 214)
- Gait of a dog with a luxated hip joint (p. 218)
- Tendovaginitis of the abductor pollicis longus – gait analysis and clinical assessment (p. 223)
- Elbow dysplasia – abnormal gait and diagnosis (p. 225)
- German Shepherd Dog showing early signs of DLSS (p. 233)
- German Shepherd Dog with degenerative myelopathy (p. 234)
- Dachshund with thoracolumbar intervertebral disc prolapse (p. 255)
- Beagle with cervical intervertebral disc prolapse (p. 237)

12 Image Attribution

Illustrations

- All illustrations in Chapter 1 and anatomical schematics in Chapter 2 were conceptualized by **Prof. Dr. Dr. h.c. Martin S. Fischer** and prepared by **Jonas Lauströer** and **Amir Andikfar**, unless otherwise indicated.
- All illustrations in Chapters 4, 5 and 8 where conceptualized by **Dr. med. vet. ECVS Daniel Koch** and prepared by **Jonas Lauströer** and **Amir Andikfar**, unless otherwise indicated.

Photographs

- The photographs in each chapter were conceptualized and commissioned by the author of the respective chapter, unless otherwise indicated.
- All photographs in Chapters 5 and 6 were taken by Gaby Ernst, Saland, Switzerland, unless otherwise indicated.
- All photographs in Chapter 7 were taken by Nicole Hollenstein, Animal Photographer. Wil, Switzerland, unless otherwise indicated.

Videos

- All videos in Chapters 3, 4 and 6 were produced by Tele D, Diessenhofen, Switzerland, unless otherwise indicated.
- All videos in Chapter 7 were produced by Nicole Hollenstein, Animal Photographer, Wil, Switzerland, unless otherwise indicated.
- The video „Patellar luxation: Information for owners" (Chapter 8) was produced by Bernhard Meier, Wald, Switzerland.

Additional images

The following individuals, institutions and publishers generously provides additional images, and gave permission for their use (in some cases, slight modifications were made to the images or corresponding legends):

- **Karin Baum**, Paphos, Cyprus: **Fig. 1.55, Fig. 7.26**
- Baumgärtner W. Pathohistologie für die Tiermedizin. Stuttgart: Enke; 2007: **Fig. 8.2**
- **Patrick Blättler Monnier**, Frenkendorf, Switzerland: **Fig. 8.40**
- **Tony Flury**, Tierklinik Lindenhof, Switzerland: **Fig. 8.14**
- **Franck Forterre**, Bern: **Fig. 9.9**
- **Ulrich Frotscher**, Meckenheim: **Aufmacher Anhang**
- **Urs Geissbühler**, Clinical radiology, Faculty of Veterinary Medicine, University of Bern, Switzerland: **Fig. 8.49, Fig. 8.80**
- **Urs Geissbühler**, Vetimage, Switzerland: **Fig. 8.86**
- **Matthias Haab**, Equine Clinic, Faculty of Veterinary Medicine, University of Bern, Switzerland: **Fig. 8.48, Fig. 8.56, Fig. 8.64, Fig. 8.88, Fig. 9.7**
- **Lisa Dargel**, Institute of Zoology and Evolutionary Research, Friedrich Schiller University Jena: **Fig. 1.1**
- Institute of Animal Pathology, Faculty of Veterinary Medicine, University of Bern, Switzerland: **Fig. 8.13**
- **Konrad Jurina**, Haar: **Fig. 9.3**
- **Dr. Alexandra Keller**, Frankfurt: **1.13**
- Small Animal Surgery Clinic, Faculty of Veterinary Medicine, University of Bern, Switzerland: **Fig. 8.18, Fig. 8.73**
- Clinical Radiology, Faculty of Veterinary Medicine, University of Bern, Switzerland: **Fig. 8.19**
- **Pierre Montavon**, Switzerland: **Fig. 8.52**
- **PD Dr. Anke Schnapper**, University of Veterinary Medicine, Hannover, Foundation: **Fig. 1.36**
- Salomon F-V, Geyer H, Gille U. Anatomie für die Tiermedizin. 3. Auflage. Stuttgart. Enke 2015: **Fig. 1.52, Fig. 1.53, Fig. 1.54, Fig. 1.56**
- **Julian Sartori**, Institute of Zoology and Evolutionary Research, Friedrich Schiller-University Jena: **Fig. 1.29**
- Schmidt MJ, Kramer M. MRT-Atlas. ZNS-Befunde bei Hund und Katze. Stuttgart: Enke; 2015: **Fig. 9.5, Fig. 9.6**
- Stoffel MH, Geiger D, Guldimann C, Kocher M. Funktionelle Neuroanatomie für die Tiermedizin. Stuttgart: Enke; 2010: **Fig. 1.51**

Index